Reeder and Felson's

# Gamuts in Bone, Joint and Spine Radiology

<small>REEDER AND FELSON'S</small>

# GAMUTS IN BONE, JOINT AND SPINE RADIOLOGY

### COMPREHENSIVE LISTS OF ROENTGEN DIFFERENTIAL DIAGNOSIS

## MAURICE M. REEDER

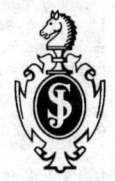

## Springer-Verlag

New York  Berlin  Heidelberg  London  Paris
Tokyo  Hong Kong  Barcelona  Budapest

Maurice M. Reeder, M.D., F.A.C.R.

Professor and Chairman, Section of Radiology, John A. Burns
School of Medicine, University of Hawaii at Manoa,
Honolulu, HI, USA;

Colonel, Medical Corps, United States Army, Retired;

Formerly Chief, Department of Radiology, Walter Reed Army
Medical Center;

Formerly Radiology Consultant to the Surgeon General, United
States Army;

Formerly Associate Radiologist, Registry of Radiologic
Pathology, Armed Forces Institute of Pathology, Washington,
DC, USA;

Founding Member, International Skeletal Society

*MRI gamuts contributed by:*
William G. Bradley, Jr., M.D., Ph.D.

Director, MRI and Radiology Research, Memorial MR
Educational Institute, Long Beach Memorial Medical Center,
Long Beach, CA, USA

Catalog records for this book are available from the U.S. Library of Congress.

Printed on acid-free paper.

Production managed by Karen Phillips; manufacturing supervised by
Jacqui Ashri.
Photocomposed copy prepared from the authors' WordPerfect file using
Ventura Publisher.
Printed and bound by Edwards Brothers, Inc., Ann Arbor, MI.
Printed in the United States of America.

9 8 7 6 5 4 3 2 1

ISBN 0-387-94016-2 Springer-Verlag New York Berlin Heidelberg
ISBN 3-540-94016-2 Springer-Verlag Berlin Heidelberg New York

# Dedication

**This book is dedicated to Colonel William LeRoy Thompson, Medical Corps, U.S. Army (1891-1975)**

Colonel Thompson, legendary teacher of morphology in radiology and originator of the Gamut concept, received his M.D. degree from the University of Pennsylvania in 1917, and began his long and illustrious career in the U.S. Army Medical Corps that same year. He had various assignments in general medicine and administration and later became one of the early Army radiologists.

It was during his last year before retirement from the Army (1951), however, that he began his most important work, his major contribution to medicine: the organization of the Registry of Radiologic Pathology at the Armed Forces Institute of Pathology. After retirement, he offered his services, without remuneration, to continue as full-time Registrar and Chief of Radiologic Pathology.

In the ensuing 16 years, Colonel Thompson worked laboriously in accessioning new material and collating the material already in the files of the Institute. He was sustained in this labor by hours of daily contact with his "students." It was here, in seminars at the viewbox, that Colonel Thompson drew upon a lifetime of accumulated knowledge and experience to educate residents, fellows, and practicing physicians from all over the world who came to study under his guidance. In this role, Colonel Thompson was the catalyst, igniting in his students a love of learning and an understanding of the vital role that pathology plays in the discipline of radiology. He was primarily a morphologist, and accepted as such by his colleagues and peers at the AFIP.

Colonel Thompson's down-to-earth nature, his éclat in interpersonal relationships, his obvious deep regard for his students as well as medicine, and his abundant and abiding warmth as a human being have made him truly beloved by all who came to know him.

# A Tribute to Ben Felson

He was certainly the greatest radiologist of his time, and perhaps of all time. He was one of the great men of this century. He was also my very close and dear friend and colleague. He was like a second father to me and his loss to me is monumental, as is his loss to all whose lives he touched in such a profound and positive manner. He lived the fullest life of anyone I ever knew. He was the quintessential student and teacher, the consummate traveler, and the most compassionate, loving, and lovable human most of us have ever known.

He was that rare combination of Will Rogers and William Osler, and wherever he went, from Cincinnati to Colombia to China, he made a lasting impact and lifelong friends. More than anyone else, he enhanced the reputation and knowledge of the fledgling speciality of Radiology through his inquisitiveness and his gift for communication with both the written and spoken word. He nurtured the careers of countless students, residents, and doctors around the world. He will live forever in the hearts and minds of all who knew and loved him.

Godspeed Ben, and continue to smile down on us from above as you did so often during your all-too-brief stay with us on earth.

Maurice Reeder, M.D.

# Foreword to *Gamuts in Radiology,* Third Edition

by *Elias G. Theros, M.D.*
I. Meschan Distinguished Professor of Radiology,
Wake Forest University Medical Center,
Winston-Salem, North Carolina, USA

Amongst the present generation of radiologists, beguiled by the glamour and excitement of the new high tech imaging and interventional modalities, too few have developed a strong sense of differential diagnosis based on radiologic pattern recognition and its correlation with clinical and laboratory findings. There is no question about the incredible contribution by the new modalities to our diagnostic armamentarium, but in the evolution of modern-day radiologic practice, the cognitive element has been neglected and our abilities as diagnosticians have suffered.

The advent of the third edition of Reeder and Felson's *Gamuts in Radiology* is timely and welcome. As always, use of the gamut lists will help evoke differential thinking, and this has been enhanced by the addition of numerous new gamuts as well as by the updating of over three-fourths of the previously existing gamuts. Interestingly, many of the new gamuts are MRI Gamuts developed by Dr. William Bradley whose enormous experience in clinical MRI has prepared him to think differentially about look-alike patterns and/or locations of lesions displayed by this modality. This is an important step forward in the use of this remarkable new diagnostic tool.

Drs. Reeder and Felson in preparing these gamuts have made a major contribution to diagnosis in radiology. This they were able to do because of the depth of their own experience and their powers of observation. Those of us who have worked closely with them know that they are radiologists of consummate skills, both in the teaching and practice settings. They are master teachers to whom we all owe much. It is radiology's great fortune that Dr. Reeder has persisted, after Dr. Felson's untimely death, in laboring long hours in gamut researching and updating. He is providing his professional colleagues with an ever improving powerful diagnostic tool. We are all in his debt.

# Table of Contents

**B**

**C**

**J**

**S**

**V**

# Preface

The word *gamut* is defined as the whole range of anything. As used in this book, it indicates a complete list of causes of a particular roentgen finding or pattern.

This book, which consists of material excerpted and reorganized from Reeder and Felson's *Gamuts in Radiology, Third Edition,* was created specifically for skeletal radiologists, orthopaedic surgeons, sports medicine physicians, and rheumatologists. If used correctly, it will become an indispensable aid to pattern recognition and differential diagnosis when interpreting radiographs in the clinical setting.

Most radiologists use the "Gamut approach" without calling it that. You see an epiphyseal lesion of bone and immediately search your memory bank for causes. You recall perhaps six causes, then eliminate two because of rarity or incompatible roentgen pattern. Then, with the clinical information at your elbow, you weed out two more that don't fit the clinical setting, leaving you with perhaps one or two likely diagnoses.

This process is the basis of the triangulation approach to radiologic diagnosis espoused by the originator of the gamut concept, Colonel William LeRoy Thompson. He taught that roentgen diagnosis begins with accurately interpreting all the nuances and data inherent in the radiograph, then using that information to derive a particular pattern. The second side of the triangle involves reference to a well-constructed list of differential diagnosis, which includes not only the common causes, responsible for over 80 percent of the entities, but also the uncommon causes, which are frequently overlooked. The triangle is then completed by reference to the pertinent clinical and laboratory data, age, sex, and other important information concerning the patient.

The purpose of this book is to provide you with complete and accurate lists of differential diagnosis. It is an unobtru-

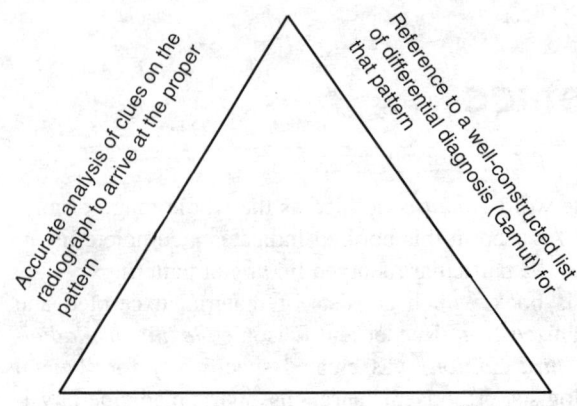

Accurate analysis of clues on the radiograph to arrive at the proper pattern

Reference to a well-constructed list of differential diagnosis (Gamut) for that pattern

Correlation of radiographic findings
and Gamut with patients clinical
and lab findings to arrive at the
most likely diagnosis

sive consultant, quickly available whenever you interpret films or prepare a presentation. In each patient, the possibilities are narrowed down to those that fit the roentgen signs and the clinical and laboratory findings. Of course, all the pertinent data on the film must be analyzed to find the appropriate roentgen sign or pattern. Study well — to identify a pattern incorrectly will land you in the wrong gamut, which could be a disaster!

Many individual gamuts that first appeared in *Gamuts in Radiology* can also be found reproduced (credited or otherwise) in a variety of publications. Many excellent texts have been published that emphasize the gamut or differential diagnosis approach, including those by Drs. Eisenberg, Swischuk, Greenfield, Poznanski, Taybi and Lachman, and Burgener and Kormano. However, residents and practitioners who use abbreviated lists from other, more watered-down, sources are deprived of the true worth of gamuts, which is to provide a comprehensive listing of the multiple causes, both common and uncommon, for a particular pattern. The point is to jog your memory to recall *all* the various possibilities for any given finding.

Dr. Felson and I were always the first to admit that the

with unerring accuracy and completeness all of the patterns which can present to the radiologist is beyond the comprehension of any two (or perhaps twenty) individuals. Nevertheless, our combined experience of over 75 years' practice in major medical centers in the United States, as well as numerous visiting professorships throughout virtually the entire world, gave us sufficient perspective to at least attempt such a prodigious endeavor. Along the way we were greatly aided by our close association with such outstanding skeletal radiologists as Colonel William Thompson, Elias (Lee) Theros, Harold Jacobson, Philip Palmer, and others who broadened our horizons and added invaluable insights in their own specialty areas.

Continuing in that collaborative tradition, I am enormously pleased that Dr. William Bradley, Jr., has contributed some twenty spine and joint MRI gamuts to this book. Although there are many experts in MRI today, I can think of no individual better qualified to develop accurate lists of differential diagnosis for the many patterns now evolving in this exciting and burgeoning modality than Bill Bradley, who has been an innovator and pioneer in the field since its inception.

While the individual gamuts are extensively referenced, you will note that the majority of current references refer to textbooks rather than journal articles. This is because today's general and subspecialty textbooks are much more likely to refer to the multiple causes for a given pattern than individual articles, which are usually focused on specific entities or procedures. Furthermore, exhaustive lists of references would increase the book's size enormously and undermine its primary goal, which is to provide a quick, efficient reference.

You may question whether a specific listed entity can give rise to a given pattern, or whether it is a common or uncommon member of that gamut. Although there may be some errors among the many thousands of entries, virtually all listed causes have appeared in the literature or have been seen by the authors or our colleagues. Obviously, what is common in one part of the world may be rare or unknown elsewhere. For example, Paget's disease is common in much of the United States but virtually unknown in most of Africa and many other areas of the tropical world, where skeletal tuberculosis and other infectious diseases are quite common. Thus, while the list of causes for a specific pattern may be quite complete within each gamut, the relative prevalence of those causes can vary widely geographically.

My first mentor in radiology, the legendary Colonel Thompson, and Dr. Lent C. Johnson, former chief of orthopaedic pathology at the AFIP, are well remembered by their former students and disciples for their insistence on the triangulation approach to radiographic interpretation. Together, these two clinically oriented physicians taught an entire generation of radiology and orthopaedics residents and fellows the nuances of interpretation and differential diagnosis of bone tumors and other skeletal lesions. In today's clinical setting, where the proliferation of new technologies is colliding with ever increasing pressures to contain costs and optimize the use of diagnostic tests (as Dr. Theros has so eloquently stated in his foreword), it is more important than ever that young radiologists and clinicians learn and apply these principles, which are summarized in these remarks by the Colonel:

"The radiograph is to the radiologist what the gross specimen is to the pathologist. It is a window on the disease, mirroring the many changes occurring within the patient during the course of an illness."

"The clues to the pattern (and often the diagnosis itself) are almost always on the film if you are observant enough and smart enough to pay attention to all the data inherent in the radiograph."

"Remember that the radiograph is only one-tenth of a second in the history of a disease process. You must always think back to what the findings looked like a day or a week or a year ago (preferably with the help of old films if available, but using intuition or deductive reasoning in their absence) and what the findings are likely to be tomorrow or next week."

"A good radiologist must be a good anatomist and morphologist and have a clear understanding of the correlation between what is seen on the radiograph and the underlying gross and microscopic pathology."

Finally, I would like to add a few of my own thoughts that I have passed on to residents over the years.

"The radiograph is only one piece of the diagnostic puzzle. It must be evaluated in light of what you know about the patient. The radiologist cannot function as an isolated island unto himself. He needs a knowledge of differential diagnosis together with clinical information and interaction with the patient's physician to arrive at the proper solution."

"The radiograph is like a single page in a mystery novel. To find out 'whodunit' you usually need more detailed information than is available at a single glance."

"Remember that what comes out of the automatic processor so often is not a diagnosis but rather a diagnostic challenge, a pattern for which there may be four or forty possible causes. It is up to us, as the physician's consultant, to interpret this pattern correctly using the triangulation approach."

And perhaps the most important advice to young residents: "Work hard and play hard. Enjoy your work and your free time. Life is short."

MMR

# Acknowledgments

In creating a project of this magnitude, the authors will inevitably borrow freely from many sources. Specific citations follow most gamuts, and a list of more general references appears at the end of this volume. For those instances where debts are not acknowledged, the reader should understand that lost notes and jaded memories, not ingratitude, are to blame.

The following outstanding radiologists made valuable additions to many of the gamuts found in this book: Drs. George B. Greenfield, Harold G. Jacobson, Andrew K. Poznanski, Leonard E. Swischuk, Hooshang Taybi, Elias G. Theros, and of course Ben Felson. I want to especially thank my long-time colleague and friend, Dr. Theros, for his insightful foreword.

Finally, this text would not be possible in its present format without the meticulous and dedicated typing and word processing skills provided by Mrs. Karen Kurihara of Honolulu.

# An Appreciation

To Barbara Reeder, whose patience, love, and perseverance made possible the timely publication of this present work, and to my sons, Dave, Dan, Bill and Robby, and stepsons Steve and Eric, and to those colleagues, mentors, and friends, past and present, who have so indelibly defined my own career.

*William LeRoy Thompson*
*Benjamin Felson*
*Elias G. Theros*
*Philip E. S. Palmer*
*Harold G. Jacobson*

# How To Use This Book

**1. SECTIONS**

This book is organized in five sections. Each section is denoted by an alphabetical letter. Thus, under V you will find all the gamuts that deal with the vertebral column or spine.

**2. TABLE OF CONTENTS**

This book has an extensive index. In addition, each section has its own table of contents, the pages of which have been black-edged for quick recognition. You can identify the appropriate table of contents by referring to page ix or by counting down the black index marks along the free edge of the closed book.

It will pay you to take a few minutes to look over the subheadings in the table of contents of each section. Gamuts are grouped in what we consider a logical manner. However, our logic may not be your logic; if you don't find a gamut where you think it belongs, scan the entire table of contents of that section or refer to the index before assuming that it is absent.

**3. SUBGAMUTS**

A subgamut amplifies some part of the gamut to which it belongs. Be sure to refer to it after you have finished with the parent gamut.

**4. INCIDENCE**

In most of the gamuts, the entities are subdivided into two groups, *Common* and *Uncommon*. These refer to the relative, rather than absolute, incidence of the disease. Although a bone blister (Gamut B-70) is an uncommon roentgen finding, if you do see one, the diagnosis will generally prove to be giant cell tumor or nonossifying fibroma or one of the other conditions listed under *Common*.

The prevalence of many disorders varies both geographically and from one type of institution to another. Skeletal tuberculosis is a common bone disease in much of the world, but it is only occasionally seen in the U.S. Histiocytosis X is much more common at Walter Reed Army Hospital than it is in a county hospital. To avoid such discrepancies, we have based our incidence estimates on our experience at Theoretical General Hospital, Midland, U.S.A.

Admittedly, some of the gamuts deal with seldom seen roentgen signs, but it is in just this type of situation that a gamut is most welcome. It substitutes someone else's experience for your own lack of it.

## 5. ALPHABETICAL LISTING

The entries in each gamut have been alphabetized for your convenience. Since the entry may not be listed in the form that first comes to your mind, be sure to scan the entire gamut before assuming that a condition is not included. Abbreviations are listed on page 463.

## 6. SUPPLEMENTARY GAMUTS

Most of the gamuts refer to a roentgen sign, pattern, or complex. However, interspersed throughout the book are classifications, anatomic and physiologic gamuts, and other information useful to the radiologist and orthopaedist. Typical examples are Gamuts B-80 (Age Range of Highest Incidence of Various Bone Neoplasms) and B-52 (Sites of Predilection and Eponyms for Avascular Necrosis).

## 7. TERMINOLOGY

We have usually selected the most widely used terms for each disease, often furnishing a synonym or eponym as well.

The term *generalized* indicates more or less diffuse involvement (eg, thalassemia of the skeleton); *widespread* means extensive but spotty involvement (eg, Paget's disease of the skeleton); *multiple* means more than one lesion but less than widespread (eg, metastatic lesions, gouty arthritis, brown tumors).

In order to shorten the gamut lists, similar or related conditions are combined, often separated by a comma or semicolon (eg, scleroderma; dermatomyositis). Inclusive group designations, such as primary anemia and lymphoma, are often utilized. In these instances you will find the subscript ₉, which tells you to look in the Glossary (page 465) if you want to know all the entities in that group. Example: Anemia, primary$_g$. If one member of a group is a more likely cause of a particular roentgen finding, it is specifically listed. To illustrate: Anemia, primary$_g$ (esp. thalassemia).

## 8. BRACKETS

Brackets are used to indicate a condition that does not actually cause the gamuted roentgen finding, but can produce roentgen changes that simulate it. In Gamut B-84C (Round Cell Lesions of Bone), *osteomyelitis*, which is not a cause, but a mimic, is bracketed.

## 9. SYNDROMES

S. stands for Syndrome. We must apologize for the great number of congenital syndromes we have included. Since the information is available, we could hardly ignore it. Lump them together? The pediatric roentgenologists had just split them apart. We had a huge tiger by the tail, an animal with variegated stripes and swollen gamuts. Seckel's bird-headed dwarfism, Cockayne, and Prader-Willi syndromes, indeed! They should have their own Gamut Book. We can only advise those of you who seldom see dwarfs and other little people to ignore these entries. For those who are interested, it will be useful to consult Taybi and Lachman's syndrome book for definitions of these congenital disorders.

## 10. REFERENCES

References are used to cite only articles, books, and other contributions that have provided a number of the disease entities listed in a gamut. To document each entity would be an impossible task. A listing of general references appears in the back of the book.

## 11. ALTERATIONS

We are fully aware that there are omissions on the Gamut lists. Very rare entities or syndromes or single case reports have been deliberately omitted. There are also some inconsistencies in terminology, coverage, and unity. There may even be occasional factual inaccuracies. We hope these flaws are neither too frequent nor too annoying.

Please correct errors if you encounter them; delete entities that you feel do not belong on a gamut; insert additional disorders and add new gamuts as you discover them in the literature or in your practice; create some gamuts yourself. Send us your changes, with documentation, so that they can be incorporated in future editions.

# B

# Bone

## I. BONE—GENERALIZED
## GROWTH OR MODELING DISORDERS

## EPIPHYSEAL DISORDERS

**B**

## OSTEOSCLEROSIS

## CYSTIC AND LYTIC LESIONS

**B**

**B** NEOPLASMS

**B**

**B**

B

B

**B**

## UPPER EXTREMITIES, SHOULDERS, AND CLAVICLES

## LOWER EXTREMITIES AND PELVIS

**B**

## RIBS AND STERNUM

## Gamut B-1

# INTERNATIONAL NOMENCLATURE OF CONSTITUTIONAL DISEASES OF BONE
## Revision, May 1983[1]

Kozlowski and Beighton have attempted to estimate the relative frequency of these conditions in terms of their own experience and a review of the literature.

| | |
|---|---|
| **** 1000+ cases | ** 20–100 cases |
| *** 100–1000 cases | * Less than 20 cases |

---

## OSTEOCHONDRODYSPLASIAS

### Abnormalities of cartilage and/or bone growth and development

**A. Defects of growth of tubular bone and/or spine**
*a. Identifiable at birth*
α. Usually lethal before or shortly after birth

| | Frequency |
|---|---|
| 1. Achondrogenesis type I (Parent-Fraccaro) | ** |
| 2. Achondrogenesis type II (Langer-Saldino) | ** |
| 3. Hypochondrogenesis | * |
| 4. Fibrochondrogenesis | * |
| 5. Thanatophoric dysplasia | *** |
| 6. Thanatophoric dysplasia with clover-leaf skull | ** |
| 7. Atelosteogenesis | * |
| 8. Short rib syndrome (with or without polydactyly) | |
|    a. type I (Saldino-Noonan) | ** |
|    b. type II (Majewski) | * |
|    c. type III (lethal thoracic dysplasia) | * |

β. *Usually non-lethal dysplasia*

| | |
|---|---|
| 9. Chondrodysplasia punctata | |
|    a. rhizomelic form autosomal recessive | ** |
|    b. dominant X-linked form (Lethal in male) | ** |
|    c. common mild form (Sheffield) | *** |
|    Exclude: symptomatic stippling (Warfarin, chromosomal aberration) | |
| 10. Campomelic dysplasia | ** |
| 11. Kyphomelic dysplasia | * |

---

12. Achondroplasia   ****
13. Diastrophic dysplasia   ***
14. Metatrophic dysplasia (several forms)   **
15. Chondro-ecto-dermal dysplasia (Ellis-Van Creveld)   ***
16. Asphyxiating thoracic dysplasia (Jeune)   **
17. Spondylo-epiphyseal dysplasia congenita
    a. autosomal dominant form   **
    b. autosomal recessive form   **
18. Kniest dysplasia
19. Dyssegmental dysplasia
20. Mesomelic dysplasia
    a. type Nievergelt   *
    b. type Langer (probable homozygous dyschondrosteosis)   *
    c. type Robinow   *
    d. type Rheinardt   *
    e. others   ***
21. Acromesomelic dysplasia   **
22. Cleido-cranial dysplasia   ****
23. Oto-palato-digital syndrome
    a. type I (Langer)   **
    b. type II (Andre)   **
24. Larsen syndrome   **
25. Other multiple dislocation syndromes (Desbuquois...)

*b. Identifiable in later life*
1. Hypochondroplasia   ***
2. Dyschondrosteosis   ***
3. Metaphyseal chondrodysplasia type Jansen   *
4. Metaphyseal chondrodysplasia type Schmid   **
5. Metaphyseal chondrodysplasia type McKusick   **
6. Metaphyseal chondrodysplasia with exocrine pancreatic insufficiency and cyclic neutropenia   **
7. Spondylo-metaphyseal dysplasia
    a. type Kozlowski   **
    b. other forms   ***
8. Multiple epiphyseal dysplasia
    a. type Fairbank   ****
    b. other forms   ***
9. Multiple epiphyseal dysplasia with early diabetes (Wolcott-Rallisson)   **
10. Arthro-ophthalmopathy (Stickler)   ***
11. Pseudo-achondroplasia
    a. dominant   ***
    b. recessive   **

12. Spondylo-epiphyseal dysplasia tarda (X-linked recessive) **
13. Progressive pseudo-rheumatoid chondrodysplasia **
14. Spondylo-epiphyseal dysplasia, other forms ***
15. Brachyolmia
    a. autosomal recessive *
    b. autosomal dominant *
16. Dyggve-Melchior-Clausen dysplasia **
17. Spondylo-epi-metaphyseal dysplasia (several forms) ***
18. Spondylo-epi-metaphyseal dysplasia with joint laxity **
19. Oto-spondylo-megaepiphyseal dysplasia (OSMED) *
20. Myotonic chondrodysplasia (Catel-Schwartz-Jampel) **
21. Parastremmatic dysplasia *
22. Tricho-rhino-phalangeal dysplasia *
23. Acrodysplasia with retinitis pigmentosa and nephropathy (Saldino-Mainzer) *

B. *Disorganized development of cartilage and fibrous components of skeleton*
1. Dysplasia epiphyseal hemimelica **
2. Multiple cartilaginous exostoses ****
3. Acrodysplasia with exostoses (Giedion-Langer) **
4. Enchondromatosis (Ollier) ***
5. Enchondromatosis with hemangioma (Maffucci) **
6. Metachondromatosis **
7. Spondyloenchondroplasia *
8. Osteoglophonic dysplasia *
9. Fibrous dysplasia (Jaffe-Lichtenstein) ***
10. Fibrous dysplasia with skin pigmentation and precocious puberty (McCune-Albright) ***
11. Cherubism (familia) fibrous dysplasia of the jaws) **

C. *Abnormalities of density of cortical diaphyseal structure and/or metaphyseal modeling*
1. Osteogenesis imperfecta (several forms) ****
2. Juvenile idiopathic osteoporosis **
3. Osteoporosis with pseudo-glioma *
4. Osteopetrosis
    a. autosomal recessive lethal **

    b.  intermediate recessive          **

    c.  autosomal dominant          ***

    d.  recessive with tubular acidosis     **

  5.  Pycnodysostosis       ***

  6.  Dominant osteosclerosis type
      Stanescu       **

  7.  Osteomesopychosis       **

  8.  Osteopoikilosis       ***

  9.  Osteopathia striata       ***

10.  Osteopathia striata with cranial sclerosis   **

11.  Melorheostosis       ***

12.  Diaphyseal dysplasia (Camurati-
      Engelmann)       ***

13.  Cranio-diaphyseal dysplasia   **

14.  Endosteal hyperostosis

    a.  autosomal dominant (Worth)   **

    b.  autosomal recessive (Van Buchem)   **

    c.  autosomal recessive (sclerosteosis)   **

15.  Tubular stenosis (Kenny-Caffey)   *

16.  Pachydermoperiostosis   **

17.  Osteodysplasty (Melnick-Needles)   **

18.  Fronto-metaphyseal dysplasia   **

19.  Cranio-metaphyseal dysplasia
      (several forms)       ***

20.  Metaphyseal dysplasia (Pyle)   **

21.  Dysosteosclerosis       **

22.  Osteo-ectasia with hyperphosphatasia   **

23.  Oculo-dento-osseous dysplasia

    a.  mild type       ***

    b.  severe type       *

24.  Infantile cortical hyperstosis (Caffey disease
      familial type)       **


## DYSOSTOSES

### Malformation of individual bones, singly or in combination

*A. Dysostoses with cranial and facial involvement*

  1.  Craniosynostosis (several forms)   ***

  2.  Cranio-facial dysostosis (Crouzon)   ***

  3.  Acrocephalo-syndactyly

    a.  type Apert       ***

    b.  type Chotzen       **

    c.  type Pfeiffer       **

    d.  other types       ***

  4.  Acrocephalo-polysyndactyly (Carpenter and
      others)       **

5. Cephalo-polysyndactyly (Greig)      *
6. First and second branchial arch syndromes
   a. mandibulo-facial dysostosis (Treacher-Collins, Franceschetti)      ***
   b. acro-facial dysostosis (Nager)      **
   c. osulo-auriculo-vertebral dysostosis (Goldenhar)      ***
   d. hemifacial microsoma      ***
   e. others      ***
   (Probably parts of a large spectrum)
7. Oculo-mandibulo-facial syndrome (Hallermann-Streff-François)      **

B. *Dysostoses with predominant axial involvement*
   1. Vertebral segmentation defects (including Klippel-Feil)      **
   2. Cervico-oculo-acoustic syndrome (Wildervanck)      ***
   3. Sprengel anomaly      ***
   4. Spondylo-costal dysostosis
      a. dominant form      **
      b. recessive forms      **
   5. Oculo-vertebral syndrome (Weyers)      *
   6. Osteo-onychodysostosis      ****
   7. Cerebro-costo-mandibular syndrome      **

C. *Dysostoses with predominant involvement of extremities*
   1. Acheira      **
   2. Apodia      **
   3. Tetraphoccomelia syndrome (Roberts) (SC pseudothalidomide syndrome)      **
   4. Ectrodactyly
      a. isolated      ***
      b. ectrodactyly-ectodermal dysplasia, cleft palate-syndrome      **
      c. ectrodactyly with scalp defects      **
   5. Oro-acral syndrome (aglossia syndrome, Hanhart syndrome)      *
   6. Familial radio-ulnar synostosis      **
   7. Brachydactyly types A, B, C, D, E (Bell's classification)      ****
   8. Symphalangism      ***
   9. Polydactyly (several forms)      ****
   10. Syndactyly (several forms)      ****
   11. Poly-syndactyly (several forms)      ***
   12. Camplodactyly      ****
   13. Manzke syndrome      *
   14. Poland syndrome      ***

15. Rubinstein-Taybi syndrome     **
16. Coffin-Siris syndrome     **
17. Pancytopenia-dysmelia syndrome (Fanconi)   ***
18. Blackfan-Diamond anemia with thumb anomalies (Aase-Syndrome)     **
19. Thrombocytopenia-radial-aplasia syndrome     **
20. Oro-digito-facial syndrome
    a. type Papillon-Leage (Lethal in males)     **
    b. type Mohr     **
21. Cardiomelic syndromes (Holt-Oram and others)   ***
22. Femoral focal deficiency (with or without facial anomalies)     **
23. Multiple synostoses (include some forms of symphalangism)   ***
24. Scapulo-iliac dysostosis (Kosenow-Sinios)     **
25. Hand foot genital syndrome     **
26. Focal dermal hypoplasia (Goltz) (Lethal in males)     **

## IDIOPATHIC OSTEOLYSES

1. Phalangeal (several forms)     **
2. Tarso-carpal
   a. including François form and others     **
   b. with nephropathy     **
3. Multicentric
   a. Hajdu-Cheney form     **
   b. Winchester form     *
   c. Torg form     *
   d. other forms     **

## MISCELLANEOUS DISORDERS WITH OSSEOUS INVOLVEMENT

1. Early acceleration of skeletal maturation
   a. Marshall-Smith syndrome     *
   b. Weaver syndrome     *
   c. other types     *
2. Marfan syndrome   ****
3. Congenital contractural arachnodactyly     **
4. Cerebro-hepato-renal syndrome (Zellweger)     **
5. Coffin-Lowry syndrome     **
6. Cockayne syndrome     **
7. Fibrodysplasia ossificans congenita   ***
8. Epidermal nevus syndrome (Solomon)     **
9. Nevoid basal cell carcinoma syndrome     **

10. Multiple hereditary fibromalosis     \*\*
11. Neurofibromatosis     \*\*\*\*

## CHROMOSOMAL ABERRATIONS:
### Primary metabolic abnormalities
*A. Calcium and/or phosphorus*
  1. Hypophosphatemic rickets     \*\*\*\*
  2. Vitamin D dependency or pseudo-deficiency
    rickets
    a. type I with probable deficiency in 25-hydroxy
       vitamin D-1-alpha-hydroxylase     \*\*
    b. type II with target-organ resistancy     \*\*
  3. Late rickets (McCance)     \*\*
  4. Idiopathic hypercalciuria     \*\*\*
  5. Hypophosphatasia (several forms)     \*\*\*
  6. Pseudo-hypoparathyroidism (normocalcemic
    and hypocalcemic forms, including
    acrodysostosis)     \*\*\*

*B. Complex carbohydrates*
  1. Mucopolysaccharidosis type I (alpha-L-
    iduronidase deficiency)
    a. Hurler form     \*\*\*
    b. Scheie form     \*\*
    c. other forms     \*\*
  2. Mucopolysaccharidosis type II—Hunter
    (sulfoiduronate sulfatase deficiency)     \*\*\*
  3. Mucopolysaccharidosis type III—Sanfilippo     \*\*\*
    a. type III A (heparin sulfamidase deficiency)
    b. type III B (N-acetyl-alpha-glucosaminidase
       deficiency)
    c. type III C (alpha-glucosaminide-N-acetyl
       transferase deficiency)
    d. type III D (N-acetyl-glucosamine-6 sulfate
       sulfatase deficiency)
  4. Mucopolysaccharidosis type IV     \*\*
    a. type IV A—Morquio )N-acetyl-galactosamine-6
       sulfate sulfatase deficiency)
    b. type IV B (beta galactosidase deficiency)
  5. Mucopolysaccharidosis type IV—Maroteaux-Lamy
    (aryl-sulfatase B deficiency)
  6. Mucopolysaccharidosis type VII (beta-
    glucuronidase deficiency)     \*\*
  7. Aspartylglucosaminuria (Aspartyl-
    glucosaminidase deficiency)     \*\*
  8. Mannosidosis (alpha-mannosidase deficiency)     \*\*
  9. Fucosidosis (alpha-fucosidase deficiency)     \*\*

10. GM1-Gangliosidosis (beta-galactosidase
    deficiency) (several forms)                    **
11. Multiple sulfatases deficiency (Austin-Thieffry)   **
12. Isolated neuraminidase deficiency, several forms
    including:
    a. mucolipidosis I
    b. nephrosialidosis
    c. cherry red spot myoclonia syndrome
13. Phosphotransferase deficiency, several forms
    including:                                    **
    a. mucolipidosis II (I cell disease)
    b. mucolipidosis III (pseudo-polydystrophy)
14. Combined neuraminidase beta-galactosidase
    deficiency                                    *
15. Salia disease                                 *

*C. Lipids*
1. Niemann-Pick disease (sphingomyelinase
   deficiency) (several forms)                    ***
2. Gaucher disease (beta-glucosidase deficiency)
   (several types)                                ****
3. Farber disease lipogranulomatosis
   (ceraminidase deficiency)                      **

*D. Nucleic acids*
1. Adenosine-deaminase deficiency and others      **

*E. Amino acids*
1. Homocystinuria and others                      ***

*F. Metals*
1. Menkes syndrome (kinky hair syndrome
   and others)                                    **

*References:*
1. Beighton P, et al: International nomenclature of constitutional diseases of bone: May 1983 revision. Ann Radiol
   1984:27:275-280
2. Kozlowski K, Beighton P: Gamut Index of Skeletal Dysplasias. Berlin: Springer-Verlag, 1984, 182-189

# CLASSIFICATION OF SCLEROSING DYSPLASIAS OF BONE

## I. DYSPLASIAS OF ENDOCHONDRAL BONE FORMATION

### A. Affecting primary spongiosa (immature bone)
1. Osteopetrosis (Albers-Schönberg disease)
   a. Autosomal-recessive type (lethal)
   b. Autosomal-dominant type
   c. Intermediate-recessive type
   d. Autosomal-recessive type with tubular acidosis (Sly disease)
2. Pyknodysotosis

### B. Affecting spongiosa (mature bone)
1. Enostosis (bone island)
2. Osteopoikilosis
3. Osteopathia striata (Voorhoeve disease)

## II. DYSPLASIAS OF INTRAMEMBRANOUS BONE FORMATION
1. Progressive diaphyseal dysplasia (Camurati-Engelmann disease)
2. Hereditary multiple diaphyseal sclerosis (Ribbing disease)
3. Endosteal hyperostosis (hyperostosis corticalis generalisata)
   a. Autosomal-recessive form
      i. Van Buchem disease
      ii. Sclerosteosis (Truswell-Hansen disease)
   b. Autosomal-dominant form
      i. Worth disease
      ii. Nakamura disease

### III. MIXED SCLEROSING DYSPLASIAS (affecting both endochondral and intramembranous ossification)

#### A. Affecting predominantly endochondral ossification
1. Dysosteosclerosis
2. Metaphyseal dysplasia (Pyle's disease)
3. Craniometaphyseal dysplasia

#### B. Affecting predominantly intramembranous ossification
1. Melorheostosis
2. Progressive diaphyseal dysplasia with skull base involvement (Neuhauser variant)
3. Craniodiaphyseal dysplasia

#### C. Coexistence of two or more sclerosing bone dysplasias (overlap syndrome)
1. Melorheostosis with osteopoikilosis and osteopathia striata
2. Osteopathia striata with cranial sclerosis (Horan-Beighton S.)
3. Osteopathia striata with osteopoikilosis and cranial sclerosis
4. Osteopathia striata with generalized cortical hyperostosis
5. Osteopathia striata with osteopetrosis
6. Osteopoikilosis with progressive diaphyseal dysplasia

*Reference:*
1. Greenspan A: Sclerosing bone dysplasias - a target-site approach. Skeletal Radiol 1991;20:561-583

## Gamut B-3

# LETHAL FORMS OF DWARFISM*

**COMMON**
1. Achondrogenesis, types I & II
2. Achondroplasia, homozygous form
3. Campomelic dysplasia
4. Chondrodysplasia punctata, rhizomelic form
5. Fetal infection (eg, cytomegalovirus, herpes simplex, or rarely rubella)
6. Hypophosphatasia, severe
7. Osteogenesis imperfecta congenita
8. Short rib syndromes (with or without polydactyly)
   a. Type I (Saldino-Noonan)
   b. Type II (Majewski)
   c. Type III (lethal thoracic dysplasia)
9. Thanatophoric dysplasia (with or without cloverleaf skull)

**UNCOMMON**
1. Asphyxiating thoracic dysplasia (Jeune S.)
2. Atelosteogenesis
3. Cephaloskeletal dysplasia (Taybi-Linder S.)
4. Diastrophic dysplasia (rarely lethal)
5. Dyssegmental dysplasia
6. Fibrochondrogenesis
7. Hypochondrogenesis
8. Metatropic dysplasia (lethal variant)
9. Neu-Laxova S.
10. Osteodysplasty (Melnick-Needles S.) (lethal male)
11. Osteopetrosis with precocious manifestations
12. Potter S.
13. Spondyloepiphyseal dysplasia congenita
14. Spondylothoracic dysostosis (Jarcho-Levin S.)
15. Warfarin embryopathy

*Death usually in neonatal period or within first year of life.

References:
1. Kozlowski K, Beighton P: Gamut Index of Skeletal Dysplasias. Berlin: Springer-Verlag, 1984, pp 27-28
2. Kozlowski K, et al: Neonatal death dwarfism. Fortschr Röntgenstr 1978;129:626-633
3. Taybi H, Lachman RS: Radiology of Syndromes, Metabolic Disorders, and Skeletal Dysplasias. (ed 3) Chicago: Year Book Medical Publ, 1990, p 885

## Gamut B-4

# LATE-ONSET DWARFISM (IDENTIFIABLE IN LATER LIFE)

**COMMON**

1. Arthro-ophthalmopathy (Stickler S.)
2. Dyschondrosteosis
3. Hypochondroplasia
4. Multiple epiphyseal dysplasia (Fairbank and other forms)
5. Pseudoachondroplasia (dominant and recessive)
6. Spondylo-epi-metaphyseal dysplasia, several forms
7. Spondyloepiphyseal dysplasia tarda and other forms
8. Spondylometaphyseal dysplasia (Kozlowski and other forms)

**UNCOMMON**

1. Acrodysplasia (Saldino-Mainzer S.)
2. Brachyolmia
3. Dyggve-Melchior-Clausen dysplasia
4. Metaphyseal chondrodysplasia (types Jansen, Schmid, McKusick); Shwachman S.
5. Myotonic chondrodystrophy (Schwartz-Jampel S.)
6. Oto-spondylo-megaepiphyseal dysplasia (OSMED)
7. Parastremmatic dysplasia
8. Progressive pseudorheumatoid chondrodysplasia
9. Spondyloperipheral dysplasia
10. Tricho-rhino-phalangeal dysplasia

B. Bone

*Reference:*
1. Beighton P, et al: International Nomenclature of Constitutional Diseases of Bone: May 1983 revision. Ann Radiol 1984;27:275-280

## Gamut B-5

# MAJOR SYNDROMES OF SHORT LIMB DWARFISM (RHIZOMELIC, MESOMELIC, AND ACROMELIC)

## RHIZOMELIC DWARFISM (PROXIMAL LIMB SHORTENING—HUMERUS, FEMUR)

1. Achondrogenesis
2. Achondroplasia
3. Chondrodysplasia punctata (Conradi's disease)
4. Femoral-facial S.
5. Metatropic dysplasia
6. Pseudoachondroplasia
7. Thanatophoric dysplasia

## MESOMELIC DWARFISM (MIDDLE SEGMENT LIMB SHORTENING—RADIUS, ULNA OR TIBIA, FIBULA)

### I. Mesomelia with Normal Hands and Feet

1. Dyschondrosteosis
2. Mesomelic dysplasia (eg, Langer and Reinhardt-Pfeiffer types)

### II. Mesomelia with Hand and Foot Abnormalities

1. Acromesomelic dysplasia (Maroteaux and Campailla-Martinelli types)
2. Campomelic dysplasia
3. Chondroectodermal dysplasia (Ellis-van Creveld S.)

4. Mesomelic dysplasia (Nievergelt, Robinow, and Werner types)

## ACROMELIC DWARFISM (DISTAL SEGMENT SHORTENING—HANDS, FEET)
1. Asphyxiating thoracic dysplasia (Jeune S.)
2. Peripheral dysostosis

*Reference:*
1. Kozlowski K, Beighton P: Gamut Index of Skeletal Dysplasias. Berlin: Springer-Verlag, 1984, p 64

## Gamut B-6

# CONGENITAL SYNDROMES WITH SHORT LIMBS

## COMMON
1. Achondroplasia, pseudoachondroplasia
2. Chondrodysplasia punctata (Conradi's disease)
3. Dyschondrosteosis; Madelung's deformity
4. Enchondromatosis (Ollier's disease); Maffucci S.
5. Hypothyroidism
6. Mucopolysaccharidoses$_g$ (eg, Hurler S.); $GM_1$ gangliosidosis
7. Multiple cartilaginous exostoses
8. Multiple epiphyseal dysplasia (Fairbank)
9. Osteogenesis imperfecta congenita

## UNCOMMON
1. Achondrogenesis; Grebe chondrodysplasia
2. Acrodysostosis
3. Acromesomelic dysplasia
4. Asphyxiating thoracic dysplasia (Jeune S.)
5. Bird-headed dwarfism (Seckel S.)

6. Bloom S.
7. Campomelic dysplasia
8. Cephaloskeletal dysplasia (Taybi-Linder S.)
9. Chondroectodermal dysplasia (Ellis-van Creveld S.)
10. Cornelia de Lange S.
11. Diastrophic dysplasia
12. Dyggve-Melchior-Clausen S.
13. Dyssegmental dysplasia
14. Fetal aminopterin S.
15. Fibrochondrogenesis
16. Holt-Oram S.
17. Hyperphosphatasia
18. Hypochondroplasia
19. Hypophosphatasia
20. Kniest dysplasia
21. Larsen S.
22. Mesomelic dysplasia (Langer, Nievergelt types)
23. Metaphyseal chondrodysplasias (Jansen, McKusick, Schmid)
24. Metatropic dysplasia
25. Mietens-Weber S.
26. Orofaciodigital S. I
27. Phocomelia (incl. maternal thalidamide ingestion, diabetes)
28. Pseudoleprechaunism (Patterson S.)
29. Roberts S.
30. Robinow S.
31. Short rib-polydactyly S.
32. Spondyloepiphyseal dysplasia congenita
33. Spondylometaphyseal dysplasia
34. Thanatophoric dysplasia
35. Turner S.
36. Warfarin embryopathy
37. Weill-Marchesani S.

*References:*
1. Felson B (ed): Dwarfs and other little people. Semin Roentgenol 1973;8:255
2. Swischuk LE: Differential Diagnosis in Pediatric Radiology. Baltimore: Williams & Wilkins, 1984, pp 165-167

3. Taybi H, Lachman RS: Radiology of Syndromes, Metabolic Disorders, and Skeletal Dysplasias. (ed 3) Chicago: Year Book Medical Publ, 1990

## Gamut B-7

## SHORT SQUAT BONES

**COMMON**
1. Achondroplasia
2. Epiphyseal-metaphyseal injury (trauma, infection, radiation, hypervitaminosis A)
3. Mucopolysaccharidoses

**UNCOMMON**
1. Achondrogenesis
2. Asphyxiating thoracic dysplasia
3. Campomelic dysplasia
4. Cleidocranial dysplasia
5. Cornelia de Lange S.
6. Diastrophic dysplasia
7. Dyschondrosteosis; Madelung's deformity
8. Hyperphosphatasia
9. Hypochondroplasia
10. Hypophosphatasia
11. Hypothyroidism
12. Kniest dysplasia
13. Larsen S.
14. Metaphyseal chondrodysplasia (Jansen)
15. Metatropic dysplasia
16. Neonatal dwarfs, other
17. Phocomelia (eg, thalidomide embryopathy)
18. Pseudoachondroplasia
19. Rickets (hypophosphatemic, type B)
20. Short rib-polydactyly S. (Majewski and Saldino-Noonan types)

21. Thanatophoric dysplasia
22. Turner S.

*Reference:*
1. Swischuk LE: Differential Diagnosis in Pediatric Radiology. Baltimore: Williams & Wilkins, 1984, pp 165-167

## Gamut B-8

# BOWED BONES, SINGLE OR MULTIPLE

## COMMON

*1. Achondroplasia
*2. Bow legs; knock-knees (See B-189, B-190)
 3. Enchondromatosis (Ollier's disease); Maffucci S.
 4. Fibrous dysplasia (incl. Albright's S.)
 5. Fracture, traumatic or pathologic (esp. greenstick or healed fracture)
 6. Hyperparathyroidism (osteitis fibrosa cystica)
*7. Neurofibromatosis (esp. tibia, fibula)
*8. Osteogenesis imperfecta
 9. Osteomalacia (See B-46)
10. Osteomyelitis, severe (eg, bacterial, tuberculous, small-pox; syphilis-saber shin; yaws-boomerang tibia)
11. Paget's disease
12. Paralysis or restricted movement during growth (eg, poliomyelitis, muscular dystrophy, juvenile rheuma-toid arthritis)
*13. Physiologic bowing
*14. Prenatal bowing of long bones
15. Rickets, all types
16. Tibia vara (Blount's disease)

## UNCOMMON

*1. Achondrogenesis, types I and II
*2. Acromesomelic dysplasia
*3. Asphyxiating thoracic dysplasia
*4. Campomelic dysplasia

 *5. Chondroectodermal dysplasia (Ellis-van Creveld S.)
 *6. Cloverleaf skull
 *7. Congenital pseudarthrosis
 *8. Contractural arachnodactyly
 *9. Cornelia de Lange S.
*10. Diastrophic dysplasia
 11. Dyschondrosteosis (radius and tibia); Madelung's deformity
*12. Dyssegmental dysplasia
 13. Epidermal nevus S.
*14. Fibrochondrogenesis
*15. Hemihypertrophy (eg, Klippel-Trenaunay S.)
 16. Homocystinuria
 17. Hydatid disease
*18. Hyperphosphatasia
*19. Hypochondroplasia
*20. Hypophosphatasia
*21. Infantile cortical hyperostosis (Caffey's disease) (late)
*22. Intrauterine positional deformity
*23. Isolated anomaly
*24. Larsen S.
*25. Mesomelic dysplasia
*26. Metaphyseal chondrodysplasias, all types
*27. Mucopolysaccharidosis VI; mucolipidosis; $GM_1$ gangliosidosis
*28. Osteodysplasty (Melnick-Needles S.)
 29. Osteolysis (Hajdu-Cheney S.)
*30. Otopalatodigital S.
*31. Parastremmatic dwarfism
*32. Pseudoachondroplasia
*33. Pseudohypoparathyroidism
 34. Renal osteodystrophy
*35. Short rib-polydactyly syndromes
*36. Spondylometaphyseal dysplasia (Kozlowski)
*37. Thanatophoric dysplasia
*38. Tibial bowing with or without absent fibula
 39. Weismann-Netter S. (saber shin)

* Bowed limbs in infancy.

*References:*
1. Swischuk LE: Differential Diagnosis in Pediatric Radiology. Baltimore: Williams & Wilkins, 1984, pp 171-178
2. Taybi H, Lachman RS: Radiology of Syndromes, Metabolic Disorders, and Skeletal Dysplasias. (ed 3) Chicago: Year Book Medical Publ, 1990, p 864

## Gamut B-9

## TWISTED BONES

### COMMON
1. Fibrous dysplasia
2. Hyperparathyroidism (osteitis fibrosa cystica)
3. Neurofibromatosis
4. Osteodysplasty (Melnick-Needles S.)
5. Osteogenesis imperfecta
6. Osteomyelitis (late sequela)
7. Posttraumatic; postoperative (esp. regenerated rib)

### UNCOMMON
1. Basal cell nevus S. (Gorlin S.)
2. Idiopathic
3. Metaphyseal dysplasia (Pyle's disease)
4. Otopalatodigital S.

*Reference:*
1. Swischuk LE: Differential Diagnosis in Pediatric Radiology. Baltimore: Williams & Wilkins, 1984, p 178

# OVERCONSTRICTION OR OVERTUBULATION (NARROW DIAMETAPHYSIS, LONG THIN BONES)

## COMMON

1. Chronic illness with hypotonia or immobilization
2. Disuse atrophy
3. Muscular disorders (eg, arthrogryposis, amyotonia congenita, progressive muscular dystrophy, Werdnig-Hoffmann S.)
4. Paralytic disorders (eg, poliomyelitis, cerebral palsy, congenital malformation of brain or spinal cord)

## UNCOMMON

1. Acromegaly (phalanges)
2. Cockayne S.
3. Congenital pseudarthrosis
4. Contractural arachnodactyly
5. Dermatomyositis
6. Epidermolysis bullosa
7. Hallermann-Streiff S.
8. Homocystinuria
9. Hypopituitarism (eg, primordial dwarfism)
10. Juvenile rheumatoid arthritis
11. Marfan S.
12. MMM S. (3-M S.)
13. Neurofibromatosis
14. Osteogenesis imperfecta
15. Prader-Willi S.
16. Progeria
17. Stickler S. (arthro-ophthalmopathy)
18. Tubular stenosis (Kenny-Caffey S.)
19. Winchester S.

*References:*
1. Greenfield GB: Radiology of Bone Diseases. (ed 5) Philadelphia: Lippincott, 1990
2. Kozlowski K, Beighton P: Gamut Index of Skeletal Dysplasias. Berlin: Springer-Verlag, 1984, p 902
3. Swischuk LE: Differential Diagnosis in Pediatric Radiology. Baltimore: Williams & Wilkins, 1984, pp 169-170

## Gamut B-11

# UNDERCONSTRICTION OR UNDERTUBULATION (WIDE DIAMETAPHYSIS), LOCALIZED OR GENERALIZED (See Gamut B-34, Subgamut B34A)

**COMMON**
1. Achondroplasia, other chondrodysplasias (See B-1)
2. Anemia$_g$ (eg, thalassemia, sickle cell anemia)
3. Bone cyst or benign expansile neoplasm
4. Fibrous dysplasia
5. Gaucher's disease; Niemann-Pick disease
6. Healing fracture; metaphyseal injury

**UNCOMMON**
1. Biliary atresia; biliary cirrhosis
2. Cleidocranial dysplasia
3. Craniometaphyseal dysplasia
4. Cystic fibrosis
5. Enchondromatosis (Ollier's disease)
6. Engelmann's disease (diaphyseal dysplasia)
7. Hyperphosphatasia
8. Hypervitaminosis D or A
9. Hypophosphatasia (adult)
10. Infantile cortical hyperostosis (Caffey's disease)
11. Lead poisoning (late)
12. Metaphyseal dysplasia (Pyle's disease)

13. Mucopolysaccharidoses (esp. Morquio S., Hurler S.); mucolipidoses
14. Multiple cartilaginous exostoses (diaphyseal aclasis)
15. Osteomyelitis, chronic productive (eg, Garré's; congenital syphilis)
16. Osteopetrosis
17. Paget's disease
18. Peripheral dysostosis
19. Rickets (healing)
20. Rubella embryopathy
21. Scurvy (healing)
22. Total lipodystrophy; membranous lipodystrophy

*References:*
1. Greenfield GB: Radiology of Bone Diseases. (ed 5) Philadelphia: Lippincott, 1990
2. Silverman FN (ed): Caffey's Pediatric X-ray Diagnosis. (ed 8) Chicago: Year Book Medical Publ, 1985, vol 1, p 484

## Gamut B-12

### WIDE DIAPHYSIS

**COMMON**
1. Anemia$_g$, severe (esp. thalassemia)
2. Bone cyst or expansile neoplasm
3. Fibrous dysplasia
4. Osteomyelitis, chronic productive (eg, Garré's, syphilis, yaws); tuberculosis; tropical ulcer
5. Paget's disease
6. Subperiosteal hemorrhage (eg, trauma, leukemia, hemophilia, scurvy)

**UNCOMMON**
1. Craniodiaphyseal dysplasia
2. Dysosteosclerosis

3. Endosteal hyperostosis (van Buchem, Worth)
4. Engelmann's disease (diaphyseal dysplasia)
5. Gaucher's disease; Niemann-Pick disease
6. Hyperphosphatasia
7. Infantile cortical hyperostosis (Caffey's disease)
8. Mastocytosis
9. Mucopolysaccharidoses
10. Oculo-dento-osseous dysplasia
11. Osteopetrosis
12. Otopalatodigital S.
13. Pachydermoperiostosis
14. Singleton-Merten S.
15. Trisomy 8 S.

*Reference:*
1. Kozlowski K, Beighton P: Gamut Index of Skeletal Dysplasias. Berlin: Springer-Verlag, 1984, p 62

## Gamut B-13

# LOCALIZED EPIPHYSEAL OR METAPHYSEAL LESION RESULTING IN PREMATURE CLOSURE OF GROWTH PLATE AND A SHORTENED BONE

**COMMON**
1. Local hyperemia (eg, infection, juvenile rheumatoid arthritis, hemophilia, AV malformation)
2. Osteomyelitis (eg, bacterial, tuberculous, yaws, smallpox, meningococcal)
3. Trauma; battered child S.; surgical trauma

**UNCOMMON**
1. Disuse (eg, immobilization, postfracture)

2. Enchondromatosis (Ollier's disease)
3. Hypervitaminosis A
4. Infarction (eg, sickle cell anemia)
5. Multiple cartilaginous exostoses
6. Neoplasm invading growth plate
7. Radiation injury
8. Rickets
9. Scurvy
10. Thermal injury (burn, frostbite)

*Reference:*
1. Greenfield GB: Radiology of Bone Diseases. (ed 5) Philadelphia: Lippincott, 1990

## Gamut B-14

## ASYMMETRY IN SIZE OF A BONE OR LIMB (HEMIHYPERTROPHY OR HEMIATROPHY), LOCALIZED OR GENERALIZED (See Gamuts B-13, B-15)

### WITH BONE DYSPLASIA, DYSOSTOSIS, OR OTHER PRIMARY BONE DISORDER

1. Chondrodysplasia punctata (Conradi's disease)
2. Chromosomal abnormalities
3. Coffin-Lowry S.
4. Dysplasia epiphysealis hemimelica (Trevor's disease)
5. Enchondromatosis (Ollier's disease)
6. Fibrous dysplasia (incl. Albright's S.)
7. Goldenhar-Gorlin S.
8. Melorheostosis
9. Multiple cartilaginous exostoses
10. Osteogenesis imperfecta

11. Phocomelia (eg, thalidomide embryopathy); other congenital limb hypoplasias
12. Prader-Willi S.
13. Proteus S.
14. Seckel S. (bird-headed dwarfism)

## WITH BONE OVERGROWTH IN THE ABSENCE OF A LOCALIZED LESION
1. Beckwith-Wiedemann S.
2. Idiopathic; congenital hemihypertrophy
3. Silver-Russell S.

## WITH VASCULAR MALFORMATIONS
1. Hemangioma; AV malformation; Klippel-Trenaunay-Weber S.; Maffucci S.
2. Lymphangioma
3. Lymphatic abnormality

## WITH NEUROCUTANEOUS OR CUTANEOUS SYNDROMES OR SOFT TISSUE ABNORMALITY
1. Ichthyosis-limb reduction S. (CHILD S.)
2. Incontinentia pigmenti
3. Macrodystrophia lipomatosa
4. Neurofibromatosis
5. Poland S. (absence of pectoral muscles)
6. Romberg S. (esp. mandible)
7. Sturge-Weber S.; von Hippel-Lindau S.
8. Tuberous sclerosis

## WITH NEOPLASM
1. Adrenal gland neoplasm (adrenocortical carcinoma, adenoma)
2. Gonadal neoplasm
3. Hepatic neoplasm (hepatoblastoma)
4. Neuroblastoma
5. Renal neoplasm (Wilms' tumor)

## ACQUIRED ASYMMETRY

1. Endocrine disorder (eg, adrenogenital S.)
2. Hyperemia, any cause (eg, from chronic infection, rheumatoid arthritis, hemophilia); also conditions leading to decreased blood supply to a limb
3. Hypospadias; cryptorchidism
4. Infantile cortical hyperostosis (Caffey's disease)
5. Lymphangiectasia (intestinal, pulmonary, extremity)
6. Medullary sponge kidney; benign renal cystic disease
7. Neuromuscular disorder; cerebral palsy; poliomyelitis
8. Osteomyelitis (eg, bacterial, yaws, smallpox)
9. Radiation therapy
10. Renal hypertrophy, unilateral or bilateral
11. Scurvy (with epiphyseal trauma)
12. Trauma (eg, burn, epiphyseal injury, impacted or distracted fracture, surgical procedure)

*References:*
1. Kozlowski K, Beighton P: Gamut Index of Skeletal Dysplasias. Berlin: Springer-Verlag, 1984, pp 22-23
2. Taybi H, Lachman RS: Radiology of Syndromes, Metabolic Disorders, and Skeletal Dysplasias. (ed 3) Chicago: Year Book Medical Publ, 1990, p 893

## Gamut B-15

### LOCALIZED ACCELERATED MATURATION, ELONGATION, OR OVERGROWTH (GIGANTISM) OF A BONE, DIGIT, OR LIMB

#### COMMON

1. AV fistula, hemangioma, lymphangioma
2. Chronic arthritis (eg, tuberculous, juvenile rheumatoid)

3. Chronic osteomyelitis (eg, Garré's, tuberculous, tropical ulcer)
4. Fracture, healing
5. Hyperemia, any cause
6. Neurofibromatosis

**UNCOMMON**
1. Congenital macrodactyly
2. Dysplasia epiphysealis hemimelica (Trevor's disease)
3. Fibrous dysplasia
4. Hemihypertrophy (See B-14)
5. Hemophilic hemarthrosis
6. Idiopathic
7. Infantile cortical hyperostosis (Caffey's disease)
8. Klippel-Trenaunay S.; Parkes-Weber S.
9. Lymphatic obstruction, chronic (eg, lymphangiectasia, congenital hypoplasia of lymphatics, filariasis, neoplasm)
10. Macrodystrophia lipomatosa
11. Maffucci S. (enchondromatosis with hemangiomas)
12. Melorheostosis
13. Neoplasm (eg, infiltrating angiolipoma)

*Reference:*
1. Greenfield GB: Radiology of Bone Diseases. (ed 5) Philadelphia: Lippincott, 1990

## Gamut B-16

## GENERALIZED OR WIDESPREAD OVERGROWTH OR ELONGATION OF THE SKELETON

1. Adrenogenital S. (prior to premature closure of epiphyses)

2. Beckwith-Wiedemann S.
3. Cerebral gigantism (Sotos S.)
4. Hemihypertrophy (See B-14)
5. Homocystinuria
6. Hyperpituitarism, pituitary gigantism, acromegaly
7. Klinefelter S.
8. Marfan S.
9. Neurofibromatosis
10. Total lipodystrophy

*References:*

1. Greenfield GB: Radiology of Bone Diseases. (ed 5) Philadelphia: Lippincott, 1990
2. Silverman FN (ed): Caffey's Pediatric X-ray Diagnosis. (ed 8) Chicago: Year Book Medical Publ, 1985, vol 1, p 494
3. Taybi H, Lachman RS: Radiology of Syndromes, Metabolic Disorders, and Skeletal Dysplasias. (ed 3) Chicago: Year Book Medical Publ, 1990

## Gamut B-17

# GENERALIZED ACCELERATED SKELETAL MATURATION (INCREASED BONE AGE)

## COMMON

1. Adrenogenital S. (adrenocortical tumor or hyperplasia)
2. Cerebral gigantism (Sotos S.)
3. Constitutional (congenital tall stature)
4. Excessive androgen or estrogen administration or production (eg, virilizing adrenal or gonadal neoplasm or hyperplasia; Cushing S.)
5. Pituitary gigantism; hyperpituitarism
6. Polyostotic fibrous dysplasia (esp. Albright's S.)

## UNCOMMON

1. Congenital syndromes, other
   a. Acrodysostosis (peripheral dysostosis)
   *b. Asphyxiating thoracic dysplasia (hips)
   *c. Beckwith-Wiedemann S. (fetal visceromegaly)
   *d. Chondroectodermal dysplasia (Ellis-van Creveld S.)
   e. Cockayne S.
   f. Contractural arachnodactyly
   g. Diastrophic dysplasia (hands)
   *h. Greig cephalopolysyndactyly S.
   *i. Larsen S.
   j. Lipoatrophic diabetes (total lipodystrophy)
   *k. Marshall-Smith S.
   l. Pseudohypoparathyroidism
   m. Trisomy 8 S.
   n. Tuberous sclerosis
   *o. Weaver-Smith S.
2. Ectopic gonadotropin production (hepatoma, choriocarcinoma, teratoma)
3. Encephalitis
4. Exogenous obesity with overgrowth and tall stature
5. Homocystinuria
*6. Hyperthyroidism (maternal or acquired)
7. Hypothalamic or parahypothalamic lesion with sexual precocity (eg, craniopharyngioma, hamartoma, optic chiasm glioma, tuberculosis)
8. Idiopathic isosexual precocious puberty
9. Pinealoma, primary or ectopic
10. Primary hyperaldosteronism (Conn S.)

* Advanced bone age in the newborn.

### References:

1. Greenfield GB: Radiology of Bone Diseases. (ed 5) Philadelphia: Lippincott, 1990
2. Poznanski AK: The Hand in Radiologic Diagnosis. (ed 2) Philadelphia: W.B. Saunders, 1984
3. Rieth KG, et al:CT of cerebral abnormalities in precocious puberty. AJR 1987;148:1231-1238
4. Taybi H, Lachman RS: Radiology of Syndromes, Metabolic Disorders, and Skeletal Dysplasias. (ed 3) Chicago: Year Book Medical Publ, 1990, p 884

5. Wesenberg RL, Gwinn JL, Barnes GR Jr: The roentgeno-graphic findings in total lipodystrophy. AJR 1968;103:154-164

## Gamut B-18

# GENERALIZED RETARDED SKELETAL MATURATION (DECREASED BONE AGE)

## COMMON

1. Congenital heart disease (esp. cyanotic)
2. Congenital syndromes of dwarfism or mental retardation (See B-19)
3. Constitutional delay of growth and adolescence; non-specific or idiopathic retardation
4. Cretinism, hypothyroidism
5. Diabetes, juvenile
6. Hypogonadism (eg, Turner S.)
7. Hypopituitarism with growth hormone deficiency (eg, idiopathic, craniopharyngioma)
8. Intrauterine growth retardation
9. Malnutrition, failure to thrive
10. Neurologic disorders; cerebral hypoplasia
11. Psychosocial (deprivation) dwarfism
12. Renal disease (eg, nephrosis, chronic renal failure, cystinosis, renal tubular acidosis)
13. Severe constitutional disease or chronic illness (eg, celiac disease, cystic fibrosis, ulcerative colitis)

## UNCOMMON

1. Addison's disease
2. Anemia, chronic$_g$ (eg, sickle cell anemia, thalassemia)
3. Congenital hyperuricosuria
4. Copper deficiency

5. Hypoparathyroidism
6. Idiopathic juvenile osteoporosis
7. Lipid storage diseases
8. Phenylketonuria
9. Rickets, all types
10. Steroid therapy; Cushing S.

*References:*
1. Dorst J: Personal communication
2. Greenfield GB: Radiology of Bone Diseases. (ed 5) Philadelphia: Lippincott, 1990
3. Poznanski AK: The Hand in Radiologic Diagnosis. (ed 2) Philadelphia: W.B. Saunders, 1984
4. Teplick JG, Haskin ME: Roentgenologic Diagnosis. (ed 3) Philadelphia: W.B. Saunders, 1976

## Gamut B-19

## CONGENITAL SYNDROMES WITH RETARDED SKELETAL MATURATION

### COMMON
1. Achondroplasia
2. Cystic fibrosis
3. Deprivation dwarfism
4. Hypothyroidism, cretinism
5. Idiopathic, familial
6. Mucopolysaccharidoses (esp. Morquio S.)
7. [Small for gestational age neonate]
8. Trisomy 21 S. (Down S.)

### UNCOMMON
1. Achondrogenesis
2. C syndrome
3. Campomelic dysplasia
4. Celiac disease (gluten-induced enteropathy)
5. Cephaloskeletal dysplasia (Taybi-Linder S.)

6. Cerebrohepatorenal S. (Zellweger S.)
7. Chondroectodermal dysplasia (Ellis-van Creveld S.)
8. Cleidocranial dysplasia
9. Cloverleaf skull S.
10. Coffin-Lowry S.; Coffin-Siris S.
11. Cornelia de Lange S.
12. Cystinosis
13. Diastrophic dysplasia
14. Dubowitz S.
15. Fanconi S. (pancytopenia-dysmelia S.)
16. Fetal aminopterin S.
17. Glycogen storage disease (von Gierke)
18. Incontinentia pigmenti
19. Infant of toxemic mother
20. Larsen S.
21. Lenz-Majewski hyperostotic dwarfism
22. LEOPARD S. (lentiginosis S.)
23. Leprechaunism; pseudoleprechaunism (Patterson S.)
24. Lesch-Nyhan S.
25. Metatropic dysplasia
26. Mucolipidosis III; fucosidosis
27. Multiple epiphyseal dysplasia (Fairbank)
28. Noonan S.
29. Oculocerebrorenal S. (Lowe S.)
30. Osteodysplasty (Melnick-Needles S.)
31. Papillon-Lefèvre S.
32. Phenylketonuria
33. Pituitary dwarfism (Levi-Lorain S.)
34. Pleonosteosis (Léri)
35. Prader-Willi S.
36. Riley-Day S.
37. Rubella S.
38. Rubinstein-Taybi S.
39. Silver-Russell S.
40. Spondylo-epi-metaphyseal dysplasia
41. Spondyloepiphyseal dysplasia
42. Spondylometaphyseal dysplasia (esp. Kozlowski)
43. Thanatophoric dysplasia
44. Trisomy 18 S.
45. Turner S.

B. Bone

46. Weill-Marchesani S.
47. Whistling face S.(Freeman-Sheldon S.)
48. Wilson's disease
49. XXXXY S.

*References:*
1. Felson B (ed): Dwarfs and other little people. Semin Roentgenol 1973;8:255
2. Kozlowski K, Beighton P: Gamut Index of Skeletal Dysplasias. Berlin:Springer-Verlag, 1984, pp 18-19
3. Swischuk LE: Differential Diagnosis in Pediatric Radiology. Baltimore: Williams & Wilkins, 1984, p 322
4. Taybi H, Lachman RS: Radiology of Syndromes, Metabolic Disorders, and Skeletal Dysplasias. (ed 3) Chicago: Year Book Medical Publ, 1990, pp 884-885

## Gamut B-20

# PSEUDOEPIPHYSES AND ACCESSORY EPIPHYSES

## COMMON
1. Cleidocranial dysplasia
2. Idiopathic; normal variant
*3. Otopalatodigital S.
*4. Trisomy 21 S. (Down S.)

## UNCOMMON
1. Brachydactyly C
2. Chromosome 4p S. (Wolf S.)
*3. Cockayne S.
4. Diastrophic dysplasia
5. Dyggve-Melchior-Clausen S.
6. Fanconi S. (pancytopenia-dysmelia S.) (thumb)
7. Fetal Dilantin S.
*8. Gordon S.
9. Hand-foot-genital S.

10. Larsen S. (esp. calcaneus)
*11. MMM S. (3-M S.)
12. Peripheral dysostosis
13. Spondyloepiphyseal dysplasia
14. Trisomy 9p S.
*15. XXXXY S.

*Affecting primarily the second metacarpal.

*References:*
1. Greenfield GB: Radiology of Bone Diseases. (ed 5) Philadelphia: Lippincott, 1990
2. Poznanski AK: The Hand in Radiologic Diagnosis. (ed 2) Philadelphia: W.B. Saunders, 1984, p 154

## Gamut B-21

# IRREGULARITY, FRAGMENTATION, OR STIPPLING OF MULTIPLE EPIPHYSEAL OSSIFICATION CENTERS

## COMMON
1. Avascular necrosis (eg, Legg-Perthes, steroid therapy, sickle cell anemia (See B-51); osteochondroses
*2. Congenital syndromes (See B-21A)
*3. Cretinism, hypothyroidism
*4. Normal, age related (eg, distal femur, capitellum)

## UNCOMMON
*1. Dysplasia epiphysealis hemimelica (Trevor's disease)
2. Frostbite
3. Hypo-hyperparathyroidism
*4. Hypopituitarism (anterior lobe) with growth hormone deficiency
5. Juvenile rheumatoid arthritis

6. Osteomyelitis (eg, *Listeria monocytogenes**); prenatal infections
7. Pituitary gigantism
8. Rickets
9. Thiemann's disease (hand)
10. Trauma

*Stippled epiphyses.

*Reference:*
1. Greenfield GB: Radiology of Bone Diseases. (ed 5) Philadelphia: Lippincott, 1990

## Subgamut B-21A

# CONGENITAL SYNDROMES WITH IRREGULARITY, FRAGMENTATION, OR STIPPLING OF MULTIPLE EPIPHYSEAL OSSIFICATION CENTERS

### COMMON
*1. Chondrodysplasia punctata (Conradi's disease)
*2. Cretinism, hypothyroidism
*3. Multiple epiphyseal dysplasia (Fairbank)
*4. Osteopoikilosis
*5. Spondyloepiphyseal dysplasia (congenita, tarda, and pseudoachondroplastic types)
*6. Trisomy 21 S. (Down S.)

### UNCOMMON
*1. Cerebrohepatorenal S. (Zellweger S.)
2. Diastrophic dysplasia
3. Dyggve-Melchior-Clausen S.
4. Enchondromatosis (Ollier's disease); Maffucci S.
*5. Homocystinuria
6. Kniest dysplasia

7. Metatropic dysplasia
*8. Meyer dysplasia of femoral head
*9. Mucolipidosis II (I-cell disease); GM$_1$ gangliosidosis
10. Mucopolysaccharidoses (eg, Morquio S.)
11. Nail-patella S. (osteo-onychodysplasia)
*12. Osteopathia striata
13. Parastremmatic dwarfism
*14. Smith-Lemli-Opitz S.
15. Smith-McCort S.
16. Spondyloepimetaphyseal dysplasia
17. Stickler S. (arthro-ophthalmopathy)
18. Tricho-rhino-phalangeal dysplasia (hips)
*19. Trisomy 18 S.
*20. Warfarin embryopathy
21. Winchester S.

*Stippled epiphyses.

*References:*
1. Felson B (ed): Dwarfs and other little people. Semin Roentgenol 1973;8:255
2. Kozlowski K. Beighton P: Gamut Index of Skeletal Dysplasias. Berlin: Springer-Verlag, 1984, pp 68-69
3. Taybi H, Lachman RS: Radiology of Syndromes, Metabolic Disorders, and Skeletal Dysplasias. (ed 3) Chicago: Year Book Medical Publ, 1990, p 871

**Gamut B-22**

## ALTERATION IN SIZE OR APPEARANCE OF MULTIPLE EPIPHYSES
### (See Gamuts B-21, B-23 to B-29)

**COMMON**
1. Achondroplasia
2. Arthritis (eg, rheumatoid, psoriatic)

3. Avascular necrosis (eg, sickle cell anemia, steroid therapy) (See B-51); osteochondroses
4. Cone-shaped epiphyses (See B-29)
5. Cretinism, hypothyroidism
6. Hemophilia
7. Normal variant
8. Trauma, including battered child S.

## UNCOMMON
1. Chondrodysplasia punctata (Conradi's disease)
2. Chondroectodermal dysplasia (Ellis-van Creveld S.)
3. Diabetes, juvenile
4. Diastrophic dysplasia
5. Dysplasia epiphysealis hemimelica (Trevor's disease)
6. Enchondromatosis (Ollier's disease)
7. Hypochondroplasia
8. Hypophosphatasia
9. Hypopituitarism
10. Infection (eg, smallpox, tuberculosis)
11. Kniest dysplasia
12. Malnutrition
13. Metaphyseal chondrodysplasias
14. Metatropic dysplasia
15. Mucopolysaccharidoses (eg, Hurler, Hunter, Morquio)
16. Multiple epiphyseal dysplasia (Fairbank)
17. Nail-patella S. (osteo-onychodysplasia)
18. Osteogenesis imperfecta
19. Parastremmatic dwarfism
20. Pseudoachondroplasia
21. Psychosocial (deprivation) dwarfism
22. Radiation therapy
23. Rickets
24. Scurvy
25. Spondyloepiphyseal dysplasia congenita
26. Stickler S. (arthro-ophthalmopathy)
27. Thermal injury (eg, frostbite, burn)
28. Thiemann's disease

## Gamut B-23

# SMALL EPIPHYSES

## Generalized

**COMMON**
1. Cretinism, hypothyroidism
2. Delayed skeletal maturation, any cause (See B-18, B-19)

**UNCOMMON**
1. Congenital heart disease, cyanotic
2. Diabetes, juvenile
3. Diastrophic dysplasia
4. Hypopituitarism (eg, idiopathic, craniopharyngioma)
5. Malnutrition, malabsorption
6. Morquio S.
7. Mucolipidosis III
8. Multiple epiphyseal dysplasia (Fairbank)
9. Psychosocial (deprivation) dwarfism
10. Rheumatoid arthritis; other chronic arthropathy
11. Rickets
12. Spondyloepiphyseal dysplasia
13. Steroid therapy, prolonged; Cushing S.

## Localized

1. Congenital dislocation of hip
2. Disuse of an extremity (eg, neuromuscular disease, arthritis)
3. Infection
4. Legg-Perthes disease, early; other aseptic necrosis
5. Trauma

*References:*

1. Oh KS, Ledesma-Medina J, Bender TM: Practical Gamuts and Differential Diagnosis in Pediatric Radiology. Chicago: Year Book Medical Publ, 1982, p 146

B. Bone

2. Swischuk LE: Differential Diagnosis in Pediatric Radiology. Baltimore: Williams & Wilkins, 1984, pp 218-220

## Gamut B-24

## LARGE EPIPHYSES

### Generalized

**COMMON**
1. [Diseases leading to thin diaphyses (eg, neurogenic diseases, osteogenesis imperfecta)] (See B-10)
2. Dwarf syndromes
3. Juvenile rheumatoid arthritis

**UNCOMMON**
1. Adrenogenital S.
2. Beckwith-Wiedemann S.
3. Cerebral gigantism (Sotos S.)
4. Hemophilia
5. Hormone-secreting neoplasm, other (eg, gonadal tumor, teratoma, pinealoma, hepatoblastoma)
6. Hyperthyroidism
7. Idiopathic precocious puberty
8. Oto-spondylo-megaepiphyseal dysplasia
9. Spondylo-megaepiphyseal-metaphyseal dysplasia

### Localized

**COMMON**
1. Chronic arthritis, other (eg, septic, tuberculous, fungal)
2. Coxa magna and plana (eg, healed Legg-Perthes disease)

3. Hemophilic hemarthrosis
4. Juvenile rheumatoid arthritis
5. Posttraumatic; healing fracture

**UNCOMMON**
1. Angioma, vascular malformation
2. Dysplasia epiphysealis hemimelica (Trevor's disease)
3. Idiopathic localized gigantism
4. Localized hyperemia, other causes
5. Neurofibromatosis
6. Postsurgical (eg, open reduction with internal fixation)

*References:*
1. Oh KS, Ledesma-Medina J, Bender TM: Practical Gamuts and Differential Diagnosis in Pediatric Radiology. Chicago: Year Book Medical Publ, 1982, pp 142-144
2. Swischuk LE: Differential Diagnosis in Pediatric Radiology. Baltimore: Williams & Wilkins, 1984, pp 216-217

## Gamut B-25

## THIN EPIPHYSES

**COMMON**
1. Renal osteodystrophy
2. Rickets

**UNCOMMON**
1. Epiphyseal acrodysplasia (Thiemann's disease)
2. Kniest dysplasia
3. Multiple epiphyseal dysplasia (Fairbank)
4. Myotonic chondrodysplasia
5. Stickler S. (arthro-ophthalmopathy)

*Reference:*
1. Poznanski AK: The Hand in Radiologic Diagnosis. (ed 2) Philadelphia: W.B. Saunders, 1984, p 900

## Gamut B-26

## INDISTINCT OR FUZZY EPIPHYSES

### COMMON
1. Hyperparathyroidism, primary or secondary (eg, renal osteodystrophy)
2. Hypothyroidism, cretinism
3. Osteomalacia
4. Rickets

### UNCOMMON
1. Hypophosphatasia
2. Metaphyseal chondrodysplasia (Jansen)
3. Mucolipidosis II (I-cell disease); $GM_1$ gangliosidosis

*Reference:*
1. Swischuk LE: Differential Diagnosis in Pediatric Radiology. Baltimore: Williams & Wilkins, 1984, pp 221-222

## Gamut B-27

## RING EPIPHYSES (DENSE CORTEX WITH LUCENT CENTER)

### COMMON
1. Osteoporosis, severe (esp. disuse atrophy)
2. Scurvy (Wimberger ring)

## UNCOMMON

1. Hyperparathyroidism, primary or secondary (healing)
2. Hypothyroidism (healing)
3. Osteogenesis imperfecta
4. Rickets (healing)

*Reference:*
1. Swischuk LE: Differential Diagnosis in Pediatric Radiology. Baltimore: Williams & Wilkins, 1984, pp 221-222

## Gamut B-28

# DENSE (IVORY) EPIPHYSES OF HANDS AND FEET

## ACQUIRED

*1. Hypopituitarism
 2. Hypothyroidism
*3. Normal variant (esp. distal phalanges)
 4. Renal osteodystrophy
*5. Retarded skeletal maturation; deprivation dwarfism

## CONGENITAL

 1. Bird-headed dwarfism (Seckel S.)
*2. Cockayne S.
 3. Coffin-Lowry S.
 4. Coffin-Siris S.
 5. Dyggve-Melchior-Clausen S.
*6. Epiphyseal acrodysplasia (Thiemann's disease)
 7. Homocystinuria
 8. Idiopathic hypercalcemia (Williams S.)
 9. Morquio S.
10. Mucolipidosis III
*11. Multiple epiphyseal dysplasia (Fairbank)
12. Robinow S.

13. Silver-Russell S.
14. Spondyloepiphyseal dysplasia
15. Stickler S. (arthro-ophthalmopathy)
*16. Tricho-rhino-phalangeal dysplasia
17. Trisomy 21 S. (Down S.)

*Common.

### References:
1. Kuhns LR, Poznanski AK, Shaw HAS, et al: Ivory epiphyses. Radiology 1973;109:643-648
2. Poznanski AK: The Hand in Radiologic Diagnosis. (ed 2) Philadelphia: W.B. Saunders, 1984, pp 147-152
3. Swischuk LE: Differential Diagnosis in Pediatric Radiology. Baltimore: Williams & Wilkins, 1984, p 216
4. Taybi H, Lachman RS: Radiology of Syndromes, Metabolic Disorders, and Skeletal Dysplasias. (ed 3) Chicago: Year Book Medical Publ, 1990, p 871

## Gamut B-29

## CONE-SHAPED EPIPHYSES

**COMMON**
1. Idiopathic or normal
2. Dactylitis (esp. sickle cell anemia, smallpox, osteomyelitis, frostbite, burn)
3. Trauma; epiphyseal-metaphyseal fracture; battered child S.

**UNCOMMON**
1. Achondroplasia
2. Acrocephalosyndactyly (Apert S.)
3. Acrodysostosis
4. Acromesomelic dysplasia
5. Asphyxiating thoracic dysplasia (Jeune S.)
6. Beckwith-Wiedemann S.
7. Bird-headed dwarfism (Seckel S.)

8. Brachydactyly S., type E
9. Chondrodysplasia punctata (Conradi's disease)
10. Chondroectodermal dysplasia (Ellis-van Creveld S.)
11. Cleidocranial dysplasia
12. Cockayne S.
13. Conorenal S.; Saldino-Mainzer S.
14. Dyggve-Melchior-Clausen S.
15. Hyperthyroidism, neonatal
16. Hypervitaminosis A, chronic
17. Hypophosphatasia (knees)
18. Infarction (eg, sickle cell anemia, vasculitis)
19. Infection (esp. meningococcemia)
20. Kashin-Beck disease
21. Metaphyseal chondrodysplasia (McKusick)
22. Multiple cartilaginous exostoses (lateral cone)
23. Multiple epiphyseal dysplasia (Fairbank)
24. Orofaciodigital S.
25. Osteoglophonic dwarfism
26. Osteopetrosis
27. Otopalatodigital S.
28. Peripheral dysostosis
29. Pseudohypoparathyroidism, pseudopseudohypoparathyroidism
30. Radiation injury
31. Spondyloepiphyseal dysplasia, pseudoachondro-plastic type
32. Tricho-rhino-phalangeal dysplasia; Langer-Giedion S.
33. Weill-Marchesani S.

*References:*
1. Giedion A: Cone-shaped epiphyses of the hands and their diagnostic value. The tricho-rhino-phalangeal syndrome. Ann Radiol 1967;10:322-329
2. Poznanski AK: The Hand in Radiologic Diagnosis. (ed 2) Philadelphia: W.B. Saunders, 1984, pp 155-161
3. Swischuk LE: Differential Diagnosis in Pediatric Radiology. Baltimore: Williams & Wilkins, 1984, p 220
4. Taybi H, Lachman RS: Radiology of Syndromes, Metabolic Disorders, and Skeletal Dysplasias. (ed 3) Chicago: Year Book Medical Publ, 1990, p 868

B. Bone

# WIDE EPIPHYSEAL PLATE (PHYSIS)

## Generalized

**COMMON**

1. Growth hormone excess (eg, pituitary tumor, gigantism, or treatment with growth hormone)
2. Hyperparathyroidism, primary or esp. secondary (renal osteodystrophy)
3. Maturation delay (endocrine, constitutional, other causes)
4. Rickets, all types (See B-46)

**UNCOMMON**

1. Aminoaciduria (eg, phenylketonuria, homocystinuria)
2. Hypophosphatasia
3. Hypothyroidism, cretinism
4. Metaphyseal chondrodysplasias
5. Mucolipidosis II (I cell disease); $GM_1$ gangliosidosis

## Localized

**COMMON**

1. Fracture, epiphyseal-metaphyseal (Salter-Harris)
2. Pathologic fracture (eg, scurvy, rickets, leukemia, lymphoma$_g$, metastasis)
3. Slipped capital femoral epiphysis

**UNCOMMON**

1. Congenital indifference to pain (fracture)
2. Infection (eg, syphilis, rubella)
3. Kirner deformity
4. Radiation therapy

*References:*
1. Greenfield GB: Radiology of Bone Diseases. (ed 5) Philadelphia: Lippincott, 1990
2. Swischuk LE: Differential Diagnosis in Pediatric Radiology. Baltimore: Williams & Wilkins, 1984, pp 241-243

## Gamut B-31

# RADIOLUCENT METAPHYSEAL BANDS

## COMMON
1. Leukemia, lymphoma$_g$
2. Metastatic neoplasm (esp. neuroblastoma)
3. Normal variant (esp. in neonate)
4. Systemic illness or stress in childhood, infancy, or in utero
5. Transplacental infection (eg, toxoplasmosis, rubella, cytomegalic inclusion disease, herpes, syphilis)
6. Trauma; battered child S.; deprivation dwarfism

## UNCOMMON
1. Chemotherapy; radiation therapy
2. Cushing S.
3. Erythroblastosis fetalis
4. Heavy metal poisoning (alternating with dense lines)
5. Hypophosphastasia
6. Infection, postnatal (eg, brucellosis)
7. Intrauterine gut perforation with meconium peritonitis
8. Juvenile rheumatoid arthritis
9. Osteopetrosis
10. Prolonged parenteral hyperalimentation
11. Rickets, healing
12. Scurvy

*References:*
1. Greenfield GB: Radiology of Bone Diseases. (ed 5) Philadelphia: Lippincott, 1990

2. Oh KS, Ledesma-Medina J, Bender TM: Practical Gamuts and Differential Diagnosis in Pediatric Radiology. Chicago: Year Book Medical Publ, 1982, pp 148-149
3. Poznanski AK: Annual oration-diagnostic clues in the growing ends of bone. J Can Assoc Radiol 1978;29:7-21
4. Swischuk LE: Differential Diagnosis in Pediatric Radiology. Baltimore: Williams & Wilkins, 1984, p 227
5. Wolfson JJ, Engel RR: Anticipating meconium peritonitis from metaphyseal bands. Radiology 1969;92:1055-1060

## Gamut B-32

# TRANSVERSE LINES OR ZONES OF INCREASED DENSITY IN THE METAPHYSES

**COMMON**
1. Chemotherapy (eg, methotrexate)
2. Chronic anemia$_g$ (eg, sickle cell anemia, thalassemia)
3. Growth arrest lines due to systemic illness or stress in infancy or childhood (eg, asthma, diabetes, cystic fibrosis, juvenile rheumatoid arthritis, malnutrition)
4. Lead poisoning
5. Leukemia, treated
6. Normal variant (esp. in neonate—dense zone of provisional calcification)
7. Rickets; renal osteodystrophy (healing)
8. Trauma; battered child S.; deprivation dwarfism; stress fracture

**UNCOMMON**
1. Aminopterin fetopathy
2. Cretinism, hypothyroidism (treated)
3. Drug or hormone therapy in high dosage (eg, steroids, parathormone, methotrexate, estrogen or heavy metal therapy to mother during pregnancy)

4. Heavy metal or chemical absorption, other (eg, bismuth, arsenic, phosphorus, fluoride, mercury, lithium, radium, thorotrast)
5. Hypervitaminosis D
6. Hypoparathyroidism, pseudohypoparathyroidism
7. Idiopathic hypercalcemia (Williams S.)
8. Meconium peritonitis (neonatal dense bands)
9. Metaphyseal chondrodysplasias (Schmid, McKusick)
10. Osteopetrosis
11. Parathormone therapy
12. Radiation therapy, including bone-seeking isotopes ($Sr^{90}$, $Y^{90}$, $P^{32}$)
13. Scurvy, healing
14. Transplacental infection, healing (eg, toxoplasmosis, rubella, cytomegalic inclusion disease, herpes, syphilis)
15. Vascular injury

*References:*

1. Follis RH Jr, Park EA: Some observations on bone growth, with particular respect to zones and transverse lines of increased density in the metaphysis. AJR 1952;68:709-724
2. Poznanski AK: The Hand in Radiologic Diagnosis. (ed 2) Philadelphia: W.B. Saunders, 1984, pp 143-144

## Gamut B-33

# DENSE VERTICAL METAPHYSEAL LINES

## COMMON

1. Epiphyseal injury (localized)
2. Osteopathia striata
3. Prenatal infections ("celery stalk" metaphyses) (eg, rubella, cytomegalovirus, syphilis)

**UNCOMMON**
1. Hypophosphatasia
2. Metaphyseal chondrodysplasias
3. Normal

*Reference:*
1. Swischuk LE: Differential Diagnosis in Pediatric Radiology. Baltimore: Williams & Wilkins, 1984, p 229

## Gamut B-34

# SPLAYING, FLARING, OR WIDENING OF THE METAPHYSES (INCLUDING ERLENMEYER FLASK DEFORMITY) (See Subgamuts B-34A, B-34B)

**COMMON**
*1. Anemia, primary$_g$ (eg, thalassemia, sickle cell anemia)
2. Bone cyst or benign expansile tumor
3. Fracture, epiphyseal-metaphyseal injury
*4. Gaucher's disease, Niemann-Pick disease
5. Normal variant
*6. Rickets, including renal osteodystrophy and biliary rickets; Dilantin therapy

**UNCOMMON**
*1. Congenital syndromes (esp. metaphyseal dysplasia, osteopetrosis, achondroplasia) (See B-34A, B-34B)
2. Histiocytosis X$_g$
3. Hypervitaminosis A
4. Immunologic disorders$_g$
*5. Lead poisoning, chronic
*6. Mastocytosis
7. Scurvy

*Erlenmeyer flask deformity.

*References:*
1. Kozlowski K, Beighton P: Gamut Index of Skeletal Dysplasias. Berlin: Springer-Verlag, 1984, p 63
2. Swischuk LE: Differential Diagnosis in Pediatric Radiology. Baltimore: Williams & Wilkins, 1984, pp 233-235

## Subgamut B-34A

# CONGENITAL SYNDROMES WITH SPLAYING, FLARING, OR WIDENING OF THE METAPHYSES

**COMMON**

1. Achondroplasia
2. Enchondromatosis (Ollier's disease)
3. Chondrodysplasia punctata (Conradi's disease)
4. Chondroectodermal dysplasia (Ellis-van Creveld S.)
*5. Hypophosphatasia (adult)
*6. Metaphyseal dysplasia (Pyle's disease)
*7. Multiple cartilaginous exostoses (diaphyseal aclasis)
*8. Osteopetrosis

**UNCOMMON**

1. Cephaloskeletal dysplasia (Taybi-Linder S.)
2. Cockayne S.
*3. Craniometaphyseal dysplasia
4. Diastrophic dysplasia
*5. Dysosteosclerosis
6. Dyssegmental dysplasia
*7. Frontometaphyseal dysplasia
8. Hypochondroplasia
*9. Kniest dysplasia
*10. Membranous lipodystrophy
11. Mesomelic dysplasia (Langer)
12. Metaphyseal chondrodysplasia (types Jansen, McKusick, Schmid)
13. Metatropic dysplasia
14. Morquio S.

15. Mucolipidosis II
*16. Osteodysplasty (Melnick-Needles S.)
17. Osteogenesis imperfecta (rare "cystic" form)
*18. Otopalatodigital S.
19. Phenylketonuria
*20. Schwarz-Lélek S.
21. Short rib-polydactyly S.
22. Spondyloepiphyseal dysplasia (congenital and pseudoachondroplastic types)
23. Spondylometaphyseal dysplasia
24. Thanatophoric dysplasia
25. Williams S. (distal femurs)

* Erlenmeyer flask deformity.

*References:*
1. Kozlowski K, Beighton P: Gamut Index of Skeletal Dysplasias. Berlin: Springer-Verlag, 1984, p 63
2. Swischuk LE: Differential Diagnosis in Pediatric Radiology. Baltimore: Williams & Wilkins, 1984, pp 233-235

## Subgamut B-34B

## ERLENMEYER FLASK DEFORMITY OF METAPHYSIS
## (See Gamut B-34, Subgamut B-34A)

**COMMON**
1. Anemia, primary$_g$ (eg, thalassemia, sickle cell anemia)
2. Gaucher's disease; Niemann-Pick disease
3. Metaphyseal dysplasia (Pyle's disease); craniometaphyseal dysplasia; frontometaphyseal dysplasia
4. Osteopetrosis

**UNCOMMON**
1. Dysosteosclerosis
2. Hypophosphatasia (adult)

---

3. Kniest dysplasia
4. Lead intoxication, chronic
5. Mastocytosis
6. Membranous lipodystrophy
7. Osteodysplasty (Melnick-Needles S.)
8. Otopalatodigital S.
9. Rickets, healing
10. Schwarz-Lélek S.

*References:*
1. Greenfield GB: Radiology of Bone Diseases. (ed 5) Philadelphia: Lippincott, 1990
2. Swischuk, LE: Differential Diagnosis in Pediatric Radiology. Baltimore: Williams & Wilkins, 1984, pp 234-235
3. Taybi H, Lachman RS: Radiology of Syndromes, Metabolic Disorders, and Skeletal Dysplasias. (ed 3) Chicago: Year Book Medical Publ, 1990, p 871

## Gamut B-35

## DUMBBELL BONES (SHORT LONG BONES WITH PRONOUNCED METAPHYSEAL FLARING)

### COMMON
1. Kniest dysplasia
2. Metatropic dysplasia
3. Pseudoachondroplasia, severe

### UNCOMMON
1. Chondroectodermal dysplasia (Ellis-van Creveld S.)
2. Diastrophic dysplasia

*Reference:*
1. Swischuk LE: Differential Diagnosis in Pediatric Radiology. Baltimore: Williams & Wilkins, 1984, p 166

## Gamut B-36

# METAPHYSEAL CUPPING

**COMMON**
1. Cone-shaped epiphyses (See B-29)
2. Normal variant (eg, distal ulna and fibula; triangular-shaped finger and toe phalanges)
3. Prolonged immobilization of joints causing distal metaphyseal cupping (eg, poliomyelitis; tuberculosis or pyarthrosis of hip; slipped femoral epiphysis; congenital hip dislocation)
4. Rickets, all types (See B-46)
5. Trauma (to cartilage); epiphyseal-metaphyseal injury

**UNCOMMON**
1. Congenital indifference to pain
2. Copper deficiency, nutritional; kinky-hair S. (Menkes S.) (spurs)
3. Hypervitaminosis A
4. Hypophosphatasia
5. Immune deficiency syndromes (eg, metaphyseal dysostosis; thymolymphopenia S.; Shwachman-Diamond S.)
6. Infarction; hypovascularity
7. Leukemia
8. Mucolipidosis II (in infants)
9. Osteochondrodysplasias (incl. achondrogenesis II; achondroplasia; hypochondroplasia; pseudoachondroplasia; chondroectodermal dysplasia; peripheral dysostosis; thanatophoric dysplasia; metaphyseal chondrodysplasias; spondylometaphyseal dysplasia (Kozlowski); dyssegmental dysplasia; metatrophic dysplasia; diastrophic dysplasia; cephaloskeletal dysplasia; tricho-rhino-phalangeal dysplasia; osteodysplasty)
10. Osteomyelitis (eg, bacterial, syphilitic, yaws, smallpox)
11. Phenylketonuria

12. Radiation therapy
13. Scurvy (after a compression fracture)
14. Sickle cell anemia$_g$
15. Thermal injury (frostbite, burn)

*References:*
1. Caffey J: Traumatic cupping of the metaphyses of growing bones. AJR 1970;108:451-460
2. Greenfield GB: Radiology of Bone Diseases. (ed 5) Philadelphia: Lippincott, 1990
3. Poznanski AK: The Hand in Radiologic Diagnosis. (ed 2) Philadelphia: W.B. Saunders, 1984, p 900
4. Swischuk LE: Differential Diagnosis in Pediatric Radiology. Baltimore: Williams & Wilkins, 1984, pp 233-235

## Gamut B-37

# INDISTINCT FRAYED METAPHYSES

**COMMON**
1. Osteomalacia
2. Rickets (See B-46)

**UNCOMMON**
1. Chronic stress (in wrists of adolescent gymnasts)
2. Copper deficiency, nutritional; kinky-hair S. (Menkes S.)
3. Hyperparathyroidism, severe
4. Hypophosphatasia
5. Metaphyseal chondrodysplasias
6. Rubella S.
7. Syphilis, congenital

*References:*
1. Carter SR, et al: Stress changes of the wrist in adolescent gymnasts. Br J Radiol 1988;61:109-112
2. Greenfield GB: Radiology of Bone Disease. (ed 5) Philadelphia: Lippincott, 1990

3. Grünebaum M, Horodniceanu C, Steinherz R: The radiographic manifestations of bone changes in copper deficiency. Pediatr Radiol 1980;9:101-104
4. Swischuk LE: Differential Diagnosis in Pediatric Radiology. Baltimore: Williams & Wilkins, 1984, p 231

## Gamut B-38

# METAPHYSEAL BEAKS, SPURS, OR FRAGMENTATION

**COMMON**
1. Blount's disease
2. Bow legs, other causes (See B-189)
3. Fracture, epiphyseal-metaphyseal (eg, normal bones, battered child S., breech delivery)
4. Normal, esp. knees with bow legs
5. Osteomyelitis; congenital infections (eg, rubella, cytomegalic inclusion disease, syphilis)
6. Rickets, all types

**UNCOMMON**
1. Copper deficiency, nutritional; kinky-hair S. (Menkes S.)
2. Hyperparathyroidism
3. Leukemia, lymphoma$_g$
4. Metaphyseal chondrodysplasias
5. Metastatic disease (esp. neuroblastoma)
6. Neurogenic disease with bone atrophy
7. Scurvy (Pelkan spurs)
8. Short rib-polydactyly S., types 2 and 3

*References:*
1. Oh KS, Ledesma-Medina J, Bender TM: Practical Gamuts and Differential Diagnosis in Pediatric Radiology. Chicago: Year Book Medical Publ, 1982, p 154
2. Swischuk LE: Differential Diagnosis in Pediatric Radiology. Baltimore: Williams & Wilkins, 1984, pp 232-233

# EROSION OF THE MEDIAL ASPECT OF THE PROXIMAL METAPHYSES OF LONG BONES (ESPECIALLY THE HUMERUS, FEMUR, AND TIBIA)

## COMMON
1. Hyperparathyroidism, primary or secondary (renal osteodystrophy)
2. Leukemia
3. Metastatic neuroblastoma
4. Rheumatoid arthritis (humeral notch)

## UNCOMMON
1. Congenital syphilis
2. Gaucher's disease; Niemann-Pick disease
3. Hurler S.
4. Normal variant
5. Rickets

*Reference:*
1. Li JKW, Birch PD, Davies AM: Proximal humerus defects in Gaucher's disease. Br J Radiol 1988;61:579-583

## Gamut B-40

# GROSS DISRUPTION OF EPIPHYSEAL-METAPHYSEAL REGION

## COMMON
1. Battered child S., other severe trauma
2. Fracture in neurogenic or neuromuscular disorder
3. Fracture in weakened bone
   a. Bone infarction (esp. sickle cell anemia)

    b. Hyperparathyroidism
    c. Metastatic disease
    d. Neonatal infection (eg, syphilis, rubella, cyto-
       megalic inclusion disease)
    e. Osteomyelitis (eg, bacterial, smallpox)
    f. Rickets
    g. Scurvy

## UNCOMMON

1. Histiocytosis $X_g$ (esp. eosinophilic granuloma)
2. Osteogenesis imperfecta
3. Primary bone sarcoma
4. Sensory neuropathy
    a. Amyotrophic lateral sclerosis
    b. Congenital indifference to pain
    c. Diabetes
    d. Leprosy
    e. Peripheral nerve injury
    f. Syphilis (tabes dorsalis)
    g. Syringomyelia, hydromyelia

*Reference:*

1. Swischuk LE: Differential Diagnosis in Pediatric Radiology.
   Baltimore: Williams & Wilkins, 1984, p 240

## Gamut B-41

# DIFFERENTIAL DIAGNOSIS OF METAPHYSEAL DISTURBANCES

| Disturbance | Epiphysis | Physis | Zone of Provisional Calcification | Fraying | Cupping | Radiolucent Metaphyseal Band | Metaphyseal Fracture | Periosteal Reaction | Age of Onset (May be present at) |
|---|---|---|---|---|---|---|---|---|---|
| Rickets | Ill-defined | Widened | Early stage—ill-defined, Healing stage—widened | + | + | | - | + | 6 months—rarely at birth (osteomalacic mothers) |
| Scurvy | Ringed | Narrow, normal | Widened | - | From infraction | + | + | + | 3 months |
| Hypophosphatasia | Ill-defined | Widened | Ill-defined | + | + | - | - | + | Birth |
| Metaphyseal dysostosis | Normal | Widened | Ill-defined | + | + | - | - | - | Birth |
| Phenylketonuria | May be retarded | Spicules of calcium protrude | Normal | - | + | - | - | - | 1 month |
| Infantile trauma | Normal | Normal | Normal | - | - | - | + | + | Birth injury |
| Rubella | Ill-defined | Normal | Absent | + | - | + | - | + | Birth |
| Lues | Normal | Widened | Widened | + | + | + | + | + | Birth |
| Leukemia | Ill-defined, destructive foci | Normal | Normal | - | - | + | - | + | Birth |

*Reference:* 1. Greenfield GB: Radiology of Bone Diseases. (ed 4) Philadelphia: Lippincott, 1986, p 254

B. Bone

# LOCALIZED OR REGIONAL OSTEOPOROSIS; BONE ATROPHY

## COMMON
1. Acro-osteolysis (See B-127)
2. Arthritis (esp. rheumatoid, pyogenic, Reiter S.) (See J-12)
3. Disuse atrophy, immobilization (eg, fracture, cast); neural or muscular paralysis
4. Hemorrhage (eg, trauma, hemophilia)
5. Infection (eg, osteomyelitis, tuberculosis, mycetoma)
6. Neoplasm, benign or malignant (esp. myeloma, osteolytic metastasis)
7. Osteonecrosis (incl. radiation); bone infarct or avascular necrosis, early
8. Sudeck's atrophy (reflex sympathetic dystrophy) (See B-43)
9. Thermal injury (eg, burn, frostbite); electroshock

## UNCOMMON
1. AV malformation, hemangioma
2. Congenital pseudarthrosis
3. Denervation or tendon transection
4. Diabetes (diabetic osteopathy)
5. Paget's disease (eg, osteoporosis circumscripta)
6. Regional transitory osteoporosis (esp. hip); regional migratory painful osteoporosis of legs
7. Sarcoidosis
8. Shoulder-hand S. (eg, myocardial infarction, scalenus anticus S.)

## SUDECK'S ATROPHY
## (SPOTTY OSTEOPOROSIS)
### (See Gamut B-42)

1. Arthritis (esp. rheumatoid, pyogenic, Reiter S.) (See J-12)
2. Burn, frostbite, electroshock
3. Idiopathic
4. Immobilization
5. Infection (eg, osteomyelitis, tuberculosis, mycetoma, human bite)
6. Shoulder-hand S. (eg, myocardial infarction, scalenus anticus S.)
7. Trauma with or without fracture; fracture complications (eg, nonunion, malposition, infection)
8. Vascular insufficiency, arterial or venous (eg, arteriosclerosis obliterans, Buerger's disease, Raynaud's disease)

## Gamut B-44

## GENERALIZED OSTEOPOROSIS

**CONGENITAL**
1. Cerebro-oculo-facio-skeletal S.
2. Cockayne S.
3. Ehlers-Danlos S.
4. Fanconi S. (pancytopenia-dysmelia S.)
5. Farber's disease (lipogranulomatosis)
6. Focal dermal hypoplasia (Goltz S.)
7. Geroderma osteodysplastica
8. Glycogen storage disease (von Gierke)
9. Gonadal dysgenesis (Turner S.)
10. Hajdu-Cheney S. (osteolysis)

11. Hypophosphatasia
12. Kinky-hair S. (Menkes S.)
13. Membranous lipodystrophy
*14. Metabolic error (eg, homocystinuria, phenylketonuria)
15. Metachromatic leukodystrophies
16. Mucopolysaccharidoses; $GM_1$ gangliosidosis
*17. Neuromuscular diseases and dystrophies$_g$
18. Oculocerebrorenal S. (Lowe S.)
19. Osteochondrodysplasias (eg, Pyle's disease, Engelmann's disease, Jansen's metaphyseal chondrodysplasia, achondrogenesis)
*20. Osteogenesis imperfecta, fibrogenesis imperfecta
21. Otopalatodigital S.
22. Parastremmatic dwarfism
23. Prader-Willi S.
24. Progeria; Werner S.
25. Pseudohypoparathyroidism, pseudopseudohypoparathyroidism
26. Singleton-Merten S.
27. Trisomy 13 S.
28. Trisomy 18 S.
29. Wilson's disease
30. Winchester S.
31. Wolman's disease

## DEFICIENCY DUE TO MALASSIMILATION
*1. Alcoholism
*2. Calcium, phosphorus deficiency
3. Copper deficiency (in infants)
*4. Malabsorption (eg, sprue, celiac disease, inflammatory small bowel disease, postgastrectomy, blind loop S.)
*5. Malnutrition, kwashiorkor, starvation, anorexia nervosa
*6. Protein deficiency
*7. Vitamin C deficiency (scurvy)
*8. [Vitamin D deficiency (rickets)]

## DISUSE ATROPHY (MUSCLE WEAKNESS; LACK OF STRESS STIMULUS OR WEIGHT BEARING)

*1. Cerebral palsy; spinal cord disease
*2. Immobilization (eg, chronic disease, major fracture, cast)
*3. Muscular dystrophy; neuromuscular disease$_g$; arthrogryposis
 4. Space flight osteoporosis


## ENDOCRINE

*1. Adrenocortical abnormality (eg, adrenal atrophy-adrenopause, Addison's disease; Cushing S.)
*2. Hypogonadism
    a. Ovarian (eg, menopause, oophorectomy, Turner S.)
    b. Testicular (eg, eunuchoidism, prepubertal castration S., Klinefelter XXY S.)
 3. Pancreatic abnormality (eg, poorly controlled diabetes, pancreatic insufficiency, cystic fibrosis)
*4. Parathyroid abnormality (eg, hyperparathyroidism-primary, secondary, or tertiary; hypoparathyroidism with steatorrhea)
 5. Pituitary abnormality (eg, acromegaly, Cushing S. due to basophilic adenoma, hypopituitarism, craniopharyngioma)
 6. Steroid-producing nonendocrine neoplasm (eg, oat cell carcinoma)
*7. Thyroid abnormality (eg, hyperthyroidism, thyrotoxicosis, hypothyroidism, cretinism)


## MISCELLANEOUS

 1. Amyloidosis; familial Mediterranean fever
*2. Anemia$_g$ (eg, sickle cell, thalassemia, spherocytosis, severe iron deficiency)
*3. Collagen disease$_g$ (eg, lupus erythematosus, scleroderma, dermatomyositis, CREST S.)
 4. Gaucher's disease; Niemann-Pick disease
 5. Hemochromatosis

6. Hemophilia
7. Histiocytic medullary reticulocytosis
8. Hypoxemia (eg, chronic pulmonary disease, congenital heart disease)
*9. Iatrogenic, drug therapy (eg, excessive steroids, heparin, vitamin A); chemotherapy; experimental hyperoxia
*10. Idiopathic (eg, idiopathic juvenile osteoporosis)
11. Idiopathic hypercalcemia (Williams S.) (late)
12. Leukemia (acute)
13. Liver disease (eg, jaundice, hepatolenticular degeneration, large or multiple liver tumors or cysts with protein disturbance, biliary atresia)
14. Mastocytosis
*15. Metastatic disease (eg, carcinomatosis)
*16. Multiple myeloma
17. Ochronosis
*18. [Osteomalacia]
19. Pregnancy
*20. Renal disease (eg, nephrosis, tubular acidosis, oxalosis, renal osteodystrophy)
*21. Rheumatoid arthritis; ankylosing spondylitis
*22. Senile or postmenopausal osteoporosis
23. Vascular tumors of bone, widespread (eg, angiomatosis, Gorham's disease)
24. Waldenström's macroglobulinemia

*Common

### References:

1. Greenfield GB: Radiology of Bone Diseases. (ed 5) Philadelphia: Lippincott, 1990
2. Kozlowski K, Beighton P: Gamut Index of Skeletal Dysplasias. Berlin: Springer-Verlag, 1984, pp 3-4
3. Poznanski AK: The Hand in Radiologic Diagnosis. (ed 2) Philadelphia: W.B. Saunders, 1984, p 922
4. Taybi H, Lachman RS: Radiology of Syndromes, Metabolic Disorders, and Skeletal Dysplasias. (ed 3) Chicago: Year Book Medical Publ, 1990
5. Teplick JG, Haskin ME: Roentgenologic Diagnosis. (ed 3) Philadelphia: W.B. Saunders, 1976

# SUBPERIOSTEAL BONE RESORPTION
## (See Gamuts B-39, B-104)

**COMMON**
1. Hyperparathyroidism, primary or secondary (eg, renal osteodystrophy)
*2. Tendon avulsion (eg, parosteal desmoid)

**UNCOMMON**
1. Lipogranulomatosis, disseminated
2. Metaphyseal chondrodysplasia (Jansen)
3. Mucolipidosis, $GM_1$ gangliosidosis
4. Pseudohypohyperparathyroidism
5. Rickets, severe
*6. Subperiosteal hematoma
*7. Subperiosteal osteomyelitis

*Focal.

*Reference:*
1. Swischuk LE: Differential Diagnosis in Pediatric Radiology. Baltimore: Williams & Wilkins, 1984, p 192

## Subgamut B-45A

# SITES OF SUBPERIOSTEAL RESORPTION IN PRIMARY HYPERPARATHYROIDISM
## (In Order of Decreasing Frequency)

1. Middle phalanges of 2nd and 3rd fingers, radial aspect
2. Clavicle, outer end
3. Femur, tibia, and humerus, upper inner aspect

4. Lamina dura of teeth
5. Ischial tuberosity
6. Pubic symphysis
7. Sacroiliac joint
8. Calcaneus, tendon insertions
9. Radius and ulna, distal end
10. Sesamoid bones
11. Rib, esp. upper border
12. Sella turcica
13. Calvarium, inner and outer table
14. Tuft of terminal phalanx

*Reference:*
1. Jacobson HG: Personal communication

## Gamut B-46

## OSTEOMALACIA AND RICKETS*

### I. DEFICIENT ABSORPTION OF CALCIUM OR PHOSPHORUS

#### A. Malabsorption states
1. Cathartic abuse (esp. oily cathartics, phenolphthalein, or magnesium sulfate)
2. Mesenteric disease
3. Pancreatic insufficiency (exocrine), pancreatitis
4. Postoperative gastric or small bowel resection; small bowel bypass
5. Primary small bowel disease (eg, celiac disease, sprue, amyloidosis, scleroderma, Crohn's disease, lymphoma, small bowel fistula, blind loop S.)
6. Steatorrhea, idiopathic

#### B. Obstructive jaundice or liver failure
1. Acquired chronic biliary obstruction
2. Biliary atresia

**C. Vitamin D deficient rickets (dietary or lack of sunshine)**

## II. DIETARY CALCIUM DEFICIENCY (Rare)

## III. ENZYME ABNORMALITY (EG, HYPOPHOSPHATASIA)

## IV. EXCESSIVE EXCRETION OF CALCIUM OR PHOSPHORUS VIA BREAST OR PLACENTA (PUERPERAL OSTEOMALACIA)

## V. EXCESSIVE RENAL EXCRETION OF CALCIUM OR PHOSPHORUS

### A. Glomerular (hyperphosphatemic)
1. Renal osteodystrophy (secondary hyper-parathyroidism)
2. Renal osteomalacia

### B. Tubular (hypophosphatemic)
1. Fanconi syndromes (glycosuria, aminoaciduria, and proteinuria)
   a. Primary (idiopathic)
      i. Childhood type, with cystinosis
      ii. Adult type, without cystinosis
   b. Acquired
      i. Beryllium poisoning
      ii. Heavy metal poisoning (eg, lead, cadmium, fluoride)
      iii. Ingestion of outdated tetracycline
      iv. Multiple myeloma
      v. Nephrotic syndrome
      vi. Neurofibromatosis
      vii. Vitamin D intoxication in adults

2. Inborn metabolic disturbances (eg, galactosemia, oxalosis, tyrosinosis, Wilson's disease, $GM_1$ gangliosidosis)
3. Vitamin D-resistant rickets (hypophosphatemic familial rickets)

## VI. EXCESSIVE UTILIZATION OF CALCIUM AS FIXED BASE

1. Chronic obstructive renal disease
2. Idiopathic hypercalciuria
3. Polycystic kidney disease
4. Renal tubular acidosis
5. Ureterosigmoidostomy (hyperchloremia)

## VII. MISCELLANEOUS

1. Aluminum-induced bone disease (eg, phosphate deficiency from aluminum hydroxide hemodialysis; antacid-induced osteomalacia and nephrolithiasis)
2. Anticonvulsant drug therapy (eg, Dilantin, tranquilizers) (accelerated hepatic degradation of vitamin $D_3$ and 25-HCC)
3. Congenital rickets (mother with osteomalacia)
4. Decreased deposition of calcium in bone (eg, diphosphonate treatment for Paget's disease)
5. Fibrogenesis imperfecta ossium; axial osteomalacia (with acquired vitamin D resistance)
6. Immunologic disorders$_g$
7. [Metaphyseal chondrodysplasia, type Schmid]
8. Paraneoplastic syndromes (humoral syndromes) (See B-46A)
9. Pernicious anemia
10. Pseudovitamin D-deficiency rickets or osteomalacia

## NOTE: In infants less than 6 months of age, consider chiefly:

1. Biliary atresia
2. Hypophosphatasia

3. Neonatal rickets (premature infants with combined dietary deficiency and impaired hepatic hydroxylation of vitamin D)
4. Vitamin D-resistant rickets (associated with severe myopathy; dietary intake of vitamin D is adequate)

*References:*
1. Greenfield GB: Radiology of Bone Diseases. (ed 5) Philadelphia: Lippincott, 1990
2. Murray RO, Jacobson HG, Stoker DJ: The Radiology of Skeletal Disorders. (ed 3) Edinburgh: Churchill Livingstone, 1990
3. Turner ML, Dalinka MK: Osteomalacia: Uncommon causes. AJR 1979;133:539-540

## Subgamut B-46A

# BONE AND SOFT TISSUE NEOPLASMS ASSOCIATED WITH OSTEOMALACIA*

1. Giant cell reparative granuloma
2. Giant cell tumor, malignant
3. Hemangioma, cavernous or sclerosing
4. Hemangiopericytoma
5. Neurinoma, malignant
6. Nonossifying fibroma; fibroxanthoma
7. Ossifying mesenchymal tumor
8. Osteoblastoma
9. Sarcoma, unspecified

*Tumor-induced osteomalacia or ectopic humoral syndrome.

*Reference:*
1. Greenfield GB: Radiology of Bone Disease. (ed 5) Philadelphia: Lippincott, 1990

# CAUSES OF ALTERED CALCIUM AND PHOSPHORUS CONCENTRATIONS

## HYPERCALCEMIA

1. Adrenal insufficiency
2. Hyperparathyroidism
3. Hyperthyroidism, hypothyroidism
4. Hypervitaminosis D
5. Hypophosphatasia
6. Idiopathic hypercalcemia (Williams S.)
7. Leukemia, lymphoma$_g$
8. Metaphyseal chondrodysplasia (Jansen)
9. Milk-alkali S.
10. Myelomatosis
11. Rapid deossification of bone
12. Reticuloses
13. Sarcoidosis
14. Secretion of parathormone-like substance from malignant neoplasms
15. Skeletal metastases
16. Wermer S. (familial multiple endocrine neoplasms - MEN S., type I)

## HYPERPHOSPHATEMIA

1. Acromegaly
2. Glomerular failure
3. Hypervitaminosis D
4. Hypoparathyroidism; pseudohypoparathyroidism
5. Skeletal metastases

## HYPOCALCEMIA

1. Acidosis
2. Hypoalbuminemic states
3. Hypoparathyroidism; pseudohypoparathyroidism
4. Malabsorption states
5. Normal neonate

6. Pancreatitis
7. Uremia; uremic osteodystrophy
8. Vitamin D deficiency

## HYPOPHOSPHATEMIA

1. Dietary deficiency
2. Hyperparathyroidism
3. Hypovitaminosis D (eg, vitamin D-deficiency rickets, osteomalacia)
4. Increased carbohydrate metabolism
5. Malabsorption states
6. Pregnancy
7. Renal tubular dysfunction (eg, Fanconi S., vitamin D-resistant rickets)
8. Skeletal metastases

## HYPERCALCIURIA

1. Acidosis
2. Active osteoporosis
3. Hypercalcemia
4. Hypervitaminosis D
5. Hyperparathyroidism, primary
6. Renal tubular disease
7. Sarcoidosis
8. Widespread bone destruction

## HYPOCALCIURIA

1. Active reconstruction of bone
2. Alkalosis
3. Decreased glomerular filtration rate
4. Hypocalcemia
5. Reduced calcium absorption from intestine
6. Vitamin D deficiency

*Reference:*
1. Greenfield GB: Radiology of Bone Diseases. (ed 5) Philadelphia: Lippincott, 1990

## WIDESPREAD OR GENERALIZED DEMINERALIZATION WITH COARSE TRABECULATION

**COMMON**
1. Anemia$_g$, primary (esp. sickle cell anemia, thalassemia)
2. Carcinomatosis
3. Hyperparathyroidism, primary or secondary
4. Multiple myeloma
5. Osteomalacia, rickets (eg, biliary atresia, alimentary tract disorder) (See B-46)
6. Osteoporosis (See B-44)
7. Paget's disease
8. Paralysis

**UNCOMMON**
1. Acromegaly
2. Fibrogenesis imperfecta ossium
3. Gaucher's disease
4. Hemophilia
5. Idiopathic axial osteomalacia
6. Leukemia
7. Osteogenesis imperfecta
8. Recalcification after disuse osteoporosis

## SCATTERED AREAS OF DECREASED AND INCREASED BONE DENSITY IN THE SKELETON

**COMMON**
1. Lymphoma$_g$, leukemia
2. Metastases (esp. breast)

3. Osteomyelitis (incl. tuberculosis and syphilis)
4. Paget's disease
5. Renal osteodystrophy

## UNCOMMON
1. Fibrous dysplasia
2. Histiocytosis $X_g$
3. Hyperparathyroidism
4. Hyperphosphatasia
5. Mastocytosis
6. Tuberous sclerosis

## Gamut B-50

# BONE INFARCT
# (DIAMETAPHYSEAL ISCHEMIA)

## COMMON
1. Idiopathic
2. Occlusive vascular disease (arteriosclerosis, Buerger's disease, thromboembolic disease)
3. Primary anemia$_g$ (esp. sickle cell)

## UNCOMMON
1. Caisson disease
2. Fat embolism (eg, alcoholism)
3. Gaucher's disease
4. Infection, osteomyelitis
5. Pancreatitis with fat necrosis
6. Polyarteritis nodosa (vasculitis)
7. Radiation therapy; radium poisoning

*Reference:*
1. Edeiken J, Hodes PJ, Libshitz HI, et al: Bone ischemia. Radiol Clin North Am 1967;5:515-529

## Gamut B-51

# AVASCULAR NECROSIS (EPIPHYSEAL ISCHEMIA)

**COMMON**

1. Idiopathic; Legg-Calvé-Perthes disease
2. Occlusive vascular disease (eg, arteriosclerosis, Leriche S., thromboembolic disease, giant cell arteritis)
3. Osteochondritis dissecans (localized form of avascular necrosis)
4. Primary anemia$_g$ (esp. sickle cell)
5. Steroid therapy; Cushing S.
6. Trauma (eg, fracture - esp. of femoral neck or proximal scaphoid; dislocation; surgical correction of congenital hip; slipped capital femoral epiphysis; hip nailing; microfracture; battered child S.; congenital indifference to pain; burn; frostbite)

**UNCOMMON**

1. Caisson disease (dysbaric osteonecrosis)
2. Charcot joint
3. Collagen disease$_g$ (eg, rheumatoid arthritis, lupus erythematosus, polyarteritis nodosa, scleroderma)
4. Diabetes
5. Drug therapy (eg, anti-inflammatory agents-Butazolidin, Indocin; immunosuppressives; cytotoxic therapy; methotrexate)
6. Fabry's disease
7. Fat embolism (eg, alcoholism, liver disease, pancreatitis, trauma)
8. Gaucher's disease
9. Gout
10. Hemophilia
11. Histiocytosis X$_g$
12. Hyperlipoproteinemia
13. Hypothyroidism
14. Infection (eg, pyogenic arthritis; osteomyelitis; subacute bacterial endocarditis)

15. Meyer dysplasia of femoral head
16. Osteoporosis, generalized
17. Polycythemia vera
18. Pregnancy
19. Radiation therapy; radium poisoning
20. Thiemann's disease (phalanges)
21. Tricho-rhino-phalangeal dysplasia I
22. Winchester S.

*References:*
1. Edeiken J, Hodes PJ, Libshitz HI, et al: Bone ischemia. Radiol Clin North Am 1967;5:515-529
2. Griffiths HJ: Etiology, pathogenesis, and early diagnosis of ischemic necrosis of the hip. JAMA 1981;246:2615-2617
3. Hunder GG, Worthington JW, Bickel WH: Avascular necrosis of the femoral head in a patient with gout. JAMA 1968; 203:47-49
4. Jacobson HG, Siegelman SS: Some miscellaneous solitary bone lesions. Semin Roentgenol 1966;1:314-335
5. Jaffe HL: Ischemic necrosis of bone. Med Radiogr Photogr 1969;45:58-86
6. Mallory TH: Avascular necrosis of the femoral head in the adult. Ohio State Med J 1975;71:548-550
7. Martel W, Sitterley BH: Roentgenologic manifestations of osteonecrosis. AJR 1969;106:509-522
8. Murray RO, Jacobson HG, Stoker DJ: The Radiology of Skeletal Disorders. (ed 3) Edinburgh: Churchill Livingstone, 1990
9. Swischuk LE: Differential Diagnosis in Pediatric Radiology. Baltimore:Williams & Wilkins, 1984, pp 212-214

## Gamut B-52

# SITES OF PREDILECTION AND EPONYMS FOR AVASCULAR NECROSIS

**COMMON**

| | |
|---|---|
| 1. Carpal lunate | Kienböck 1910 |
| 2. Femoral capital epiphysis | Legg-Calvé-Perthes 1910 |

3. Medial femoral condyle
   (occasionally lateral
   femoral condyle)
4. Medial tibial condyle      Blount 1937
5. [Osteochondrosis dissecans]      König 1887
6. Second metatarsal head      Freiberg 1914
   (occasionally third or fourth)
7. Secondary patellar center      Sinding-Larsen 1921
   (at its inferior aspect)
8. Talus (trochlea)      Diaz 1928
9. Tarsal navicular      Köhler 1908
10. Tibial tubercle      Osgood-Schlatter
                                    1903
11. Vertebral body      Calvé and Kümmell
                                    1925
12. Vertebral epiphysis      Scheuermann 1921

**UNCOMMON**

1. Bases of phalanges      Thiemann 1909
*2. Calcaneal apophysis      Sever 1912
3. Capitulum of humerus      Panner 1927
4. Carpal scaphoid      Preiser 1911
5. Distal tibial epiphysis      Liffert and Arkin 1950
6. Distal ulna      Burns 1921
7. Entire carpus bilaterally      Caffey 1945
8. Fifth metatarsal base      Iselin 1912
9. Greater trochanter of femur      Mandl 1922
10. Head of humerus      Hass 1921
11. Head of radius      Brailsford
12. Heads of metacarpals      Mauclaire 1927;
                                    Dietrich 1932
*13. Iliac crest      Buchman 1927
14. Intercondylar spines of tibia      Caffey 1956
15. Ischial apophysis      Milch 1953
*16. Ischiopubic synchondrosis      Van Neck 1924
17. Os tibiale externum      Haglund 1908
18. Primary patellar center      Köhler 1908
19. Symphysis pubis      Pierson 1929

* Now considered a normal variant.

*Reference:*
1. Greenfield GB: Radiology of Bone Diseases. (ed 5) Philadelphia: Lippincott, 1990

## Gamut B-53

# "BONE WITHIN A BONE" APPEARANCE

**COMMON**
1. Bone infarction (eg, sickle cell anemia)
2. [Growth arrest and recovery, "growth lines" (eg, due to severe childhood disease, infection, scurvy, rickets, stress, immobilization, leukemia, chemotherapy)]
3. Idiopathic
4. Normal neonate (esp. spine)
5. Osteopetrosis
6. Paget's disease

**UNCOMMON**
1. Acromegaly
2. Bone diseases with a split or double-layer cortex (See B-102)
3. Chronic osteomyelitis with sequestrum and involucrum (eg, pyogenic, syphilis)
4. Heavy metal intoxication (eg, lead, phosphorus, bismuth, cadmium, fluoride)
5. Hypervitaminosis D
6. Oxalosis
7. Subcortical osteoporosis (eg, Sudeck's atrophy involving carpals or tarsals; leukemia; metastatic disease)
8. Subperiosteal hemorrhage
9. Thorotrast, radiation osteitis

*References:*
1. Brill PW, Baker DH, Ewing ML: Bone-within bone in the neonatal spine. Radiology 1973;108:363-366
2. Frager DH, Subbarao K: The "bone within a bone." JAMA 1983;249:77-79

---

3. Greenfield GB: Radiology of Bone Diseases. (ed 5) Philadelphia: Lippincott, 1990
4. Murray RO, Jacobson HG, Stoker DJ: The Radiology of Skeletal Disorders. (ed 3) Edinburgh: Churchill Livingstone, 1990
5. O'Brien JP: The manifestations of arrested bone growth: The appearance of a vertebra within a vertebra. J Bone Joint Surg 1969;51A:1376-1378
6. Sutton D: A Textbook of Radiology and Imaging. (ed 4) Edinburgh: Churchill Livingstone, 1987

## Gamut B-54

# LOCALIZED BONE SCLEROSIS WITH RADIOLUCENT NIDUS OR SEQUESTRUM

**COMMON**
1. Brodie's abscess, osteomyelitis
2. Osteoid osteoma

**UNCOMMON**
1. Eosinophilic granuloma
2. Osteoblastoma
3. Syphilis, yaws
4. Tropical ulcer
5. Tuberculosis

## Gamut B-55

# SCLEROTIC FOCI OR CALCIFIC STREAKING IN INFANTS AND CHILDREN

## NEONATES AND INFANTS

1. Cerebrohepatorenal S. (Zellweger S.)
2. Chondrodysplasia punctata (Conradi's disease)

3. Chromosomal disorders
4. GM$_1$ gangliosidosis
5. Healed fractures (eg, battered child S.)
6. Smith-Lemli-Opitz S.
7. Warfarin embryopathy

# OLDER CHILDREN

1. Bone islands
2. Cystic angiomatosis
3. Enchondromatosis (Ollier's disease)
4. Healed fractures (incl. osteogenesis imperfecta)
5. Lymphoma$_g$
6. Mastocytosis
7. Melorheostosis
8. Metaphyseal chondrodysplasia (Jansen)
9. Osteopathia striata
10. Osteopetrosis
11. Osteopoikilosis
12. Osteosarcomatosis, osteoblastic metastases
13. Parastremmatic dwarfism
14. Tuberous sclerosis

*Reference:*

1. Kozlowski K, Beighton P: Gamut Index of Skeletal Dysplasias. Berlin: Springer-Verlag, 1984, pp 9,61

## Gamut B-56

# SOLITARY OSTEOSCLEROTIC BONE LESION
# (See Gamut B-57)

## COMMON

1. Avascular necrosis (See B-51)
2. Bone infarct (See B-50)
3. Bone island or enostoma; idiopathic sclerosis

4. Callus (healed or healing fracture); stress fracture
5. Chondroid lesion (eg, enchondroma, osteochondroma)
6. Healed or healing benign bone lesion (eg, bone cyst, nonossifying fibroma, fibrous cortical defect, histiocytosis $X_g$, brown tumor)
7. Hyperostosis frontalis interna (skull)
8. Osteoblastic metastasis (esp. breast, prostate) (See B-88)
9. Osteochondritis dissecans
10. Osteoid osteoma
11. Osteoma
12. Osteomyelitis, chronic, healed, or sclerosing (eg, Garré's; Brodie's abscess; granuloma; mycetoma; tropical ulcer)
13. Osteonecrosis (eg, radiation)
14. Paget's disease

## UNCOMMON

1. Bone sarcoma (eg, osteosarcoma, chondrosarcoma, Ewing's, parosteal sarcoma)
2. Fibrous dysplasia; ossifying fibroma
3. Lymphoma$_g$
4. Lytic metastasis following radiation or chemotherapy
5. Medullary calcification in a long bone following removal of intramedullary rod
6. Melorheostosis
7. Meningioma (skull)
8. Osteitis condensans ilii (unilateral)
9. Osteoblastoma
10. Plasma cell granuloma
11. Syphilis; yaws

*References:*

1. Burgener FA, Kormano M: Differential Diagnosis in Conventional Radiology. (ed 2) New York: Thieme Medical Publ, 1991
2. Swee RG, McLeod RA, Beabout JW: Osteoid osteoma: Detection, diagnosis, and localization. Radiology 1979;130: 117-123

3. Swischuk LE: Differential Diagnosis in Pediatric Radiology. Baltimore:Williams & Wilkins, 1984, p 203

## Gamut B-57

# MULTIPLE OSTEOSCLEROTIC BONE LESIONS

## COMMON

1. Bone infarcts
2. Bone islands
3. Callus (eg, healed rib fractures, battered child S.)
4. Osteitis condensans ilii
5. Osteoblastic metastases (See B-88)
6. Osteomyelitis, chronic or healed (eg, tuberculous, fungal)
7. Paget's disease

## UNCOMMON

1. Avascular necroses
2. Chester-Erdheim disease
3. Chondrodysplasia punctata (Conradi's disease); other causes of stippled epiphyses (eg, multiple epiphyseal dysplasia - see B-21, B-21A)
4. Enchondromatosis (Ollier's disease)
5. Fibrous dysplasia
6. Heavy metal intoxication (eg, phosphorus, bismuth, lead, cadmium, fluoride)
7. Infantile cortical hyperostosis (Caffey's disease)
8. Lipoatrophic diabetes (total lipodystrophy)
9. Lymphoma$_g$, leukemia
10. Lytic metastases or myeloma following radiation or chemotherapy
11. Mastocytosis
12. Melorheostosis
13. Multiple cartilaginous exostoses

14. Multiple enchondromas, osteochondromas
15. Multiple healed or healing benign bone lesions (eg, nonossifying fibromas, fibrous cortical defects, brown tumors, Gaucher's disease, histiocytosis $X_g$, cystic angiomatosis)
16. Multiple myeloma (rare)
17. Osteomas (eg, Gardner S.)
18. Osteopathia striata (Voorhoeve's disease)
19. Osteopoikilosis
20. Osteosarcomatosis
21. Plasma cell granulomas; POEMS S.
22. Pyknodysostosis
23. Sarcoidosis
24. Syphilis; yaws
25. Tuberous sclerosis

*References:*

1. Burgener FA, Kormano M: Differential Diagnosis in Conventional Radiology. (ed 2) New York: Thieme Medical Publ, 1991
2. Griffiths HJ, Rossini AA: A case of lipoatrophic diabetes. Radiology 1975;114:329-330
3. Resnick D, Greenway GD, Bardwick PA, et al: Plasma-cell dyscrasia with polyneuropathy, organomegaly, endocrinopathy, M-protein, and skin changes. The POEMS syndrome. Radiology 1981;140:17-22

## Gamut B-58

# GENERALIZED OR WIDESPREAD OSTEOSCLEROSIS

**COMMON**

1. Fluorosis
2. Myelosclerosis, myeloid metaplasia
3. Osteoblastic metastases (esp. breast, prostate)
4. Paget's disease

5. Physiologic osteosclerosis of newborn (normal variant, esp. in prematures)
6. Renal osteodystrophy (esp. healing phase)
7. Sickle cell anemia (rarely other anemias)

## UNCOMMON

1. Chester-Erdheim disease
2. Congenital cyanotic heart disease
3. Congenital syndromes, other (See B-58A)
4. Diffuse idiopathic skeletal hyperostosis (DISH)
5. Endosteal hyperostosis (van Buchem, Worth)
6. Engelmann's disease (diaphyseal dysplasia)
7. Erythroblastosis fetalis
8. Fibrous dysplasia, polyostotic
9. Gaucher's disease
10. Heavy metal intoxication (eg, lead, phosphorus, bismuth, cadmium poisoning); thorotrast injection
11. Hyperparathyroidism, primary or secondary (esp. treated or in the young)
12. Hyperphosphatasia
13. Hypertrophic osteoarthropathy (See B-98)
14. Hypervitaminosis D, chronic
15. Hypoparathyroidism, pseudohypoparathyroidism, pseudopseudohypoparathyroidism
16. Hypothyroidism, cretinism
17. Idiopathic hypercalcemia (Williams S.)
18. Idiopathic osteosclerosis (familial)
19. Infantile cortical hyperostosis (Caffey's disease)
20. Intrauterine infection (eg, congenital syphilis, rubella, toxoplasmosis, cytomegalovirus)
21. Lymphoma$_g$, leukemia (treated)
22. Mastocytosis
23. Melorheostosis
24. Metaphyseal dysplasia (Pyle's disease) in infancy; craniometaphyseal dysplasia
25. Multiple myeloma (rare)
26. Neurofibromatosis
27. Osteodysplasty (Melnick-Needles S.)
28. Osteomalacia, rickets (healing)

29. Osteopathia striata
30. Osteopetrosis
31. Osteopoikilosis
32. Osteosarcomatosis
33. Oxalosis
34. Pachydermoperiostosis
35. Pyknodysostosis
36. Syphilis; yaws
37. Tuberous sclerosis
38. Tubular stenosis (Kenny-Caffey S.)

*References:*
1. Brancaccio D, Poggi A, Ciccarelli C, et al: Bone changes in end-stage oxalosis. AJR 1981;136:935-939
2. Burgener FA, Kormano M: Differential Diagnosis in Conventional Radiology. (ed 2) New York: Thieme Medical Publ, 1991
3. Greenfield GB: Radiology of Bone Diseases. (ed 5) Philadelphia: Lippincott, 1990
4. Griffiths HJ, Rossini AA: A case of lipoatrophic diabetes. Radiology 1975;114:329-330
5. Kozlowski K, Beighton P: Gamut Index of Skeletal Dysplasias. Berlin: Springer-Verlag, 1984, pp 7-9
6. Taybi H, Lachman RS: Radiology of Syndromes, Metabolic Disorders, and Skeletal Dysplasias. (ed 3) Chicago: Year Book Medical Publ, 1990
7. Teplick JG, Haskin ME: Roentgenologic Diagnosis. (ed 3) Philadelphia: W.B. Saunders, 1976

## Subgamut B-58A

## CONGENITAL SYNDROMES WITH GENERALIZED OR WIDESPREAD OSTEOSCLEROSIS

**COMMON**
1. Congenital cyanotic heart disease
2. Endosteal hyperostosis (van Buchem, Worth)
3. Engelmann's disease (diaphyseal dysplasia)

---

4. Erythroblastosis fetalis
5. Fibrous dysplasia
6. Gaucher's disease
7. Hyperphosphatasia
8. Hypothyroidism, cretinism
9. Idiopathic hypercalcemia (Williams S.)
10. Idiopathic osteosclerosis (familial)
11. Infantile cortical hyperostosis (Caffey's disease)
12. Melorheostosis
13. Metaphyseal dysplasia (Pyle's disease) in infancy; craniometaphyseal dysplasia; frontometaphyseal dysplasia; craniodiaphyseal dysplasia
14. Neurofibromatosis
15. Osteodysplasty (Melnick-Needles S.)
16. Osteopathia striata
17. Osteopetrosis
18. Osteopoikilosis
19. Pachydermoperiostosis
20. [Physiologic osteosclerosis of newborn]
21. Pseudohypoparathyroidism
22. Pyknodysostosis
23. Tuberous sclerosis

**UNCOMMON**
1. Dysosteosclerosis
2. Lenz-Majewski hyperostotic dwarfism
3. Lipoatrophic diabetes (total lipodystrophy)
4. Oculo-dento-osseous dysplasia
5. Osteomesopyknosis
6. Otopalatodigital S.
7. Peripheral osteosclerosis
8. POEMS S.
9. Pseudoleprechaunism (Patterson S.)
10. Robinow S.
11. Rothmund-Thomson S.
12. Schwarz-Lélek S.
13. Sclerosteosis
14. Stanescu dyostasis
15. Tricho-dento-osseous S.

16. Tubular stenosis (Kenny-Caffey S.)
17. Weismann-Netter S.

*References:*
1. Beighton P, Cremin BJ: Sclerosing Bone Dysplasias. Berlin: Springer-Verlag, 1980
2. Kozlowski K, Beighton P: Gamut Index of Skeletal Dysplasias. Berlin: Springer-Verlag, 1984, pp 7-9
3. Taybi H, Lachman RS: Radiology of Syndromes, Metabolic Disorders, and Skeletal Dysplasias. (ed 3) Chicago: Year Book Medical Publ, 1990, pp 887-888

## Gamut B-59

# GENERALIZED OSTEOSCLEROSIS: A CLASSIFICATION BASED ON ITS LOCATION WITHIN BONE

## PREDOMINANTLY IN SPONGY TRABECULAR BONE

1. Fluorosis
2. Hyperparathyroidism, primary (esp. in children)
3. Hypervitaminosis D
4. Lymphoma$_g$, leukemia
5. Mastocytosis
6. Multiple myeloma
7. Myelofibrosis
8. Osteoblastic metastases (See B-88)
9. Polycythemia vera
10. Renal osteodystrophy
11. Rickets (hypophosphatemic vitamin D-resistant in adults)
12. Sickle cell anemia and variants$_g$

## PREDOMINANTLY IN COMPACT CORTICAL BONE

1. Autosomal dominant osteosclerosis

---

2. Endosteal hyperostosis (van Buchem, Worth)
3. Engelmann's disease
4. Hypertrophic osteoarthropathy (See B-98)
5. Metaphyseal dysplasia (Pyle's disease);
   craniometaphyseal dysplasia; craniodiaphyseal
   dysplasia
6. Pachydermoperiostosis
7. Ribbing's disease

## INVOLVING TRABECULAR AND CORTICAL BONE

1. Dysosteosclerosis
2. Idiopathic hypercalcemia (Williams S.)
3. Osteopetrosis
4. Osteosclerosis with dentine dysplasia
5. Pyknodysostosis
6. Sclerosteosis

*Reference:*
1. Genant HK: Review of the osteoscleroses. In: Diagnostic
   Radiology Proceedings of the Annual Postgraduate Course in
   Diagnostic Radiology. San Francisco: U. of California School
   of Medicine, 1981, pp 109-122

## Gamut B-60

# PREFERENTIAL SITE WITHIN BONE OF VARIOUS OSSEOUS LESIONS
# (See Gamuts B-60A to B-63)

## EPIPHYSIS

1. Chondroblastoma
2. Giant cell tumor (after fusion of epiphyseal plate;
   originates in metaphysis)

## METAPHYSIS

1. Aneurysmal bone cyst

2. Bone cyst
3. Chondrosarcoma
4. Desmoplastic fibroma
5. Fibrosarcoma
6. Giant cell tumor
7. Malignant fibrous histiocytoma
8. Ossifying fibroma
9. Osteoblastoma
10. Osteochondroma, exostosis
11. Osteosarcoma (75%)
12. Parosteal (cortical) desmoid
13. Parosteal sarcoma

**DIAMETAPHYSIS**
1. Bone cyst (late)
2. Bone infarct
3. Chondromyxoid fibroma
4. Fibrosarcoma
5. Hemangioma
6. Lipoma
7. Nonossifying fibroma; benign cortical defect
8. Osteomyelitis
9. Periosteal chondroma or fibroma

**DIAPHYSIS**
1. Adamantinoma (esp. tibia)
2. Cortical fibrous dysplasia (tibia)
3. Enchondroma
4. Ewing's tumor
5. Fibrous dysplasia
6. Histiocytosis $X_g$
7. Lymphoma$_g$
8. Myeloma
9. Osteoid osteoma
10. Osteosarcoma (25%)

## Subgamut B-60A

# FAVORED SITES OF ORIGIN OF VARIOUS BONE LESIONS (THE "FIELD THEORY" OF THE ORIGIN OF BONE TUMORS)

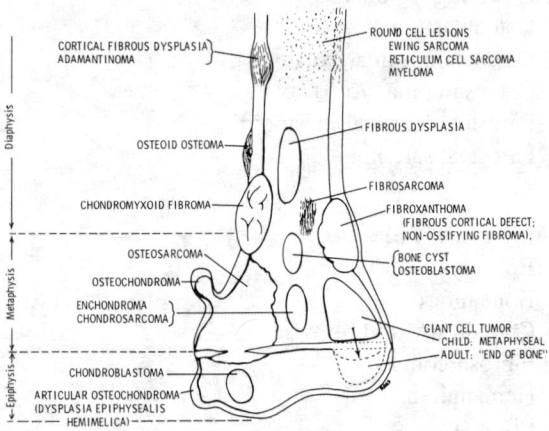

Composite diagram illustrating frequent sites of bone tumors. The diagram depicts the end of a long bone that has been divided into the epiphysis, metaphysis, and diaphysis. The typical sites of common primary bone tumors are labeled. Bone tumors tend to predominate in those ends of long bones that undergo the greatest growth and remodeling, and hence have the greatest number of cells and amount of cell activity (shoulder and knee regions). When small tumors, presumably detected early, are analyzed, preferential sites of tumor origin become apparent within each bone, as shown in this illustration. This suggests a relationship between the type of tumor and the anatomic site affected. In general, a tumor of a given cell type arises in the field where the homologous normal cells are most active. These regional variations suggest that the composition of the tumor is affected or may be determined by the metabolic field in which it arises.

*References:*

1. Johnson LC: A general theory of bone tumors. Bull NY Acad Med 1953;29:164-171.
2. Madewell JE, Ragsdale BD, Sweet DE: Radiologic and pathologic analysis of solitary bone lesions. Part I: Internal margins. Radiol Clin North Am 1981;19:715-748.

# SOLITARY LYTIC EPIPHYSEAL OR EPIPHYSEAL-METAPHYSEAL LESION OF BONE

## COMMON

1. Arthritic lesion (eg, gout, rheumatoid arthritis, tuberculosis, hemophilia, pseudogout, osteoarthritis with degenerative cyst or geode)
2. Chondroblastoma (Codman tumor)
*3. Cystic osteomyelitis (esp. tuberculous, poorly treated bacterial); Brodie's abscess
*4. Giant cell tumor
5. [Normal femoral condylar or femoral head defect (eg, fovea centralis)]
6. Osteochondrosis dissecans (See B-61A); avascular necrosis
7. Synovial lesion (eg, pigmented villonodular synovitis); synovial erosion or pit in metaphysis of femoral neck

## UNCOMMON

1. Amyloidosis
*2. Aneurysmal bone cyst
*3. Angioma
*4. Bone cyst
5. Defect from avulsion fracture (esp. knee)
*6. Enchondroma
7. Eosinophilic granuloma (histiocytosis $X_g$)
*8. Hydatid cyst
9. Intraosseous ganglion
*10. Lipoma
*11. Metastasis
12. Myeloma, plasmacytoma
*13. Osteoid osteoma
*14. Sarcoma (eg, arising in benign fibrous or chondroid lesion; clear cell chondrosarcoma)

* Epiphyseal-metaphyseal location.

*Reference:*
1. Bullough PG, Bansal M: The differential diagnosis of geodes. Radiol Clin North Am 1988;26:1165-1184

## Subgamut B-61A

## OSTEOCHONDROSIS DISSECANS— SITES OF PREDILECTION

### COMMON
1. Medial femoral condyle
2. Talus (trochlear surface)

### UNCOMMON
1. Elbow (capitellum of humerus)
2. Femoral head
3. Humeral head
4. Lateral femoral condyle
5. Metatarsal head (esp. first)
6. Patella
7. Tibial plateau (lateral portion)

*Reference:*
1. Greenfield GB: Radiology of Bone Diseases. (ed 5) Philadelphia: Lippincott, 1990

## Gamut B-62

## SOLITARY LYTIC METAPHYSEAL OR DIAMETAPHYSEAL LESION OF BONE

### WELL-DEFINED GEOGRAPHIC LESION
1. Angioma; AV fistula
2. Bone cyst

3. Bone infarct
4. Brown tumor of hyperparathyroidism
5. Chondromyxoid fibroma
6. Cortical desmoid
7. Cystic osteomyelitis
8. Enchondroma
9. Giant cell tumor
10. Histiocytosis $X_g$
11. Lipoma
12. Metastasis
13. Multiple myeloma (punched out lesion)
14. Nonossifying fibroma; fibrous cortical defect
15. Ossifying fibroma
16. Osteoblastoma
17. Osteochondroma, exostosis
18. Periosteal chondroma or fibroma

## ILL-DEFINED GEOGRAPHIC LESION

1. Adamantinoma (esp. tibia)
2. Bone infarct (eg, in sickle cell anemia)
3. Cortical desmoid
4. Desmoplastic fibroma
5. Giant cell reparative granuloma
6. Giant cell tumor
7. Histiocytosis $X_g$
8. Hydatid cyst
9. Lymphoma$_g$
10. Malignant fibrous histiocytoma
11. Metastasis
12. Multiple myeloma; plasmacytoma
13. Osteomyelitis
14. Sarcoma (eg, osteosarcoma, chondrosarcoma, fibrosarcoma)
15. Syphilis (eg, Wimberger sign)

## MOTH-EATEN OR PERMEATIVE LESION

1. Histiocytosis $X_g$ (esp. eosinophilic granuloma)
2. Lymphoma$_g$
3. Malignant fibrous histiocytoma

4. Metastasis
5. Multiple myeloma
6. Osteomyelitis
7. Sarcoma (esp. Ewing's, osteosarcoma, chondro-sarcoma, fibrosarcoma, reticulum cell sarcoma)

## Gamut B-63

## SOLITARY LYTIC DIAPHYSEAL LESION

**COMMON**
1. Bone cyst
2. Bone infarct
3. Diametaphyseal lesion extending into diaphysis (eg, nonossifying fibroma, fibrosarcoma*) (See B-62)
4. Enchondroma
5. Fibrous dysplasia
*6. Histiocytosis $X_g$ (esp. eosinophilic granuloma)
*7. Metastasis
*8. Osteomyelitis
*9. Plasmacytoma, myeloma
*10. Round cell sarcoma (esp. Ewing's tumor)

**UNCOMMON**
*1. Adamantinoma (esp. tibia)
2. Brown tumor of hyperparathyroidism
3. Cortical fibrous dysplasia (tibia)
4. Hemophilic pseudotumor
*5. Hydatid cyst
*6. Lymphoma$_g$
*7. Osteosarcoma
8. Paget's disease (osteoporosis circumscripta)
*9. Syphilis, yaws

* May be moth-eaten or permeative pattern.

## Gamut B-64

# DIAGRAM OF PATTERNS OF BONE DESTRUCTION

1A: GEOGRAPHIC DESTRUCTION WELL-DEFINED WITH SCLEROSIS IN MARGIN

1B: GEOGRAPHIC DESTRUCTION WELL-DEFINED BUT NO SCLEROSIS IN MARGIN

1C: GEOGRAPHIC DESTRUCTION WITH ILL-DEFINED MARGIN

CHANGING 1A MARGIN (DESTRUCTION OF RIND)

CHANGING 1B MARGIN (CORTICAL BREAKOUT)

CHANGING 1B MARGIN (TRANSITION TO II)

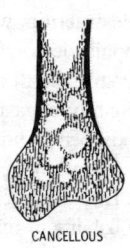

CANCELLOUS

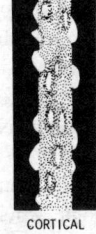

CORTICAL

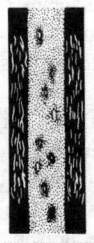

III: PERMEATED

II: MOTHEATEN

Schematic diagram of patterns of bone destruction (types IA, IB, IC, II, III) and their margins. Arrows indicate the most frequent transitions or combinations of these margins. Transitions imply increased activity and a greater probability of malignancy.

*Reference:*

1. Madewell JE, Ragsdale BD, Sweet DE: Radiologic and pathologic analysis of solitary bone lesions. Part I: Internal margins. Radiol Clin North Am 1981;19:715-748.

## Gamut B-65

# COMMON BONE LESIONS AND THEIR TYPICAL PATTERNS OF BONE DESTRUCTION

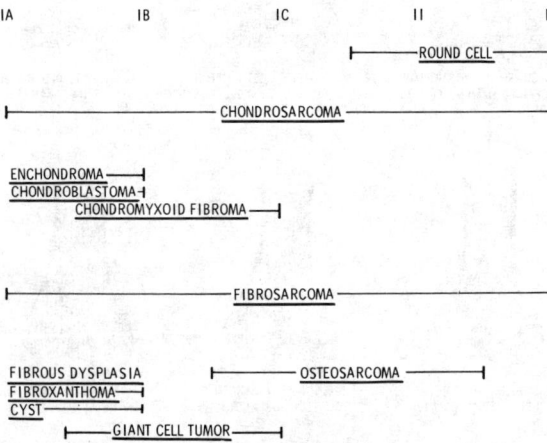

This diagram delineates common bone tumors and their typical patterns of bone destruction. IA, Geographic destruction, well-defined, with sclerosis in margin. IB, Geographic destruction, well-defined, but no sclerosis in margin. IC, Geographic destruction with ill-defined margin. II, Moth-eaten (regionally invasive). III. Permeative (diffusely invasive). Note that most benign tumors occur on the left-hand side, from IA to IC, whereas most malignant tumors occur on the right-hand side, from IC to III. This illustrates the general principle that the biologic activity and probability of malignancy increase from left to right. Chondrosarcoma and fibrosarcoma can present with any of the five patterns. In our experience, they frequently arise in preexisting benign lesions. In such cases, the radiographic pattern may lag behind the histologic activity, producing a radiographic discrepancy (slow-appearing lesions with malignant histology).

### Reference:

1. Madewell JE, Ragsdale BD, Sweet DE: Radiologic and pathologic analysis of solitary bone lesions. Part I: Internal margins. Radiol Clin North Am 1981;19:715-748.

## RELATIONSHIP OF BIOLOGIC ACTIVITY (GROWTH RATE) TO TYPE OF BONE MARGIN AND PERIOSTEAL REACTION

| Growth Rate | Internal Margins | Periosteal Reaction |
|---|---|---|
| Slow | Geographic (I) IA IB IC | Solid or Shells Ridged, lobulated, or smooth |
| Intermediate | Moth-eaten (II) | Codman Triangle Shells or lamellated |
| Fast | Permeative (III) | Lamellated or spiculated |
| Fastest | Nonvisible | Spiculated or none |

## LUCENT LESION OF BONE SURROUNDED BY MARKED SCLEROTIC REACTION OR RIM

**COMMON**

1. Bone infarct
2. Brodie's abscess
3. Chondroid lesion, benign (eg, chondroblastoma, enchondroma)
4. Cortical (parosteal) desmoid
5. Cystic osteomyelitis (esp. tuberculous)
6. Degenerative osteoarthritic cyst or geode

7. Healed or healing benign bone cyst or fibrocystic lesion (eg, nonossifying fibroma, fibrous cortical defect, fibrous dysplasia)
8. Osteoid osteoma

**UNCOMMON**
1. Eosinophilic granuloma (occasionally)
2. Lipoma
3. Osteoblastoma
4. Syphilis, yaws

## Gamut B-67

# SOLITARY WELL-DEMARCATED LYTIC LESION OF BONE

**COMMON**
*1. Arthritic or synovial lesion (eg, osteoarthritic cyst or geode, gouty tophus, rheumatoid nodule or synovial cyst, intraosseous ganglion, amyloidosis)
*2. Bone cyst
*3. Bone infarct
 4. Brown tumor of hyperparathyroidism
*5. Cortical desmoid
*6. Enchondroma
*7. Fibrous dysplasia
 8. Giant cell tumor
*9. Histiocytosis $X_g$ (esp. eosinophilic granuloma)
10. Metastasis
*11. Nonossifying fibroma; fibrous cortical defect
*12. Osteomyelitis, cystic; Brodie's abscess

**UNCOMMON**
1. Adamantinoma
2. Aneurysmal bone cyst
3. Angioma
*4. Chondroblastoma
*5. Chondromyxoid fibroma

6. Epidermoid inclusion cyst (phalanx)
*7. Granuloma (esp. tuberculous, fungal)
8. Hemophilic pseudotumor
9. Hydatid cyst
*10. Lipoma
11. Neurofibroma
*12. Osteoblastoma
*13. Osteoid osteoma
14. Paget's disease (osteoporosis circumscripta)
*15. Periosteal (juxtacortical) chondroma or fibroma
16. Plasmacytoma, myeloma
17. Sarcoidosis
*18. Sarcoma arising in previously benign lesion (eg, chondrosarcoma fibrosarcoma)
*19. Tropical ulcer, benign
*20. Tuberculosis
21. Villonodular synovitis

* Often has sclerotic rim.

## Subgamut B-67A

## WELL-DEFINED, OFTEN CYST-LIKE, INFECTIOUS LESION OF BONE

1. Blastomycosis
2. Brodie's abscess (bacterial, usually *Staph. aureus*)
3. Coccidioidomycosis
4. Cystic osteomyelitis (partially or inadequately treated bone infection)
5. Histoplasmosis duboisii
6. Hydatid disease
7. Leprosy (lepromas)
8. Spina ventosa, other cyst-like dactylitis (incl. yaws) (See B-132)
9. Tuberculosis; atypical mycobacterial infections

## Gamut B-68

# SOLITARY CYST-LIKE
# LESION OF BONE

**COMMON**
1. Bone cyst
2. Enchondroma
3. Fibrous dysplasia (monostotic, cortical)
4. Nonossifying fibroma; fibrous cortical defect
5. Osteoarthritic degenerative cyst or geode

**UNCOMMON**
1. Aneurysmal bone cyst
2. Angioma (eg, hemangioma, lymphangioma)
3. Bone infarct
4. Brown tumor of hyperparathyroidism
5. Chondroblastoma
6. Chondromyxoid fibroma
7. Cortical (periosteal) desmoid
8. Cystic osteomyelitis (incl. tuberculosis); Brodie's abscess
9. Desmoplastic fibroma
10. Epidermoid inclusion cyst
11. Fibrosarcoma, chondrosarcoma (slow growing)
12. Fungal infection (esp. blastomycosis, coccidioidomycosis)
13. Gaucher's disease
14. Giant cell tumor
15. Glomus tumor
16. Gouty tophus
17. Hemophilic pseudotumor
18. Histiocytosis $X_g$ (esp. eosinophilic granuloma)
19. Hydatid cyst
20. Intraosseous ganglion
21. Lipoma
22. Lymphoma$_g$ (rare)
23. Metastatic carcinoma (esp. from kidney or thyroid carcinoma)

24. Ossifying fibroma
25. Osteoblastoma
26. Periosteal chondroma or fibroma
27. Plasmacytoma, myeloma
28. Sarcoidosis
29. Villonodular synovitis

## Gamut B-69

## SOLITARY EXPANSILE LESION OF BONE

### BENIGN NEOPLASM OF BONE

1. Angioma
2. Chondroblastoma
3. Chondromyxoid fibroma
4. Desmoplastic fibroma
*5. Enchondroma
6. Giant cell tumor
7. Lipoma
*8. Nonossifying fibroma
9. Osteoblastoma
10. Periosteal chondroma or fibroma

### MALIGNANT NEOPLASM OF BONE

1. Adamantinoma
*2. Chondrosarcoma
3. Fibrosarcoma
4. Hemangiopericytoma; angiosarcoma
5. Malignant fibrous histiocytoma
6. Malignant giant cell tumor
*7. Metastasis (esp. carcinoma of kidney, thyroid, lung; melanoma)
8. Osteosarcoma, telangiectatic
*9. Plasmacytoma, myeloma

## TUMOR-LIKE LESION OF BONE

1. Aneurysmal bone cyst
*2. Bone cyst
*3. Brown tumor of hyperparathyroidism
 4. Epidermoid inclusion cyst
*5. Fibrous dysplasia; cortical fibrous dysplasia (tibia)
 6. Gaucher's disease
*7. Gouty tophus
 8. Hemophilic pseudotumor
 9. Histiocytosis $X_g$ (esp. eosinophilic granuloma)
10. Hydatid cyst

*Common.

### Reference:

1. Greenfield GB: Radiology of Bone Diseases. (ed 5) Philadelphia: Lippincott, 1990

## Gamut B-70

# BONE BLISTER
# (SOLITARY CYST-LIKE LESION
# EXPANDING BONE ECCENTRICALLY)

## COMMON

1. Aneurysmal bone cyst
2. Chondroid lesion (eg, osteochondroma, enchondroma)
3. Giant cell tumor
4. Nonossifying fibroma; fibrous cortical defect

## UNCOMMON

1. Angioma
2. Brown tumor of hyperparathyroidism
3. Chondromyxoid fibroma
4. Desmoplastic fibroma

5. Fibrosarcoma (esp. arising in benign fibrous lesion)
6. Fibrous dysplasia (skull); cortical fibrous dysplasia (tibia)
7. Gouty tophus
8. Metastasis to cortex (esp. lung)
9. Osteoblastoma
10. Periosteal chondroma or fibroma

## Gamut B-71

### BLOW-OUT LESION OF BONE (SOLITARY GROSSLY EXPANSILE LESION, OFTEN CYST-LIKE) (See Gamut B-72)

**COMMON**
1. Aneurysmal bone cyst
2. Chondrosarcoma
3. Fibrous dysplasia
4. Giant cell tumor
5. Metastatic carcinoma (esp. kidney, thyroid, lung)
6. Plasmacytoma, myeloma

**UNCOMMON**
1. Adamantinoma
2. Brown tumor of hyperparathyroidism
3. Burkitt's lymphoma
4. Chondromyxoid fibroma
5. Chordoma; parachordoma
6. Enchondroma
7. Fibrosarcoma
8. Gouty tophus
9. Hemangiopericytoma, angiosarcoma
10. Hemophilic pseudotumor
11. Hydatid cyst

12. Malignant fibrous histiocytoma
13. Meningocele; sacrococcygeal teratoma
14. Osteoblastoma
15. Osteosarcoma (telangiectatic)

## Gamut B-72

# LARGE DESTRUCTIVE BONE LESION (OVER 5 CM IN DIAMETER)

**COMMON**
1. Aneurysmal bone cyst
2. Angioma; AV fistula; hemangiopericytoma; Gorham's vanishing bone disease
3. Bone cyst
4. Enchondroma
5. Fibrous dysplasia
6. Giant cell tumor
7. Histiocytosis $X_g$
8. Lymphoma$_g$, Burkitt's tumor
9. Metastasis
10. Osteomyelitis; mycetoma
11. Paget's disease (osteoporosis circumscripta)
12. Plasmacytoma, multiple myeloma
13. Primary sarcoma (eg, osteosarcoma, chondrosarcoma, fibrosarcoma, Ewing's, angiosarcoma, reticulum cell sarcoma)

**UNCOMMON**
1. Adamantinoma
2. Brown tumor of hyperparathyroidism
3. Chondromyxoid fibroma
4. Chordoma; parachordoma
5. Desmoplastic fibroma
6. Gaucher's disease
7. Hemophilic pseudotumor

8. Hydatid disease
9. [Lesion arising in spinal canal (eg, meningocele, ependymoma, neurofibroma, sacrococcygeal teratoma)]
10. Malignant fibrous histiocytoma
11. Osteoblastoma
12. [Soft tissue tumor destroying bone (eg, synovioma)]
13. Syphilis, yaws
14. Tropical ulcer, malignant

## Gamut B-73

## SOLITARY POORLY DEMARCATED LYTIC LESION OF BONE

**COMMON**

1. Histiocytosis $X_g$
2. Lymphoma$_g$
3. Metastasis
4. Osteomyelitis (eg, tuberculous, fungal, bacterial)
5. Plasmacytoma, myeloma
6. Sarcoma (esp. Ewing's, osteosarcoma, chondrosarcoma, fibrosarcoma, angiosarcoma, reticulum cell sarcoma)

**UNCOMMON**

1. Adamantinoma
2. Aneurysmal bone cyst
3. Angioma
4. Brown tumor of hyperparathyroidism
5. Chordoma
6. Fibrous dysplasia
7. Giant cell tumor
8. Hemangiopericytoma
9. Hydatid cyst
10. Malignant fibrous histiocytoma
11. Paget's disease (osteoporosis circumscripta)
12. Syphilis, yaws

# MOTH-EATEN OR PERMEATIVE OSTEOLYTIC LESION, SOLITARY OR MULTIPLE

**COMMON**
1. Ewing's sarcoma
2. Metastasis, including neuroblastoma
3. Multiple myeloma
4. Osteomyelitis, including syphilis, yaws
5. Osteosarcoma

**UNCOMMON**
1. Adamantinoma
2. Angiosarcoma
3. Chondrosarcoma
4. Fibrosarcoma
5. Giant cell tumor (at margins)
6. Histiocytosis $X_g$ (esp. eosinophilic granuloma)
7. Landing-Shirkey disease (multifocal granulomatous osteomyelitis in a compromised child)
8. Lymphoma$_g$, leukemia
9. Malignant fibrous histiocytoma
10. Reticulum cell sarcoma
11. Rhabdomyosarcoma

## Gamut B-75

# LYTIC LESION OF BONE CONTAINING CALCIUM OR BONE DENSITY OR MATRIX

**COMMON**
1. Avascular necrosis; osteochondrosis dissecans
2. Bone infarct
*3. Chondrosarcoma
*4. Enchondroma

  5. Fibrous dysplasia
  6. Lymphoma$_g$
  7. Metastasis (esp. breast)
  8. Osteomyelitis with sequestrum
*9. Osteosarcoma
 10. Paget's disease

**UNCOMMON**
  1. Button sequestrum of skull
*2. Chondroblastoma
*3. Chondromyxoid fibroma
  4. Eosinophilic granuloma with sequestrum
  5. Ewing's sarcoma (with reactive bone)
  6. Fibrosarcoma with sequestrum
  7. Lipoma
  8. Osteoid osteoma
*9. Osteoblastoma
 10. Tropical ulcer with sequestrum

* Matrix-containing lesions.

## Gamut B-76

**MULTIPLE RADIOLUCENT LESIONS OF BONE (See Gamut B-106)**

**COMMON**
  1. Arthritis (eg, gout; rheumatoid; osteoarthritic cysts or geodes)
  2. Metastases
  3. Multiple myeloma

**UNCOMMON**
  1. Amyloidosis
  2. Brown tumors of hyperparathyroidism

3. Congenital multiple fibromatosis
4. Electrical injury
5. Enchondromatosis (Ollier's disease); Maffucci S.
6. Fibrous dysplasia, polyostotic
7. Fungus disease$_g$ (esp. blastomycosis, coccidioidomycosis, histoplasmosis duboisii)
8. Gaucher's disease; Niemann-Pick disease
9. Hemangiomatosis, lymphangiomatosis, cystic angiomatosis
10. Hemophilia
11. Histiocytosis X$_g$
12. Hydatid disease
13. Jackhammer operator's (driller's) disease of wrists
14. Kaposi sarcoma
15. Landing-Shirkey disease
16. Leprosy (lepromas)
17. Leukemia, lymphoma$_g$, Burkitt's tumor
18. Lipomatosis
19. Massive osteolysis (Gorham's disease)
20. Mastocytosis
21. Membranous lipodystrophy
22. Multiple nonossifying fibromas (familial)
23. Neurofibromatosis
24. Osteoglophonic dwarfism
25. Osteomyelitis, multiple (eg, cystic tuberculosis, septic)
26. Polycystic osteodysplasia with progressive dementia (hands and feet)
27. Polyvinyl chloride osteolysis
28. Primary bone neoplasm, multiple
29. Radium poisoning
30. Rothmund-Thomson S.
31. Sarcoidosis
32. Tuberous sclerosis
33. Weber-Christian disease

*Reference:*

1. Greenfield GB: Radiology of Bone Diseases. (ed 5) Philadelphia: Lippincott, 1990

# WIDESPREAD AREAS OF BONE DESTRUCTION

## COMMON
1. Arthritis (esp. rheumatoid, gout)
2. Lymphoma$_g$, leukemia, Burkitt's tumor
3. Osteomyelitis (pyogenic, tuberculous)
4. Metastases (carcinomatosis)
5. Multiple myeloma (myelomatosis)
6. Paget's disease

## UNCOMMON
1. Fibrous dysplasia, polyostotic (Albright's S.)
2. Fungus disease$_g$ (eg, blastomycosis, histoplasmosis duboisii)
3. Gaucher's disease
4. Hemangiomatosis; cystic (lymph) angiomatosis; congenital scattered fibromatosis
5. Hemophilia with pseudotumors
6. Histiocytosis $X_g$
7. Hydatid disease
8. Leprosy
9. Massive osteolysis (Gorham's vanishing bone disease)
10. Membranous lipodystrophy
11. Neuroblastoma metastases
12. Osteitis fibrosa cystica (hyperparathyroidism)
13. Sarcoidosis
14. Sarcoma, multicentric (eg, Ewing's, osteosarcoma)
15. Syphilis, yaws
16. Waldenström's macroglobulinemia; pseudomyeloma
17. Weber-Christian disease

### Reference
1. Burgener FA, Kormano M: Differential Diagnosis in Conventional Radiology. (ed 2) New York: Thieme Medical Publ, 1991

## Gamut B-78

## OSTEOLYSIS

**COMMON**
1. Acro-osteolysis (See B-127)
2. Chronic articular disorder (eg, psoriasis, multicentric reticulohistiocytosis, neuropathic arthropathy)
3. Collagen disease$_g$ (eg, scleroderma, lupus, dermatomyositis)
4. Hyperparathyroidism
5. Traumatic

**UNCOMMON**
1. Gorham's disease (massive osteolysis)
2. Idiopathic osteolyses
    a. Phalangeal (incl. ainhum)
    b. Tarsocarpal
        i. Francois form and others
        ii. With nephropathy
    c. Multicentric
        i. Hajdu-Cheney S.
        ii. Torg S.
        iii. Winchester S.
3. Osteolysis with detritic synovitis
4. Sarcoidosis
5. Thermal injury (eg, burn, frostbite, electrical)

*Reference:*
1. Rsenick D, Weisman M, Goergen TG, et al: Osteolysis with detritic synovitis: A new syndrome. Arch Intern Med 1978; 138:1003-1005

# BONE NEOPLASMS CLASSIFIED BY TUMOR MATRIX OR TISSUE OF ORIGIN

## I. Chondroid (Cartilage-Forming) Tumors

**BENIGN**
1. Chondroblastoma (Codman tumor)
2. Chondromyxoid fibroma
3. Enchondroma (incl. enchondromatosis - Ollier's disease)
4. Osteochondroma (incl. multiple cartilaginous exostoses)
5. Parosteal (juxtacortical) chondroma

**MALIGNANT**
1. Chondrosarcoma (multiple types) (See B-84)

## II. Osteoid (Bone-Forming) Tumors

**BENIGN**
1. Ossifying fibroma
2. Osteoblastoma
3. [Osteoid osteoma]
4. Osteoma

**MALIGNANT**
1. Osteosarcoma (multiple types) (See B-84B)

## III. Fibrous Connective Tissue Tumors

**BENIGN**
1. Congenital scattered fibromatosis
2. [Cortical desmoid]
3. Desmoplastic fibroma

4. Fibromyxoma
5. Nonossifying fibroma, fibroxanthoma

**MALIGNANT**
1. Fibrosarcoma
2. Malignant fibrous histiocytoma

# IV. Tumors of Fatty Tissue Origin

**BENIGN**
1. Lipoma, intraosseous or parosteal

**MALIGNANT**
1. Liposarcoma

# V. Tumors of Vascular Origin

**BENIGN**
1. Cystic angiomatosis and lymphangiomatosis
2. Glomus tumor
3. Hemangioma
4. Hemangiopericytoma
5. Lymphangioma
6. Vanishing bone disease (Gorham's disease)

**MALIGNANT**
1. Angiosarcoma; hemangioendothelioma
2. Malignant hemangiopericytoma

# VI. Tumors of Neural Origin

**BENIGN**
1. Neurilemoma (schwannoma)
2. Neurofibroma (incl. neurofibromatosis)

**MALIGNANT**
1. Neurofibrosarcoma; malignant schwannoma

## VII. Giant Cell-Containing Tumors

**BENIGN**
1. Aneurysmal bone cyst
2. Brown tumor of hyperparathyroidism
3. Chondroblastoma (Codman tumor)
4. Chondromyxoid fibroma
5. [Giant cell reparative granuloma]
6. Giant cell tumor (osteoclastoma)

**MALIGNANT**
1. Giant cell-containing osteosarcoma
2. Malignant giant cell tumor

*References:*
1. Dahnert W: Radiology Review Manual. Baltimore: Williams & Wilkins, 1991, p 5
2. Sutton D, Young JWR: A Short Textbook of Clinical Imaging. London: Springer-Verlag, 1990, pp 295-312

## Gamut B-80

# AGE RANGE OF HIGHEST INCIDENCE OF VARIOUS BONE NEOPLASMS AND TUMOR-LIKE LESIONS

| Tumor | Age (Years) |
|---|---|
| 1. Adamantinoma | 15-35 |
| 2. Aneurysmal bone cyst | 10-30 |
| 3. Bone cyst | 5-20 |
| 4. Chondroblastoma | 10-25 |

| Tumor | Age (Years) |
|---|---|
| 5. Chondromyxoid fibroma | 10-30 |
| 6. Chondrosarcoma | 30-60 |
| 7. Chordoma | 30-70 |
| 8. Desmoplastic fibroma | 10-40 |
| 9. Enchondroma | 5-50 |
| 10. Ewing's sarcoma | 5-20 |
| 11. Fibrosarcoma | 10-70 |
| 12. Giant cell tumor | 20-45 |
| 13. Hemangioma | 30-70 |
| 14. Lymphoma$_g$ (incl. reticulum cell sarcoma of bone) | 25-40 |
| 15. Malignant fibrous histiocytoma | 20-60 |
| 16. Metastasis | 40-80 |
| 17. Multiple myeloma | 40-80 |
| 18. Neuroblastoma | 0-10 |
| 19. Nonossifying fibroma; fibrous cortical defect | 5-20 |
| 20. Ossifying fibroma | 5-30 |
| 21. Osteoblastoma | 10-25 |
| 22. Osteochondroma | 10-25 |
| 23. Osteoid osteoma | 10-30 |
| 24. Osteoma | 30-50 |
| 25. Osteosarcoma | 10-25, 60-75 |
| 26. Parosteal sarcoma | 30-50 |
| 27. Parosteal (cortical) desmoid | 10-20 |

*Reference:*

1. Greenfield GB: Radiology of Bone Diseases. (ed 5) Philadelphia: Lippincott, 1990

## Gamut B-81

# BENIGN BONE NEOPLASMS

**COMMON**
1. Enchondroma
2. Hemangioma

   3. Nonossifying fibroma
   4. Osteochondroma (osteocartilaginous exostosis)
   5. [Osteoid osteoma]
   6. Osteoma

**UNCOMMON**
   1. Ameloblastoma (jaws)
   2. Aneurysmal bone cyst
   3. Benign fibrous histiocytoma
   4. Chondroblastoma
   5. Chondromyxoid fibroma
   6. Cystic angiomatosis; lymphangiomatosis
   7. Desmoplastic fibroma
   8. Fibromatosis, juvenile
   9. Fibromyxoma
 10. Giant cell tumor
 11. Glomus tumor
 12. Hemangiopericytoma, benign
 13. [Histiocytosis $X_g$]
 14. Lipoma, intraosseous or periosteal
 15. Lymphangioma
 16. Neurofibroma
 17. Osteoblastoma
 18. Osteofibrous dysplasia (ossifying fibroma)
 19. Parosteal (cortical) desmoid
 20. Parosteal osteoma
 21. Periosteal (juxtacortical) chondroma or fibroma

## Gamut B-82

# BENIGN TUMOR-LIKE LESIONS OF BONE (NONNEOPLASTIC) (See Subgamut B-82A)

**COMMON**
   1. Bone cyst
   2. Bone infarct

3. Bone island (enostoma)
4. Brown tumor of hyperparathyroidism
5. Fibrous cortical defect
6. Fibrous dysplasia
7. Gouty tophus
8. Histiocytosis $X_g$
9. Myositis ossificans (parosteal)
10. Osteoarthritic cyst (geode)
11. Osteochondrosis dissecans; avascular necrosis
12. Osteoid osteoma
13. Osteomyelitis (eg, bacterial, tuberculous, fungal)
14. Paget's disease (esp. osteoporosis circumscripta)
15. Parosteal (cortical) desmoid
16. Stress fracture, healing

## UNCOMMON

1. Aneurysmal bone cyst (See B-82C)
2. Cortical fibrous dysplasia (tibia)
3. Epidermoid, dermoid (skull)
4. Epidermoid inclusion cyst; foreign body or "thorn" granuloma
5. Fibromatosis, juvenile
6. Giant cell reparative granuloma
7. Hemophilic pseudotumor
8. Hydatid cyst
9. Intraosseous ganglion
10. Plasma cell granuloma
11. Sarcoidosis
12. [Soft tissue lesion involving bone (eg, amyloidosis, glomus tumor, giant cell tumor of tendon sheath, pigmented villonodular synovitis)]
13. Xanthoma (See B-82B)

## Subgamut B-82A

# FIBROCYSTIC LESIONS OF BONE

1. Bone cyst
2. Cherubism
3. Chondromyxoid fibroma
4. Cortical fibrous dysplasia (tibia, calvarium)
5. Desmoplastic fibroma
6. Fibrocystic changes of degenerative arthritis (esp. in hip)
7. Fibrogenesis imperfecta ossium
8. Fibromatosis, juvenile
9. Fibromyxoma
10. Fibrous cortical defect
11. Fibrous dysplasia, monostotic or polyostotic (Jaffe-Lichtenstein; Albright's S.)
12. [Intraosseous ganglion]
13. Nonossifying fibroma
14. Osteofibrous dysplasia (ossifying fibroma)
15. Xanthoma (xanthofibroma, benign histiocytic fibroma)

## Subgamut B-82B

# XANTHOMATOUS LESIONS OF BONE

### PRIMARY XANTHOMA

1. Chester-Erdheim disease (multiple sclerotic lipogranulomatous lesions or xanthofibromas of bone)
2. Xanthoma (xanthofibroma, benign histiocytic fibroma)

### SECONDARY XANTHOMATOUS REACTION

1. Aneurysmal bone cyst
2. Bone abscess
3. Eosinophilic granuloma

4. Fibrous dysplasia
5. Giant cell tumor
6. Nonossifying fibroma
7. Solitary bone cyst

*Reference:*
1. Dorfman H: International Skeletal Society Lecture, 1984

## Subgamut B-82C

# PRECURSOR LESIONS OF ANEURYSMAL BONE CYST

## COMMON

1. Giant cell tumor (esp. subperiosteal)
2. Osteoblastoma
3. [Primary]

## UNCOMMON

1. Bone cyst
2. Chondroblastoma
3. Chondromyxoid fibroma
4. Fibrous dysplasia
5. Giant cell reparative granuloma
6. Hemangioma, hemangiopericytoma
7. Metastatic carcinoma
8. Nonossifying fibroma
9. Osteosarcoma (telangiectatic)
10. Trauma (ossifying hematoma)

## Gamut B-83

# SURFACE LESION OF BONE (PERIOSTEAL OR PAROSTEAL NEOPLASM OR TUMOR-LIKE LESION)

## COMMON
1. Florid reactive periostitis (ossifying fasciitis, parosteal fasciitis)
2. Juxtacortical myositis ossificans
3. Osteocartilaginous exostosis
4. Parosteal (cortical) desmoid
5. Periosteal osteosarcoma
6. Subperiosteal osteoid osteoma
7. Turret exostosis

## UNCOMMON
1. High-grade surface osteosarcoma
2. Parosteal hemangioma
3. Parosteal lipoma
4. Parosteal osteoma
5. Parosteal osteosarcoma
6. Periosteal chondrosarcoma
7. Periosteal fibroma
8. Periosteal (juxtacortical) chondroma
9. Periosteal or subperiosteal ganglion
10. [Soft tissue tumor in a parosteal location (eg, synovioma, giant cell tumor of tendon sheath, glomus tumor, Kaposi sarcoma)]
11. Subperiosteal aneurysmal bone cyst
12. Subperiosteal osteoblastoma

*References:*
1. Dorfman H: Minisymposium on Bone-Surface Lesions Terminology. Presented at International Skeletal Society 18th Annual Refresher Course, San Diego, 1991
2. Greenfield GB: Radiology of Bone Diseases. (ed 5) Philadelphia: Lippincott, 1990

# PRIMARY MALIGNANT BONE NEOPLASM

## COMMON

1. Chondrosarcoma (classical or central, juxtacortical or periosteal, dedifferentiated, clear cell, mesenchymal)
2. Ewing's sarcoma
3. Fibrosarcoma
4. Lymphoma$_g$ (incl. Burkitt's tumor)
5. Malignant fibrous histiocytoma
6. Multiple myeloma
7. Osteosarcoma (See B-84B)
8. Undifferentiated sarcoma

## UNCOMMON

1. Adamantinoma
2. Angiosarcoma; hemangioendothelioma
3. Chordoma
4. Giant cell tumor, malignant
5. Kaposi sarcoma
6. Liposarcoma
7. Malignant hemangiopericytoma, perithelioma
8. Neurogenic sarcoma
9. Reticulum cell sarcoma

Subgamut B-84A

# RADIOLOGIC CRITERIA SUGGESTING MALIGNANT BONE NEOPLASM

1. Bone destruction (esp. moth-eaten or permeative, but may be geographic)
2. Irregular ill-defined margins of lesion ("wide transition zone" between normal and abnormal bone)

3. Cortical erosion or destruction
4. Codman triangle
5. Periosteal lamellation ("onion skin")
6. Periosteal right angle spiculation ("sunburst" or "hair-on-end")
7. Soft tissue mass adjacent to bone destruction
8. Chondroid or osteoid matrix (esp. in extraosseous tissues)
9. Metastasis to distant site

*References:*
1. Madewell JE, Ragsdale BD, Sweet DE: Radiologic and pathologic analysis of solitary bone lesions. Radiol Clin North Am 1981;19:715-748
2. Nelson SW: Some fundamentals in the radiologic differential diagnosis of solitary bone lesions. Semin Roentgenol 1966;1:244-267

## Subgamut B-84B

## TYPES OF OSTEOSARCOMA

### PRIMARY
1. Central (low-grade intramedullary)
2. Chondroblastic (chondrogenic)
3. Classical
4. Fibroblastic (fibrogenic)
5. High-grade surface
6. Intracortical
7. Mandibular
8. Multicentric osteosarcomatosis
9. Osteoclast-rich
10. Parosteal (juxtacortical)
11. Periosteal
12. Small-cell
13. Soft tissue
14. Telangiectatic

## SECONDARY, ARISING IN
1. Bone following radiation therapy
2. Bone infarct
3. Fibrous dysplasia
4. Fracture (healed)
5. Osteoblastoma
6. Osteogenesis imperfecta
7. Osteomyelitis
8. Paget's disease

*Reference:*
1. Murray RO, Jacobson HG, Stoker DJ: The Radiology of Skeletal Disorders. (ed 3) London: Churchill Livingstone, 1990, S49-S52

### Subgamut B-84C

# ROUND CELL LESIONS OF BONE

## COMMON
1. Eosinophilic granuloma
2. Ewing's sarcoma
3. Leukemia, lymphoma$_g$
4. Multiple myeloma, plasmacytoma
5. Neuroblastoma
6. [Osteomyelitis]

## UNCOMMON
1. Burkitt's tumor
2. Reticulum cell sarcoma

# MALIGNANT BONE NEOPLASM WITH GROSS DESTRUCTION AND LITTLE OR NO PERIOSTEAL REACTION

**COMMON**
1. Chondrosarcoma
2. Fibrosarcoma
3. Lymphoma$_g$; leukemia in an adult
4. Metastasis
5. Multiple myeloma
6. Osteosarcoma (osteolytic type)

**UNCOMMON**
1. Adamantinoma
2. Angiosarcoma; hemangioendothelioma
3. Chordoma
4. Ewing's sarcoma (occasionally)
5. Giant cell tumor, malignant
6. Liposarcoma
7. Malignant fibrous histiocytoma
8. Malignant hemangiopericytoma

## Gamut B-86

# MALIGNANT BONE NEOPLASM WITH MARKED PERIOSTEAL REACTION

## (May be confused with osteomyelitis)

1. Burkitt's tumor
*2. Ewing's sarcoma
3. Leukemia in a child
4. Neuroblastoma metastasis
*5. Osteosarcoma

* Often onion-skin periosteal reaction.

## Gamut B-87

# MALIGNANT BONE NEOPLASM WITH MARKED MINERALIZATION RELATIVE TO DESTRUCTION

1. Chondrosarcoma (esp. arising in benign cartilaginous lesion)
2. Osteoblastic metastasis
3. Osteosarcoma (mature)
4. Parosteal or periosteal osteosarcoma or chondro-sarcoma
5. Sarcoma or carcinoma superimposed on chronic osteomyelitis
6. Sarcoma (previously treated) with recurrence

## Gamut B-88

### OSTEOBLASTIC METASTASES

**COMMON**
1. Breast carcinoma
2. Lymphoma$_g$
3. Prostate carcinoma

**UNCOMMON**
1. Carcinoid, pulmonary
2. Cerebellar medulloblastoma or sarcoma
3. Meningiosarcoma
4. [Osteosarcomatosis]
5. Other carcinoma (esp. lung, nasopharynx, stomach, colon, pancreas, urinary bladder)

## Gamut B-89

# OSTEOLYTIC METASTASES

### COMMON
1. Carcinoma of breast
*2. Carcinoma of kidney
3. Carcinoma of lung
4. Leukemia, lymphoma$_g$

### UNCOMMON
*1. Carcinoma of adrenal; pheochromocytoma*
2. Carcinoma of gastrointestinal tract (eg, esophagus, stomach, colon, rectum)
3. Carcinoma of prostate
*4. Carcinoma of thyroid
5. Carcinoma of uterus or cervix
*6. Malignant melanoma; squamous cell carcinoma of skin
7. Neuroblastoma
8. Sarcoma of bone (eg, Ewing's)
9. Other primary neoplasms (eg, bladder, Wilms' tumor, ovary, testis)

\* Often expansile lytic lesion.

## Subgamut B-89A

# RATE OF FREQUENCY OF METASTASES TO BONE FROM VARIOUS PRIMARY CARCINOMAS

| 1. Breast | 35% (incl. osteoblastic) |
|---|---|
| 2. Prostate | 30% (incl. osteoblastic) |

| | |
|---|---|
| 3. Lung | 10% |
| 4. Kidney | 5% |
| 5. Stomach | 2% |
| 6. Thyroid | 2% |
| 7. Uterus | 2% |
| 8. Colon | 1% |
| 9. Other organs | 13% |

*Reference:*
1. Greenfield GB: Radiology of Bone Diseases. (ed 5) Philadelphia: Lippincott, 1990

## Subgamut B-89B

# DISTRIBUTION OF METASTATIC BONE DISEASE

| | |
|---|---|
| Axial skeleton | 75% |
| (incl. dorsolumbar spine, | (32%) |
| sacroiliac joints) | (5%) |
| Skull | 10% |
| Upper and lower extremities | 11% |
| Forearm, hand, leg, foot | 4% |

*Reference:*
1. Greenfield GB: Radiology of Bone Diseases. (ed 5) Philadelphia: Lippincott, 1990

## Gamut B-90

# DIAGRAM OF VARIOUS PERIOSTEAL REACTIONS

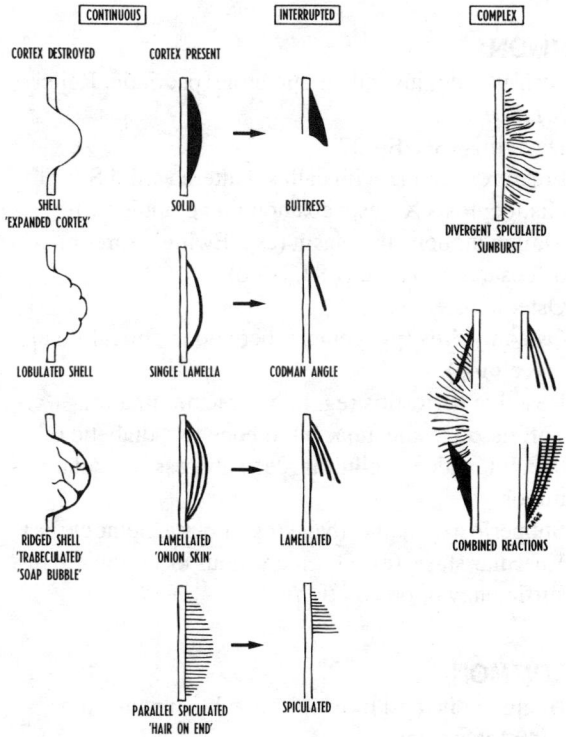

Schematic diagram of periosteal reactions. The arrows indicate that the continuous reactions may be interrupted.

### Reference:

1. Ragsdale BD, Madewell JE, Sweet DE: Radiologic and pathologic analysis of solitary bone lesions. Part II: Periosteal reactions. Radiol Clin North Am 1981;19:749-783.

## Gamut B-91

# LOCALIZED PERIOSTEAL REACTION
## (See Gamuts B-92 to B-99)

**COMMON**

1. Arthritis (eg, juvenile rheumatoid, psoriatic, Reiter S.) (See J-16)
2. Dactylitis (See B-132)
3. Fracture, healing with callus; battered child S.
4. Histiocytosis $X_g$ (esp. eosinophilic granuloma)
5. Malignant bone neoplasm (esp. Ewing's sarcoma, osteosarcoma) (See B-84, B-86)
6. Osteoid osteoma
7. Osteomyelitis (pyogenic, tuberculous, fungal - incl. mycetoma)
8. Reactive periostitis (eg, idiopathic, traumatic)
9. Soft tissue lesion adjacent to bone (eg, diabetic or decubitus ulcer, cellulitis, deep abscess, vascular tumor)
10. Subperiosteal hemorrhage (eg, trauma, hemophilia)
11. Vascular stasis (eg, chronic venous or lymphatic insufficiency or obstruction)

**UNCOMMON**

1. Benign bone cyst or neoplasm with expansion or pathologic fracture
2. Bone infarct (esp. in sickle cell disease)
3. Chondroblastoma invading metaphysis
4. Hypertrophic osteoarthropathy (See B-98)
5. Infantile cortical hyperostosis (Caffey's disease)
6. Leukemia, lymphoma$_g$
7. Melorheostosis
8. Metastasis (eg, neuroblastoma)
9. Radiation therapy
10. Syphilis, yaws
11. Thermal injury (eg, burn, frostbite, electrical)
12. Tropical ulcer ("ivory osteoma")

## Gamut B-92

## CODMAN TRIANGLE

**COMMON**
1. Malignant bone neoplasm, primary (See B-84)

**UNCOMMON**
1. Aneurysmal bone cyst
2. Healing fracture
3. Metastasis
4. Osteomyelitis (incl. mycetoma)
5. Subperiosteal hemorrhage (eg, hemophilia)

*References:*
1. Nelson SW: Some fundamentals in the radiologic differential diagnosis of solitary bone lesions. Semin Roentgenol 1966;1:244-267
2. Ragsdale BD, Madewell JE, Sweet DE: Radiologic and pathologic analysis of solitary bone lesions. Part II: Periosteal reactions. Radiol Clin North Am 1981;19:749-783

## Gamut B-93

## PARALLEL SPICULATED ("HAIR-ON-END") OR DIVERGENT SPICULATED ("SUNRAY") PERIOSTEAL REACTION

**COMMON**
1. Anemia$_g$ (eg, thalassemia or sickle cell anemia involving cranial vault with "hair-on-end" pattern)
2. Ewing's sarcoma
3. Osteosarcoma

**UNCOMMON**

1. Adamantinoma
2. Bone sarcoma, other (See B-84)
3. Healing fracture (esp. march fracture)
4. Hemangioma (esp. skull)
5. Infantile cortical hyperostosis (Caffey's disease)
6. Leukemia
7. Meningioma
8. Metastasis
9. Neuroblastoma metastasis (in skull)
10. Osteomyelitis (incl. mycetoma)
11. Thyroid acropachy

*Reference:*

1. Ragsdale BD, Madewell JE, Sweet DE: Radiologic and pathologic analysis of solitary bone lesions. Part II: Periosteal reactions. Radiol Clin North Am 1981;19:749-783

## Gamut B-94

# WIDESPREAD OR GENERALIZED PERIOSTEAL REACTION (USUALLY LAYERED AND OFTEN SYMMETRICAL)

**COMMON**

1. Arthritis (eg, juvenile rheumatoid, psoriatic, Reiter S.) (See J-16)
2. Fractures, traumatic or pathologic; battered child S.
3. Prematurity; physiologic periostitis of newborn
4. Venous or lymphatic stasis

**UNCOMMON**

1. Acromegaly (hands, feet)
2. Bone infarction, multiple (esp. hand-foot S. in sickle cell anemia)

---

3. Collagen disease with arteritis (eg, lupus erythematosus, polyarteritis nodosa)
4. Cushing S. with excess callus
5. Engelmann's disease
6. Florid reactive periostitis of the phalanges
7. Fluorosis
8. Gaucher's disease; Niemann-Pick disease
9. Hemophilia; Christmas disease
10. Histiocytosis $X_g$
11. Hyperphosphatasia
12. Hypertrophic osteoarthropathy (See B-98)
13. Hypervitaminosis A or D
14. Idiopathic
15. Infantile cortical hyperostosis (Caffey's disease)
16. Infection, neonatal (eg, syphilis, rubella, cytomegalovirus)
17. Kinky-hair S. (Menkes S.); infantile nutritional copper deficiency
18. Leukemia, lymphoma$_g$, Burkitt's tumor
19. Mastocytosis (early)
20. Metastases (eg, neuroblastoma, Ewing's sarcoma)
21. Mucolipidosis II (I-cell disease); $GM_1$ gangliosidosis
22. Neurofibromatosis (subperiosteal hemorrhages)
23. Neurogenic disorder (eg, congenital insensitivity to pain, spinal cord injury, meningomyelocele, leprosy)
24. Osteomalacia with fractures (eg, Milkman's S., aluminum-induced bone disease)
25. Osteomyelitis, widespread (eg, pyogenic, tuberculous, fungal)
26. Pachydermoperiostosis
27. Prostaglandin E therapy
28. Renal osteodystrophy
29. Rickets, healing
30. Scurvy
31. Syphilis, yaws
32. Thermal injury (frostbite, burn, electrical)
33. Thyroid acropachy (hands, feet)
34. Tuberous sclerosis

*References:*
1. Greenfield GB: Radiology of Bone Diseases. (ed 5) Philadelphia: Lippincott, 1990
2. Kozlowski K, Beighton P: Gamut Index of Skeletal Dysplasias. Berlin: Springer-Verlag, 1984, pp 11-13
3. Swischuk LE: Differential Diagnosis in Pediatric Radiology. Baltimore: Williams & Wilkins, 1984, pp 302-308

## Gamut B-95

## PERIOSTITIS IN A CHILD

### COMMON
1. Dactylitis (See B-132)
2. Histiocytosis $X_g$ (esp. eosinophilic granuloma)
3. Infection, neonatal (eg, syphilis, rubella, cytomegalovirus)
4. Juvenile rheumatoid arthritis
5. Leukemia, lymphoma$_g$, Burkitt's tumor
6. Metastasis (eg, neuroblastoma, retinoblastoma, embryonal rhabdomyosarcoma)
7. Osteomyelitis (pyogenic, tuberculous, fungal, smallpox)
8. Prematurity; physiologic periostitis of newborn (up to 6 months)
9. Rickets, healing, all types
10. Scurvy
11. Sickle cell anemia (hand-foot S.)
12. Trauma (eg, callus, traumatic periostitis, battered child S., stress fracture, osteogenesis imperfecta)

### UNCOMMON
1. Benign bone cyst or neoplasm with expansion or pathologic fracture
2. Cornelia de Lange S. II (pseudomuscular hypertrophy)
3. Engelmann's disease

4. Gaucher's disease; Niemann-Pick disease
5. Hemophilia; Christmas disease
6. Hyperphosphatasia
7. Hypertrophic osteoarthropathy (See B-98)
8. Hypervitaminosis A or D
9. Idiopathic
10. Infantile cortical hyperostosis (Caffey's disease)
11. Kinky-hair S. (Menkes S.); infantile nutritional copper deficiency
12. Melorheostosis
13. Mucolipidosis II (I-cell disease); $GM_1$ gangliosidosis
14. Osteoid osteoma
15. Pachydermoperiostosis
16. Prostaglandin-induced
17. Radiation therapy
18. Sarcoma of bone (eg, Ewing's, osteosarcoma)
19. Soft tissue ulcer, cellulitis, deep abscess, vascular tumor
20. Thermal injury (eg, burn, frostbite, electrical)
21. Tuberous sclerosis
22. Yaws

*References:*
1. Kozlowski K, Beighton P: Gamut Index of Skeletal Dysplasias. Berlin: Springer-Verlag, 1984, pp 11-13
2. Swischuk LE: Differential Diagnosis in Pediatric Radiology. Baltimore: Williams & Wilkins, 1984, pp 302-308

## Subgamut B-95A

## CLUES TO THE BATTERED CHILD

1. Unsuspected or inadequately explained fractures
2. Multiple fractures at different stages of healing
3. "Bucket-handle" sign of metaphyseal fracture
4. Excessive callus formation
5. Subdural hematoma

6. Thoracic findings consistent with contusion (eg, local alveolar infiltrate without fever, pneumothorax, pneumomediastinum)
7. Intramural hematoma of intestine
8. Underdevelopment, failure to thrive

## EXCESS CALLUS FORMATION

**COMMON**
1. Steroid therapy; Cushing S.
2. Trauma, unrecognized; battered child S.; stress or march fracture (esp. metatarsal)

**UNCOMMON**
1. Charcot joint (neuropathic arthropathy)
2. Congenital insensitivity to pain
3. Familial
4. Paralytic states
5. Osteogenesis imperfecta
6. Renal osteodystrophy

## Gamut B-97

## SCLEROSIS OF BONE WITH PERIOSTEAL REACTION

**COMMON**
1. Healing fracture with callus
2. Malignant neoplasm (eg, Ewing's sarcoma, osteosarcoma, chondrosarcoma, lymphoma$_g$)

3. Osteoid osteoma
4. Osteomyelitis (incl. Garré's sclerosing osteomyelitis, Brodie's abscess)

**UNCOMMON**
1. Infantile cortical hyperostosis (Caffey's disease)
2. Melorheostosis
3. Mycetoma, fungus disease$_g$
4. Osteoblastic metastasis (esp. prostate)
5. Syphilis
6. Tropical ulcer
7. Tuberculosis
8. Tuberous sclerosis
9. Yaws

## Gamut B-98

# HYPERTROPHIC OSTEOARTHROPATHY

**COMMON**
1. Carcinoma of lung

**UNCOMMON**
1. Abscess of lung
2. AV fistula of lung
3. Bronchial adenoma
4. Chronic gastrointestinal disease (eg, carcinoma, lymphoma, celiac disease, Crohn's disease, ulcerative colitis, Whipple's disease, dysentery, juvenile polyposis)
5. Chronic liver disease, cirrhosis (esp. biliary)
6. Chronic pulmonary infection (eg, tuberculosis, fungus disease$_g$, bronchiectasis, cystic fibrosis, empyema)

7. Cyanotic congenital heart disease
8. Emphysema; chronic obstructive pulmonary disease (COPD)
9. Familial
10. Idiopathic
11. Lymphoma$_g$ of lung
12. Mesothelioma or fibroma of pleura
13. Metastasis to lung (esp. from osteosarcoma)
14. Nasopharyngeal carcinoma (Schmincke tumor)
15. Pachydermoperiostosis (primary hypertrophic osteoarthropathy)
16. Polyarteritis nodosa
17. Renal osteodystrophy
18. Thyroid acropachy

*Reference:*
1. Pineda CJ, Sartoris DJ, Clopton P, Resnick D: Periostitis in hypertrophic osteoarthropathy: Relationship to disease duration. AJR 1987;148:773-778

## Gamut B-99

## MARKED CORTICAL HYPEROSTOSIS AND/OR THICK, SOLID, WAVY, OR BALLOONED PERIOSTEAL REACTION INVOLVING THE SHAFT OF A BONE

### COMMON
1. Fracture (eg, ordinary, stress or march fracture; battered child S.; neurogenic fracture; osteogenesis imperfecta)
2. Osteoid osteoma
3. Osteomyelitis (esp. chronic, low grade, or subperiosteal; Garré's sclerosing osteomyelitis; mycetoma)
4. Reactive periostitis (idiopathic - usually due to trauma)

5. Subperiosteal hemorrhage (eg, trauma, hemophilia or other bleeding disorder$_g$, leukemia, scurvy, neurofibromatosis)
6. Venous or lymphatic stasis

**UNCOMMON**
1. Cellulitis, adjacent soft tissue inflammation
2. Cortical fibrous dysplasia (tibia)
3. Fluorosis
4. Histiocytosis X$_g$
5. Hyperphosphatasia
6. Hypertrophic osteoarthropathy (See B-98)
7. Infantile cortical hyperostosis (Caffey's disease)
8. Melorheostosis
9. Mucolipidosis II (I-cell disease); GM$_1$ gangliosidosis
10. Pachydermoperiostosis
11. Rickets, healing (esp. ribs)
12. Sickle cell anemia with bone infarction (esp. hand-foot S.); other dactylitis (See B-132)
13. Syphilis; yaws (healing)
14. Thyroid acropachy
15. Tropical ulcer osteoma
16. Tuberous sclerosis (esp. rib)

## Gamut B-100

# LOCALIZED CORTICAL THICKENING (ONE OR A FEW BONES) (See Gamut B-101)

**COMMON**
1. Bowed bones (See B-8)
2. Fracture, healing or healed; traumatic periostitis; battered child S.
3. Hypertrophic osteoarthropathy (See B-98)

4. Osteoid osteoma
5. Osteomyelitis with involucrum; Garré's sclerosing osteomyelitis; mycetoma; syphilis, yaws (healing)
6. Paget's disease
7. Venous or lymphatic stasis

**UNCOMMON**

1. Bone neoplasm (esp. enchondroma, low-grade chondrosarcoma, benign tumor after pathological fracture)
2. Fibrous dysplasia
3. Hypervitaminosis A (esp. ulna)
4. Infantile cortical hyperostosis (Caffey's disease)
5. Klippel-Trenaunay S.
6. Melorheostosis
7. Pachydermoperiostosis
8. Sickle cell anemia (eg, with infarction or osteomyelitis)
9. Subperiosteal hemorrhage, old (eg, trauma, hemophilia, scurvy)
10. Thyroid acropachy
11. Tropical ulcer osteoma

## Gamut B-101

# WIDESPREAD CORTICAL THICKENING

**COMMON**

1. Conditions in which periosteal new bone has blended with the cortex (esp. widespread osteomyelitis or trauma) (See B-99)
2. Fibrous dysplasia, polyostotic
3. Paget's disease

**UNCOMMON**
1. Acromegaly, gigantism
2. Beckwith-Wiedemann S.
3. Chester-Erdheim disease
4. Craniodiaphyseal dysplasia (ribs, clavicles)
5. Dentino-osseous dysplasias (esp. tricho-dento-osseous S.)
6. Dubowitz S.
7. Endosteal hyperostosis (van Buchem, Worth)
8. Engelmann's disease (diaphyseal dysplasia)
9. Fluorosis
10. Frontometaphyseal dysplasia
11. Hyperphosphatasia
12. Hypertrophic osteoarthropathy (See B-98)
13. Hypervitaminosis A or D
14. Infantile cortical hyperostosis (Caffey's disease)
15. Melorheostosis
16. Pachydermoperiostosis
17. Physiologic osteosclerosis of newborn
18. Pyknodysostosis
19. Ribbing's disease (hereditary multiple diaphyseal sclerosis)
20. Stanescu dysostosis
21. Tuberous sclerosis
22. Tubular stenosis (Kenny-Caffey S.)
23. Weismann-Netter S.

*References:*
1. Greenfield GB: Radiology of Bone Diseases. (ed 5) Philadelphia: Lippincott, 1990
2. Taybi H, Lachman RS: Radiology of Syndromes, Metabolic Disorders, and Skeletal Dysplasias. (ed 3) Chicago: Year Book Medical Publ, 1990, p 869

## Gamut B-102

# "SPLIT" OR DOUBLE-LAYER CORTEX

**COMMON**
1. Bone infarct (eg, sickle cell anemia)
2. Healing fracture; battered child S.
3. Osteomyelitis
4. Osteoporosis (esp. disuse, immobilization)

**UNCOMMON**
1. Bone graft (local)
2. Gaucher's disease
3. Hyperphosphatasia
4. Osteopetrosis
5. Postsurgical removal of intramedullary rod
6. Scurvy

*Reference:*
1. Greenfield GB: Radiology of Bone Diseases. (ed 5) Philadelphia: Lippincott, 1990

## Gamut B-103

# SCALLOPING, EROSION, OR RESORPTION OF THE INNER CORTICAL MARGIN

**COMMON**
*1. Bone cyst
*2. Chondroid lesion (eg, enchondroma, chondroblastoma, chondromyxoid fibroma, chondrosarcoma, periosteal chondroma)
*3. Fibrous dysplasia
4. Histiocytosis $X_g$
5. Hyperparathyroidism
6. Leukemia, lymphoma$_g$

---

7. Metastasis
8. Multiple myeloma
*9. Nonossifying fibroma; fibrous cortical defect

## UNCOMMON

1. Anemia, primary$_g$ (esp. thalassemia, sickle cell anemia)
2. Gaucher's disease
3. Mastocytosis

*Usually with well-defined, often sclerotic margin.

*Reference:*

1. Greenfield GB: Radiology of Bone Diseases. (ed 5) Philadelphia: Lippincott, 1990

## Gamut B-104

# DESTRUCTION OR EROSION OF THE EXTERNAL CORTICAL SURFACE OF A BONE
## (See Gamuts B-39, B-45)

## COMMON

1. Absorption of terminal phalanx (See B-127, B-127A)
2. Aneurysm or AV fistula adjacent to bone (esp. traumatic)
3. Gouty tophus
4. Hyperparathyroidism, primary or secondary
5. Juxta-articular erosion from rheumatoid or other arthritis or amyloidosis
6. Leukemia, lymphoma$_g$
7. Metastasis (esp. carcinoma of lung, neuroblastoma)
8. Nonossifying fibroma; fibrous cortical defect

9. Parosteal (cortical) desmoid (esp. lower posterior femur)
10. Soft tissue neoplasm (eg, hemangioma, neuro-fibroma, fibroma, lipoma, chondroma, sarcoma)
11. Subperiosteal bone resorption (See B-45)
12. Subperiosteal osteomyelitis; syphilis; yaws; mycetoma; adjacent soft tissue infection (incl. tuberculosis)
13. Synovial lesion (eg, giant cell tumor of tendon sheath, pigmented villonodular synovitis, synovioma)
14. Tendon avulsion

**UNCOMMON**
1. Foreign body or thorn granuloma
2. Glomus tumor
3. Kaposi sarcoma
4. Periosteal chondroma or fibroma
5. Periosteal or parosteal neoplasm, other (See B-83)
6. Primary bone neoplasm
7. Squamous cell carcinoma of skin; malignant tropical ulcer
8. Subperiosteal hematoma

## Gamut B-105

# BONY WHISKERING (PROLIFERATION OF NEW BONE AT TENDON AND LIGAMENT INSERTIONS)

**COMMON**
1. Ankylosing spondylitis
2. DISH

**UNCOMMON**
1. Fluorosis
2. Hypoparathyroidism
3. Plasma cell dyscrasia, POEMS S.

*Reference:*
1. Resnick D, Greenway GD, Bardwick PA, et al: Plasma-cell dyscrasia with polyneuropathy, organomegaly, endocrinopathy, M-protein, and skin changes: The POEMS syndrome. Radiology 1981;140:17-22

## Gamut B-106

## POLYOSTOTIC BONE LESIONS AT DIFFERENT AGES
## (See Gamut B-76)

## Adults

**COMMON**
1. Arthritic or synovial cystic lesions
2. Hyperparathyroidism (brown tumors); renal osteodystrophy
3. Metastases
4. Multiple myeloma
5. Osteomyelitis (bacterial, tuberculous, fungal$_g$, smallpox)
6. Paget's disease

**UNCOMMON**
1. Acro-osteolysis (See B-127)
2. Amyloidosis
3. Anemia, primary$_g$
4. Bone infarcts; aseptic necroses
5. Fibrocystic lesions (eg, polyostotic fibrous dysplasia, nonossifying fibromas)
6. Gaucher's disease, Niemann-Pick disease
7. Hemangiomas, lymphangiomas
8. Histiocytosis X$_g$ (eosinophilic granuloma)
9. Hydatid disease
10. Hypertrophic osteoarthropathy (See B-98)

11. Jackhammer operator's (driller's) disease of wrists
12. Kaposi sarcoma
13. Leprosy
14. Lymphoma$_g$
15. Mastocytosis
16. Membranous lipodystrophy
17. Radium poisoning
18. Sarcoidosis
19. Syphilis, yaws
20. Thyroid acropachy
21. Tuberous sclerosis
22. Weber-Christian disease; pancreatitis with bone lesions

# Children 5-15 Years

**COMMON**
1. Anemia, primary$_g$
2. Fibrocystic lesions (eg, polyostotic fibrous dysplasia, nonossifying fibromas)
3. Histiocytosis X$_g$
4. Leukemia, lymphoma$_g$, Burkitt's tumor
5. Osteochondrodysplasias and dysostoses (See B-1)
6. Osteomyelitis (bacterial, tuberculous, fungal, smallpox)
7. Renal osteodystrophy

**UNCOMMON**
1. Bone infarcts (esp. sickle cell anemia)
2. Chronic granulomatous disease of childhood (Landing-Shirkey S.)
3. Dactylitis (See B-132)
4. Enchondromatosis (Ollier's disease); Maffucci S.
5. Ewing's sarcoma
6. Gaucher's disease, Niemann-Pick disease
7. Hemangiomatosis, lymphangiomatosis
8. Hemophilia
9. Hypervitaminosis A or D
10. Leprosy
11. Mastocytosis

12. Melorheostosis
13. Metastases
14. Mucopolysaccharidoses; mucolipidoses
15. Multiple cartilaginous exostoses
16. Neurofibromatosis
17. Osteosarcomatosis
18. Pachydermoperiostosis
19. Parosteal (cortical) desmoids
20. Rheumatoid arthritis, juvenile
21. Syphilis, yaws
22. Tuberous sclerosis

# Infants and Children Up to 5 Years

## COMMON

1. Anemia$_g$, primary
2. Battered child S.
3. Histiocytosis X$_g$
4. Leukemia, lymphoma$_g$
5. Metastases (esp. neuroblastoma)
6. Osteochondrodysplasias and dysostoses (See B-1)
7. Osteomyelitis
8. Physiologic periostitis (up to 6 months)
9. Rickets
10. Transplacental infection (toxoplasmosis, rubella, cytomegalic inclusion disease, herpes, syphilis)

## UNCOMMON

1. Congenital fibromatosis
2. Hypervitaminosis A
3. Infantile cortical hyperostosis (Caffey's disease)
4. Macrodystrophia lipomatosis
5. Mucopolysaccharidoses, mucolipidoses
6. Neurofibromatosis
7. Osteogenesis imperfecta
8. Osteopetrosis
9. Scurvy
10. Yaws

---

B. Bone

## Gamut B-107

# BALLOONED BONES (WIDE SHAFTS, USUALLY THIN CORTICES), LOCALIZED OR GENERALIZED

### COMMON
*1. Anemia, severe (esp. thalassemia)
*2. Blow-out lesion (See B-71)
*3. Bone cyst
*4. Enchondroma
*5. Fibrous dysplasia
 6. Paget's disease
 7. [Subperiosteal hemorrhage, healing stage (eg, severe trauma, battered child S., neurogenic disease, scurvy, hemophilia)]

### UNCOMMON
*1. Gaucher's disease (esp. diametaphyses)
*2. Hyperparathyroidism, severe (eg, brown tumor)
 3. Hyperphosphatasia
*4. Mastocytosis
*5. Metaphyseal dysplasia (Pyle's disease)
 6. Osteomyelitis (eg, spina ventosa)
*7. Otopalatodigital S.

* Thin cortices.

### Reference:
1. Swischuk LE: Differential Diagnosis in Pediatric Radiology. Baltimore: Williams & Wilkins, 1984, pp 168-169

# MULTIPLE FRACTURES

## SKELETAL DYSPLASIAS WITH PREDOMINANT BONE FRAGILITY
1. Achondrogenesis
2. Juvenile idiopathic osteoporosis
*3. Osteogenesis imperfecta

## OTHER RARE FRAGILE BONE DISORDERS
1. Glycogen storage disease
2. Homocystinuria
3. Metaphyseal chondrodysplasia (Jansen)
4. Mucolipidosis II (I-cell disease)
5. Osteopetrosis
6. Pyknodysostosis

## METABOLIC DISORDERS
1. Copper deficiency, nutritional; kinky-hair S. (Menkes S.)
2. Hyperparathyroidism, osteitis fibrosa cystica
3. Hyperphosphatasia
4. Hypophosphatasia
5. Rickets, severe (multiple types)
6. Scurvy (metaphyseal chip fractures)

## OTHER SKELETAL DISORDERS IN WHICH FRACTURES MAY OCCUR
1. Angiomatosis
2. Arthrogryposis
3. Enchondromatosis
4. Fibrous dysplasia
5. Histiocytosis $X_g$
6. Leukemia, lymphoma$_g$
*7. Metastases
*8. Multiple myeloma
*9. Osteomalacia (See B-46)

10. Osteomyelitis, diffuse (eg, congenital syphilis)
*11. Osteoporosis (See B-44)
*12. Paget's disease
*13. Steroid therapy; Cushing's S.

## SKELETAL FRACTURES IN OTHERWISE NORMAL BONES

1. Seizures; electroshock therapy
2. Tetanus
*3. Trauma; battered child S.

* Common.

### Reference:

1. Kozlowski K, Beighton P: Gamut Index of Skeletal Dysplasias. Berlin: Springer-Verlag, 1984, pp 5-6

## Gamut B-109

# SITES OF AVULSION INJURIES

## COMMON

1. Iliac crest
2. Iliac spines (anterior superior and inferior)
3. Ischial tuberosity (hamstrings and abductor muscle origins)
4. Knee (eg, cruciate ligament origin or insertion)
5. Symphysis pubis (eg, separation of symphysis or avulsion of fragment inferiorly at insertion of gracilis)

## UNCOMMON

1. Calcaneus (achilles tendon)
2. Foot (eg, site of external digitorum brevis, peroneus brevis, plantar aponeurosis, and sesamoid of great toe - "turf toe")
3. Lesser trochanter of femur

*Reference:*
1. Pavlov H: Avulsion injuries - Presented at the International Skeletal Society 18th Annual Refresher Course, San Diego, 1991

## Gamut B-110

## PSEUDOFRACTURE

**COMMON**
1. Osteomalacia
2. Paget's disease
3. Rickets
4. [Spondylolysis]
5. [Stress fracture] (See B-111)

**UNCOMMON**
1. Fibrous dysplasia (incl. Albright's S.)
2. Hyperphosphatasia
3. Hypophosphatasia
4. Idiopathic
5. Neuropathic disorder (eg, leprosy)
6. Osteogenesis imperfecta
7. Osteopetrosis
8. Osteoporosis
9. Postoperative (eg, graft donor site)
10. Pyknodysostosis
11. Radiation osteitis
12. Renal osteodystrophy
13. Rheumatoid arthritis
14. Steroid therapy, Cushing S.

*References:*
1. Greenfield GB: Radiology of Bone Diseases. (ed 5) Philadelphia: Lippincott, 1990
2. Grusd R: Pseudofractures and stress fractures. Semin Roentgenol 1978;13:81-82

3. Murray RO, Jacobson HG, Stoker DJ: The Radiology of Skeletal Disorders. (ed 3) London: Churchill Livingstone, 1990
4. Schneider R, Kaye JJ: Insufficiency and stress fractures of the long bones occurring in patients with rheumatoid arthritis. Radiology 1975;116:595-599

## Subgamut B-110A

## SITES OF PSEUDOFRACTURES (LOOSER'S ZONES OR MILKMAN'S SYNDROME)

1. Femur (neck and shaft)
2. Ischial and pubic rami
3. Scapula, outer margin
4. Clavicle
5. Ribs
6. Other long bones (esp. proximal ulna shaft, distal radius shaft)
7. Metatarsals and phalanges

*Reference:*
1. Burgener FA, Kormano M: Differential Diagnosis in Conventional Radiology. (ed 2) New York: Thieme Medical Publ, 1991

## Gamut B-111

## STRESS FRACTURE (SITES OF PREDILECTION AND CAUSATIVE ACTIVITIES)

1. Athlete (midtibia-shinsplints, pubis)
2. Ballet dancer (midtibia)
3. Chronic coughing (lower ribs); dyspnea (first rib)
4. Clay-shoveler (cervicodorsal spinous process)
5. Golfer (ribs)

6. Heavy pack-bearer (first rib)
7. Long-distance runner (distal fibula, midtibia)
8. March fracture (metatarsals, proximal phalanges)
9. Parachutist (proximal fibula)
10. Pitchfork-handler (ulna)
11. Standing (calcaneus, metatarsal, sesamoid)
12. Stooping (obturator ring)
13. Tic (clavicle)
14. Trapshooter (coracoid)

*References:*

1. Burgener FA, Kormano M: Differential Diagnosis in Conventional Radiology. (ed 2) New York: Thieme Medical Publ, 1991
2. Grusd R: Pseudofractures and stress fractures. Semin Roentgenol 1978;13:81-82

## Gamut B-112

## PSEUDARTHROSIS

**COMMON**
1. Neurofibromatosis (tibia and fibula)
2. Pathologic fracture (eg, neoplasm, cyst, osteomyelitis, postradiation)
3. Ununited fracture in a normal bone

**UNCOMMON**
1. Amniotic band S.
2. Ankylosing spondylitis (in fused bamboo spine)
3. Cleidocranial dysplasia (esp. femur)
4. Congenital (esp. clavicle, tibia, and long bones); proximal focal femoral deficiency
5. Fibrous dysplasia
6. Idiopathic; isolated anomaly
7. Increased bone fragility (eg, osteogenesis imperfecta, osteoporosis, osteomalacia)
8. Kuskokwim S. (clavicle)

*References:*
1. Greenfield GB: Radiology of Bone Diseases. (ed 5) Philadelphia: Lippincott, 1990
2. Park WM, Spencer DG, McCall IW, et al: The detection of spinal pseudarthrosis in ankylosing spondylitis. Br J Radiol 1981;54:467-472
3. Swischuk LE: Differential Diagnosis in Pediatric Radiology. Baltimore: Williams & Wilkins, 1984, pp 191-192
4. Taybi H, Lachman RS: Radiology of Syndromes, Metabolic Disorders, and Skeletal Dysplasias. (ed 3) Chicago: Year Book Medical Publ, 1990, p 875

## Gamut B-113

## PENCIL-POINTING (VASCULAR DEOSSIFICATION OF BONE)<sup>*</sup>

1. Diabetes
2. Leprosy, other neurotrophic arthropathy
3. Psoriatic arthritis
4. Reiter S.
5. Rheumatoid arthritis
6. Sarcoidosis
7. Septic arthritis

* Results from combination of metaphyseal cutback and epiphyseal articular deossification.

*Reference:*
1. Allman RM, Brower A: Radiological Society of North America Scientific Exhibit, 1982

## Gamut B-114

## EXOSTOSIS

**COMMON**
1. Bunion
2. Calcaneal spur (See J-17)

3. [Fracture fragment, healed]
4. [Hypertrophic spur, degenerative arthritis]
5. Multiple cartilaginous exostoses
6. Myositis ossificans (traumatic exostosis)
7. Osteochondroma (metaphyseal)

**UNCOMMON**

1. Acrodysostosis (proximal tibia)
2. Acromegaly
3. Arteriohepatic S. (Alagille S.)
4. Blount's disease (tibia vara)
5. Campomelic dysplasia (calcaneal spur)
6. Chondroectodermal dysplasia (Ellis-van Creveld S.) (tibia, humerus)
7. [Costoclavicular ligament exostosis]
8. Fluorosis
9. Iliac spur with tethered cord-sacral lipoma S.
10. Intracapsular osteochondroma; dysplasia epiphysealis hemimelica (Trevor's disease) (esp. knee and ankle epiphyses)
11. Metachondromatosis (hands, feet, knees)
12. Myositis (fibrodysplasia) ossificans progressiva
13. Nail-patella S. (Fong S.) (iliac horns)
14. Occipital horn S. (Ehlers-Danlos S., type IX)
15. Pachydermoperiostosis
16. Posthemorrhagic (eg, hemophilia)
17. Pseudohypoparathyroidism, pseudopseudohypoparathyroidism
18. Radiation injury
19. Spondylo-epi-metaphyseal dysplasia with joint laxity
20. Subungual exostosis
21. Supracondylar spur of humerus
22. Trichorhinophalangeal S., type II (Langer-Giedion S.)
23. Tuberous sclerosis
24. Turner S. (medial tibial condyle)
25. Turret exostosis (phalanx)

*References:*
1. Greenfield GB: Radiology of Bone Diseases. (ed 5) Philadelphia: Lippincott, 1990
2. Kozlowski K, Beighton P: Gamut Index of Skeletal Dysplasias. Berlin: Springer-Verlag, 1984, p 14
3. Poznanski AK: The Hand in Radiologic Diagnosis. (ed 2) Philadelphia: W.B. Saunders, 1984, p 920
4. Swischuk LE: Differential Diagnosis in Pediatric Radiology. Baltimore: Williams & Wilkins, 1984, pp 207-210
5. Taybi H, Lachman RS: Radiology of Syndromes, Metabolic Disorders, and Skeletal Dysplasias. (ed 3) Chicago: Year Book Medical Publ, 1990, p 885

## Gamut B-115

# SYNOSTOSIS OF TUBULAR BONES
## (See Gamut B-166)

1. Cloverleaf skull S.
2. Ehlers-Danlos S.
3. Fetal alcohol S.
4. Holt-Oram S.
5. Humeroradial-humeroulnar synostosis
6. Inflammatory periostitis, severe (eg, Caffey's infantile cortical hyperostosis)
7. Klinefelter S. (XXY S.)
8. Mesomelic dysplasia
9. Multiple cartilaginous exostoses
10. Multiple synostosis S.
11. Posttraumatic (esp. following severe bleeding)
12. Radioulnar synostosis (See B-166)
13. XXXXY S.

*References:*
1. Swischuk LE: Differential Diagnosis in Pediatric Radiology. Baltimore: Williams & Wilkins, 1984, p 190
2. Taybi H, Lachman RS: Radiology of Syndromes, Metabolic Disorders, and Skeletal Dysplasias. (ed 3) Chicago: Year Book Medical Publ, 1990, p 877

## Gamut B-116

### GAS WITHIN BONE
### (ESPECIALLY ON CT)

1. Bone cyst adjacent to sacroiliac joint ("vacuum cyst")
2. Methylmethacrylate prosthesis
3. Neoplasm
4. Osteomyelitis (gas forming organism)
5. Osteonecrosis
6. Postoperative; posttraumatic

*References:*
1. Greenfield GB: Radiology of Bone Diseases. (ed 5) Philadelphia: Lippincott, 1990
2. Ramirez H Jr, Blatt ES, Cable HF, et al: Intraosseous pneumatocysts of the ilium: Findings on radiographs and CT scans. Radiology 1984;150:503-505

## Gamut B-117

### CONGENITAL ABNORMALITIES OF THE THUMB
### (ABSENT, SHORT, WIDE, ENLARGED, ECTOPIC, OR TRIPHALANGEAL THUMB)

#### ABSENT THUMB
1. Bird-headed dwarfism (Seckel S.)
2. Fanconi S. (pancytopenia-dysmelia S.)
3. Franceschetti S.
4. Holt-Oram S.
5. Phocomelia (eg, thalidomide embryopathy)
6. Ring D chromosome S.
7. Rothmund-Thomson S.
8. Trisomy 18 S.

## HYPOPLASTIC OR SHORT THUMB

1. Acrocephalosyndactyly
2. Aminopterin fetopathy
3. Basal cell nevus S. (Gorlin S.)
4. Brachydactyly C or D; hereditary shortness of thumbs
5. Christian brachydactyly
6. Chromosome 18 q- S.
7. Cornelia de Lange S.
8. Diastrophic dysplasia
9. Dyggve-Melchior-Clausen S.
10. Dyssegmental dysplasia
11. Ectodermal dysplasia
12. Fanconi S. (pancytopenia-dysmelia S.)
13. Hand-foot-genital S.
14. Holt-Oram S.
15. Isolated anomaly
16. IVIC S.
17. Juberg-Hayward S.
18. Myositis (fibrodysplasia) ossificans progressiva
19. Otopalatodigital S.
20. Phocomelia (eg, thalidomide embryopathy)
21. Popliteal pterygium S.
22. Radial hypoplasia syndromes
23. Rubinstein-Taybi S.
24. Taybi-Linder S.
25. Thrombocytopenia-absent radius (TAR) S.
26. Trisomy 9p S.
27. Trisomy 18 S.
28. VATER association
29. Werner S.
30. WL symphalangism - brachydactyly

## WIDE THUMB

1. Acrocephalopolysyndactyly (Carpenter S.)
2. Acrocephalosyndactyly (Pfeiffer)
3. Diastrophic dysplasia
4. FG syndrome
5. Frontodigital S.

6. Hand-foot-genital S.
7. Larsen S.
8. Léri's pleonosteosis
9. Meckel S.
10. Myositis (fibrodysplasia) ossificans progressiva
11. Otopalatodigital S.
12. Rubinstein-Taybi S.
13. Weaver-Smith S.

## ENLARGED THUMB

1. Angioma, arteriovenous malformation (Klippel-Trenaunay-Weber S.)
2. Isolated anomaly
3. Lipoma; macrodystrophia lipomatosa
4. Neurofibromatosis
5. Triphalangeal thumb (eg, Blackfan-Diamond S.)

## ECTOPIC THUMB (ABNORMAL POSITION)

1. Cornelia de Lange S. (proximally placed thumb)
2. Diastrophic dysplasia ("hitchhiker thumb")
3. Freeman-Sheldon S. (whistling face S.) (flexed thumb overlaps palm)
4. Rubinstein-Taybi S. (radially curved or "hitchhiker thumb")

## TRIPHALANGEAL THUMB

1. Aase S.
2. Blackfan-Diamond S.
3. DOOR S.
4. Duane S.
5. Goodman S.
6. Holt-Oram S.
7. IVIC S.
8. Juberg-Hayward S.
9. LADD S.
10. Normal variant, isolated anomaly
11. Poland S.
12. Thalidomide embryopathy

13. Townes-Brocks S.
14. Trisomy 13 S.
15. Trisomy 22 S.
16. VATER association

*References:*
1. Jones KL: Smith's Recognizable Patterns of Human Malformation. Philadelphia: W.B. Saunders, 1988
2. Poznanski AK: The Hand in Radiologic Diagnosis. (ed 2) Philadelphia: W.B. Saunders, 1984, p 912
3. Poznanski AK, Garn SM, Holt JF: The thumb in the congenital malformation syndromes. Radiology 1971;100:115-129
4. Silverman F (ed): Caffey's Pediatric X-ray Diagnosis. (ed 8) Chicago: Year Book Medical Publ, 1985
5. Swischuk LE: Differential Diagnosis in Pediatric Radiology. Baltimore: Williams & Wilkins, 1984, p 250
6. Taybi H, Lachman RS: Radiology of Syndromes, Metabolic Disorders, and Skeletal Dysplasias. (ed 3) Chicago: Year Book Medical Publ, 1990

B. Bone

## Subgamut B-117A

# THUMB APPEARANCE IN VARIOUS SYNDROMES*

| | Distal Phalanx | | | | Proximal Phalanx | | | | Metacarpal | | | | | | |
|---|---|---|---|---|---|---|---|---|---|---|---|---|---|---|---|
| | Cone Epiphysis | Short D1 Met 2 | Broad | Triphalangeal Thumb | Short P1 Met 2 | Long D1 Met 2 | Triangular | Thin Short | Wide Met 2 Met 1 | Long Met 2 Met 1 | Pseudo-epiphysis | Clasped Thumb | "Hitchhiker" Thumb | Duplication | Absent Thumb |
| Apert's and other acrocephalosyndactyly | | X | X | | X | | X | | | | | | O | O | |
| Arthrogryposis | | | | | | | | | | | | | | | |
| Cardiomelic (Holt-Oram) | | X | | X | | | | X | | X | | | | | X |
| Cornelia de Lange | | X | | | | | | | | | | X | | | |
| Diastrophic dwarfism | | O | | | O | | | | X | | | | X | | |
| Hand-foot-genital | X | O | | | O | | | | X | | X | | | | |
| Myositis ossificans | | X | | | O | O | | | X | | O | | | | |
| Otopalatodigital | X | X | | | | | | | | | | | | | |
| Pancytopenia-dysmelia (Fanconi's anemia) | | X | | | | | | X | | | | | | | X |
| Rubinstein-Taybi | | X | X | | X | X | | | | | | | X | O | |
| Thalidomide embryopathy | | | | X | | | | | | | | | | | O |
| Trisomy 18 | | O | | | | | | | | | | | | | O |

(Modified from Poznanski AK, Garn SM, Holt JF: Radiology 1971;100:115-129)

* O = occasional; X = frequent; P1 = proximal phalanx of thumb; D1 = distal phalanx of thumb

## Gamut B-118

# SHORT DISTAL PHALANX OF THE THUMB

**SHORT AND BROAD**
1. Acrocephalopolysyndactyly (Carpenter S.)
2. Acrocephalosyndactyly (Apert S., Pfeiffer S.)
3. Brachydactyly A-4 and D
4. Christian brachydactyly
5. Diastrophic dysplasia
6. Hand-foot-genital S.
7. Myositis (fibrodysplasia) ossificans progressiva
8. Osteodysplasty (Melnick-Needles S.)
9. Otopalatodigital S.
10. Pseudohypoparathyroidism, pseudopseudohypoparathyroidism
11. Robinow S.
12. Rubinstein-Taybi S.

**THIN AND SMALL**
1. Cornelia de Lange S.
2. Fanconi S. (pancytopenia-dysmelia S.)
3. Holt-Oram S.
4. Myositis (fibrodysplasia) ossificans progressiva
5. Radial hypoplasia syndromes (See B-164)
6. Trisomy 18 S.

*Reference:*
1. Poznanski AK: The Hand in Radiologic Diagnosis. (ed 2) Philadelphia: W.B. Saunders, 1984, p 905

B. Bone

## SHORT PROXIMAL PHALANGES OF THE THUMB AND/OR OTHER DIGITS

### ACQUIRED
1. Arthritis
2. Infection (eg, osteomyelitis, yaws, smallpox)
3. Neoplasm
4. Trauma
5. Sickle cell disease

### CONGENITAL
1. Acrocephalopolysyndactyly (Carpenter S.)
2. Acrocephalosyndactyly (Apert S., Pfeiffer S.)
3. Basal cell nevus S.
4. Brachydactyly A-1, A-2, and C
5. Diastrophic dysplasia
6. Myositis (fibrodysplasia) ossificans progressiva
7. Rubinstein-Taybi S.
8. Trisomy 18 S.

### Gamut B-120

## BROAD PHALANGES OF THE THUMB AND/OR OTHER DIGITS

### BROAD DISTAL PHALANX OF THUMBS
1. Acrocephalopolysyndactyly (Carpenter S.)
2. Acrocephalosyndactyly (Apert S., Pfeiffer S.)
3. Brachydactyly B and D
4. Mesomelic dysplasia (Robinow type)
5. Otopalatodigital S.
6. Rubinstein-Taybi S.
7. Syndactyly

## OTHER BROAD DISTAL PHALANGES

1. Distal brachydactyly
2. Larsen S.
3. Pachyonychia congenita
4. Warfarin embryopathy

## BROAD MIDDLE PHALANGES

1. Achondroplasia (infant)
2. Acrodysostosis
3. Acromesomelic dysplasia
4. Brachydactyly A-1
5. Campomelic dysplasia
6. Chondrodysplasia punctata (infant)
7. Chondroectodermal dysplasia (infant)
8. Frontometaphyseal dysplasia
9. Marshall S.
10. Mucolipidosis III
11. Noonan S.
12. Pseudoachondroplasia
13. Saldino-Mainzer S.
14. Tricho-rhino-phalangeal S. I and II

*Reference:*
1. Poznanski AK: The Hand in Radiologic Diagnosis. (ed 2) Philadelphia: W.B. Saunders, 1984, p 901

### Gamut B-121

# CONGENITAL ABNORMALITY OF THE GREAT TOE

## COMMON

1. Acrocephalosyndactyly (Apert, Pfeiffer types)
2. Cornelia de Lange S.
3. Myositis (fibrodysplasia) ossificans progressiva
4. Otopalatodigital S.
5. Rubinstein-Taybi S.

**UNCOMMON**
1. Acrocephalopolysyndactyly (Carpenter S.)
2. Cleidocranial dysplasia
3. Diastrophic dysplasia
4. Freeman-Sheldon S. (whistling face S.)
5. Frontodigital S.
6. Greig cephalopolydactyly S.
7. Hand-foot-genital S.
8. Larsen S.
9. Léri's pleonosteosis
10. Orofaciodigital S.
11. Popliteal pterygium S.
12. Trisomy 13 S.
13. Trisomy 18 S.
14. XXXXY S.

*Reference:*
1. Poznanski AK: Foot manifestations of the congenital malformation syndromes. Semin Roentgenol 1970;5:354-366

## Gamut B-122

## CLINODACTYLY OF THE FIFTH FINGER (INCURVING OF FIFTH DIGIT WITH HYPOPLASTIC MIDDLE PHALANX)

**COMMON**
1. Brachydactyly A-1, A-2, A-3, C
2. Cornelia de Lange S.
3. Fetal alcohol S.
4. Hand-foot-genital S.
5. Holt-Oram S.
6. [Kirner's deformity (distal phalanx - seen as isolated anomaly or in Cornelia de Lange S., Silver-Russell S.)]

7. Local disorder (eg, trauma, arthritis, contracture)
8. Nail-patella S. (osteo-onychodysplasia)
9. Noonan S.
10. Normal variant; isolated anomaly
11. Oculo-dento-osseous dysplasia
12. Orofaciodigital S.
13. Otopalatodigital S.
14. Shwachman S.
15. Thrombocytopenia-absent radius (TAR) S.
16. Trisomy 21 S. (Down S.)
17. Williams S. (idiopathic hypercalcemia)

## UNCOMMON

1. Aarskog S.
2. Acrocephalosyndactyly (Saethre-Chotzen type)
3. Aminopterin fetopathy
4. Bird-headed dwarfism (Seckel S.)
5. Bloom S.
6. Campomelic dysplasia
7. Cerebrohepatorenal S. (Zellweger S.)
8. Chromosome 4p- S. (Wolf S.)
9. Cohen S.
10. Cri du chat S. (Cat's cry S.)
11. EEC S.
12. Ehlers-Danlos S.
13. Fanconi S. (pancytopenia-dysmelia S.)
14. Focal dermal hypoplasia (Goltz S.)
15. Klinefelter S. (XXY S.)
16. LADD S. (Levy-Hollister S.)
17. Laurence-Moon-Biedl S.
18. Marfan S.
19. Mesomelic dysplasia (Nievergelt type)
20. Mitral valve prolapse S.
21. Myositis ossificans progressiva
22. Poland S.
23. Popliteal pterygium S.
24. Prader-Willi S.
25. Pseudothalidomide S.
26. Rieger S.

27. Roberts S.
28. Robinow S.
29. Silver-Russell S.
30. Symphalangism
31. Treacher Collins S.
32. Tricho-rhino-phalangeal dysplasia
33. Trisomy syndromes (8, 9p, 13, 18)
34. XXXX S.; XXXXX S.; XXXXY S.

*References:*
1. Edeiken J, Dalinka M, Karasick D: Edeiken's Roentgen Diagnosis of Diseases of Bone. (ed 4) Baltimore: Williams & Wilkins, 1989
2. Jones KL: Smith's Recognizable Patterns of Human Malformation. Philadelphia: W.B. Saunders, 1988
3. Poznanski AK: The Hand in Radiologic Diagnosis. (ed 2) Philadelphia: W.B. Saunders, 1984, p 915
4. Poznanski AK, Pratt GB, Manson G, et al: Clinodactyly, camptodactyly, Kirner's deformity, and other crooked fingers. Radiology 1969;93:573-582
5. Swischuk LE: Differential Diagnosis in Pediatric Radiology. Baltimore: Williams & Wilkins, 1984, pp 252-253
6. Taybi H, Lachman RS: Radiology of Syndromes, Metabolic Disorders, and Skeletal Dysplasias. (ed 3) Chicago: Year Book Medical Publ, 1990, p 867

## Gamut B-123

# CONGENITAL SYNDROMES WITH SHORT MIDDLE PHALANX OF FIFTH FINGER

**COMMON**
1. Brachydactyly A-1, A-3, A-4
2. Holt-Oram S.
3. Myositis (fibrodysplasia) ossificans progressiva
4. Noonan S.
5. Trisomy 21 S. (Down S.)

## UNCOMMON

1. Aarskog S.
2. Bird-headed dwarfism (Seckel S.)
3. Bloom S.
4. Chromosome 4p- S. (Wolf S.)
5. Coffin-Siris S.
6. Focal dermal hypoplasia (Goltz S.)
7. Hand-foot-genital S.
8. Laurence-Moon-Biedl S.
9. Oculo-dento-osseous dysplasia
10. Orofaciodigital S. I and II
11. Otopalatodigital S.
12. Poland S.
13. Popliteal pterygium S.
14. Pseudothalidomide S.
15. Shwachman S.
16. Silver-Russell S.
17. Symphalangism
18. Thrombocytopenia-absent radius (TAR) S.
19. Tricho-rhino-phalangeal dysplasia
20. Trisomy 9p S.
21. Trisomy 18 S.
22. Williams S. (idiopathic hypercalcemia)
23. XXXXX S.
24. XXXXY S.

*References:*
1. Poznanski AK: The Hand in Radiologic Diagnosis. (ed 2) Philadelphia: W.B. Saunders, 1984, p 907
2. Taybi H, Lachman RS: Radiology of Syndromes, Metabolic Disorders, and Skeletal Dysplasias. (ed 3) Chicago: Year Book Medical Publ, 1990

B. Bone

## Gamut B-124

# CONGENITAL SYNDROMES WITH ONE OR MORE SHORT MIDDLE PHALANGES (OTHER THAN FIFTH FINGER) (See Gamut B-123)

1. Aarskog S.
2. Acrocephalopolysyndactyly (Carpenter S.)
3. Acrocephalosyndactyly (Apert S.)
4. Campomelic dysplasia
5. Cloverleaf skull
6. Familial brachydactylies A-1, A-4, B, and C (A-2 and A-3 - second finger)
7. Hunter S. (Ruvalcaba S.)
8. Levy-Hollister S. (LADD S.)
9. Poland S.
10. Pseudohypoparathyroidism, pseudopseudohypoparathyroidism (second finger)
11. Saldino-Mainzer S.
12. Sclerosteosis (second finger)
13. Symphalangism syndromes (eg, WL symphalangism-brachydactyly S.)
14. Tricho-rhino-phalangeal dysplasia

*References:*
1. Poznanski AK: The Hand in Radiologic Diagnosis. (ed 2) Philadelphia: W.B. Saunders, 1984, p 907
2. Taybi H, Lachman RS: Radiology of Syndromes, Metabolic Disorders, and Skeletal Dysplasias. (ed 3) Chicago: Year Book Medical Publ, 1990

## Gamut B-125

# GENERALIZED SHORT DISTAL PHALANGES OF THE HAND

## SHORT AND BROAD

1. Acrodysostosis
2. [Acro-osteolysis (eg, frostbite, leprosy, trauma) (See B-127)]
3. Asphyxiating thoracic dysplasia (Jeune S.)
4. Cleidocranial dysplasia
5. Coffin-Lowry S.
6. Diastrophic dysplasia
7. DOOR S.
8. Larsen S.
9. Metaphyseal chondrodysplasia (Jansen)
10. Pachydermoperiostosis
11. Pseudoachondroplasia
12. Pseudohypoparathyroidism, pseudo-pseudohypoparathyroidism
13. Robinow S.
14. Warfarin embryopathy

## THIN AND SMALL

1. Acrocephalopolysyndactyly (Carpenter S.)
2. [Acro-osteolysis (eg, frostbite) (See B-127)]
3. Asphyxiating thoracic dysplasia (Jeune S.)
4. C syndrome
5. Chondroectodermal dysplasia (Ellis-van Creveld S.)
6. Christian S.
7. Coffin-Siris S.
8. Fetal alcohol S.
9. Fetal Dilantin S.
10. Hypoplastic nails S.
11. Marshall S.
12. Mucolipidosis II
13. Osteodysplasty (Melnick-Needles S.)
14. Pseudohypoparathyroidism
15. Symphalangism

16. Trisomy 9p S.
17. Trisomy 13 S.
18. Trisomy 18 S.
19. Warfarin embryopathy

*Reference:*
  1. Poznanski AK: The Hand in Radiologic Diagnosis. (ed 2) Philadelphia: W.B. Saunders, 1984, pp 905-906

**Gamut B-126**

## HYPOPLASTIC (SPINDLE-SHAPED OR STUBBY) TERMINAL PHALANGES

**COMMON**
  1. Cleidocranial dysplasia
  2. Congenital indifference to pain
  3. Cornelia de Lange S.
  4. Fanconi S. (pancytopenia-dysmelia S.)
  5. Holt-Oram S.
  6. Myositis (fibrodysplasia) ossificans progressiva
  7. Normal (foot)
  8. Pseudohypoparathyroidism, pseudopseudohypoparathyroidism
  9. Pyknodysostosis
10. Spade hand

**UNCOMMON**
  1. Aarskog S.
  2. Acrocephalopolysyndactyly (Carpenter S.)
  3. Acrocephalosyndactyly (Apert S.)
  4. Arteriohepatic dysplasia
  5. Asphyxiating thoracic dysplasia (Jeune S.)
  6. Chondroectodermal dysplasia (Ellis-van Creveld S.)
  7. Coffin-Lowry S.
  8. Coffin-Siris S.
  9. Diastrophic dysplasia

10. Fetal hydantoin S. (Dilantin embryopathy)
11. Hand-foot-genital S.
12. Hypoplasia or aplasia of fingernails
13. Larsen S.
14. Otopalatodigital S.
15. Progeria
16. Pseudoxanthoma elasticum
17. Rothmund-Thomson S.
18. Rubinstein-Taybi S.
19. Trisomy 13 S.
20. Trisomy 18 S.
21. Warfarin embryopathy

*References:*
1. Poznanski AK: The Hand in Radiologic Diagnosis. (ed 2) Philadelphia: W.B. Saunders, 1984, pp 214-215
2. Swischuk LE: Differential Diagnosis in Pediatric Radiology. Baltimore: Williams & Wilkins, 1984, p 245
3. Taybi H, Lachman RS: Radiology of Syndromes, Metabolic Disorders, and Skeletal Dysplasias. (ed 3) Chicago: Year Book Medical Publ, 1990, pp 464-465

## Gamut B-127

# ACRO-OSTEOLYSIS
## (EROSION OF MULTIPLE TERMINAL PHALANGEAL TUFTS)

**COMMON**
1. Arteriosclerosis obliterans
2. Diabetic gangrene
*3. Hyperparathyroidism, primary or secondary (renal osteodystrophy)
4. Infection, osteitis
5. Neurotrophic disease (esp. diabetes, leprosy, tabes dorsalis, syringomyelia, meningomyelocele) (See B-153)
6. Psoriatic arthritis

7. Raynaud's disease
8. Rheumatoid arthritis
*9. Scleroderma, dermatomyositis, MCTD
10. Thermal injury (eg, burn, frostbite, electrical)
11. Trauma (biomechanical stress, guitar player)

**UNCOMMON**

1. Brachydactyly B
2. Cleidocranial dysplasia
3. Clubbing of fingers (See B-133)
+4. Congenital (familial or idiopathic) acro-osteolysis
    (eg, Hajdu-Cheney S.)
*5. Congenital indifference to pain
6. Disseminated lipogranulomatosis
7. Drug therapy (eg, Dilantin, phenobarbital, ergot)
8. Dysosteosclerosis
9. Ectodermal dysplasia
*10. Ehlers-Danlos S.
*11. Epidermolysis bullosa
*12. Gout
13. Hunger osteopathy
14. Hypertrophic osteoarthropathy
15. Lesch-Nyhan S.
16. Metastasis
17. Multicentric reticulohistiocytosis (lipoid
    dermatoarthritis)
18. Osteomalacia (eg, malabsorption syndromes)
19. Osteopetrosis
20. Osteopoikilosis
21. Pachydermoperiostosis
22. Pityriasis rubra
23. Plantar warts
+24. Polyvinyl chloride osteolysis; chemical
    acro-osteolysis
25. Porphyria
26. Progeria; Werner S.
27. Pseudoxanthoma elasticum
28. Pyknodysostosis
29. Radiation injury

*30. Rothmund-Thomson S.
31. Sarcoidosis
32. Singleton-Merten S.
33. Sjögren S.
34. Snake or scorpion venom
35. Streeter's congenital amniotic bands
36. Thromboangiitis obliterans (Buerger's disease)
37. Winchester S.

* May be associated with calcification.
+ Resorption of midportion of phalanx.

*References:*

1. Destouet JM, Murphy WA: Acquired acroosteolysis and acronecrosis. Arthritis Rheum 1983;26:1150-1154
2. Greenfield GB: Radiology of Bone Diseases. (ed 5) Philadelphia: Lippincott, 1990
3. Jones SN, Stoker DJ: Radiology at your fingertips; lesions of the terminal phalanx. Clin Radiol 1988; 39:478-485
4. Kozlowski K, Beighton P: Gamut Index of Skeletal Dysplasias. Berlin: Springer-Verlag, 1984, pp 76-77
5. Moss AA, Mainzer F: Osteopetrosis: An unusual cause of terminal-tuft erosion. Radiology 1970;97:631-632
6. Poznanski AK: The Hand in Radiologic Diagnosis. (ed 2) Philadelphia: W.B. Saunders, 1984, p 170
7. Taybi H, Lachman RS: Radiology of Syndromes, Metabolic Disorders, and Skeletal Dysplasias. (ed 3) Chicago: Year Book Medical Publ, 1990, p 863

## Subgamut B-127A

### ACQUIRED ACRO-OSTEOLYSIS CONFINED TO ONE DIGIT

1. Angioma$_g$
2. Carcinoma of nail bed
3. Epidermoid inclusion cyst
4. Fibroma
5. Giant cell tumor of tendon sheath
6. Glomus tumor

7. Infection (eg, osteomyelitis, paronychia)
8. Lymphoma$_g$
9. Metastasis
10. Neurofibroma
11. Subungual exostosis
12. Thermal injury (eg, burn, frostbite)

## BAND-LIKE DESTRUCTION OR EROSION OF THE MIDPORTION OF A TERMINAL PHALANX

1. Chemical acro-osteolysis (eg, polyvinyl chloride)
2. Cleidocranial dysplasia
3. Congenital or familial acro-osteolysis (Hajdu-Cheney S.)
4. Hyperparathyroidism, primary or secondary (renal osteodystrophy)
5. Juvenile rheumatoid arthritis

*Reference:*
1. Burgener FA, Kormano M: Differential Diagnosis in Conventional Radiology. New York: Thieme Medical Publ, 1991, p 280

## ACRO-OSTEOSCLEROSIS (TERMINAL PHALANGEAL SCLEROSIS)

**COMMON**
1. Idiopathic, normal variant
2. Rheumatoid arthritis

**UNCOMMON**
1. Lupus erythematosus
2. Melorheostosis
3. Osteopetrosis
4. Osteopoikilosis
5. Sarcoidosis
6. Scleroderma

*References:*
1. Burgener FA, Kormano M: Differential Diagnosis in Conventional Radiology. New York: Thieme Medical Publ, 1991, p 276
2. Goodman N: The significance of terminal phalangeal osteosclerosis. Radiology 1967;89:709-712
3. Williams M, Barton E: Terminal phalangeal sclerosis in rheumatoid arthritis. Clin Radiol 1984;35:237-238

## Gamut B-129

# AMPUTATION OR ABSENCE OF A PHALANX, DIGIT, HAND, OR FOOT

## ACQUIRED

1. Ainhum
2. Congenital indifference to pain
3. Constriction (eg, bandages, bands, strings, hair)
*4. Diabetes
*5. Infection; severe osteomyelitis (eg, mycetoma)
6. Intravascular coagulation (eg, meningococcemia)
*7. Leprosy
8. Lesch-Nyhan S.
*9. Neurologic disorder
10. Psoriasis, severe
11. Psychotic states
12. Radiation, radium injury
*13. Scleroderma
*14. Surgical amputation

\*15. Thermal injury (eg, frostbite, burn, electrical)
\*16. Trauma; battered child S.
\*17. Vascular insufficiency (eg, arteriosclerosis, ergot re-
action, gangrene)

## CONGENITAL

1. Aglossia-adactylia S.
\*2. Amniotic band S. (Streeter's bands)
3. Arthrogryposis (toe)
4. [Clawhand; radial or ulnar ray syndromes]
5. Cornelia de Lange S.
6. Fetal Dilantin S.
7. Grebe chondrodysplasia
8. Keratoderma palmaris et plantaris familiaris (tylosis)
9. Möbius S.
10. Poland S.
11. Popliteal pterygium S.
12. Roberts S.
13. Scalp defect S.
\*14. Thalidomide embryopathy; pseudothalidomide S.

\* Common.

*References:*

1. Poznanski AK: The Hand in Radiologic Diagnosis. (ed 2)
Philadelphia: W.B. Saunders, 1984, p 912
2. Swischuk LE: Differential Diagnosis in Pediatric Radiology.
Baltimore: Williams & Wilkins, 1984, p 258

### Subgamut B-129A

## SELF-MUTILATION OF DIGITS

1. Congenital indifference to pain
2. Congenital sensory neuropathy with or without
anhidrosis
3. Diabetic neuropathy

4. Leprosy
5. Lesch-Nyhan S.
6. Psychotic states
7. Riley-Day S. (familial dysautonomia)

# GANGRENE OF A FINGER OR TOE

## COMMON
1. Arteriosclerosis obliterans
2. Arteritis (eg, hypersensitivity angiitis, Kawasaki's disease, ergot intoxication)
3. Collagen disease$_g$ (eg, scleroderma, polyarteritis nodosa)
4. Diabetes
5. Neurotrophic disease (eg, leprosy) (See B-153)
6. Trauma, external or postoperative

## UNCOMMON
1. Autoimmune disorder, macroglobulinemia (Waldenström's disease, tumor-produced globulins)
2. Blood disorder (eg, leukemia, myeloid metaplasia, polycythemia vera)
3. Burn; electrical or chemical injury
4. Constriction (eg, bandage, baby mittens, hair ring or band, ainhum)
5. Disseminated intravasular coagulation (eg, sepsis, meningococcemia)
6. Frostbite
7. Iatrogenic (eg, radial artery catheterization)
8. Infection, osteomyelitis
9. Raynaud's disease
10. Thromboangiitis obliterans (Buerger's disease)
11. Trench foot
12. Trophic ulcer with underlying destruction

*Reference:*
1. Poznanski AK: The Hand in Radiologic Diagnosis. (ed 2) Philadelphia: W.B. Saunders, 1984, pp 888-890

## Gamut B-131

## CYST-LIKE LESION IN A PHALANX (SOLITARY OR MULTIPLE)

**COMMON**

*1. Arthritis (esp. gout, rheumatoid arthritis, osteoarthritis)
 2. Bone cyst
*3. Enchondroma

**UNCOMMON**

 1. Aneurysmal bone cyst
 2. Angioma_g
 3. [Carcinoma of nail bed]
 4. Chondroblastoma
 5. Chondromyxoid fibroma
 6. Chondrosarcoma (slow growing)
 7. Cystic osteomyelitis
 8. Epidermoid inclusion cyst (distal phalanx)
 9. Fibrous dysplasia
10. Giant cell tumor
*11. [Glomus tumor (distal phalanx)]
*12. Hemophilic pseudotumor
*13. Leprosy (leproma)
*14. Metastasis (esp. lung, breast)
*15. Myeloma
16. Osteoblastoma; osteoid osteoma
17. Periosteal chondroma or fibroma
*18. Sarcoidosis
*19. [Synovial lesion (eg, villonodular synovitis, giant cell tumor of tendon sheath)]
20. Thorn granuloma

21. Tuberculosis ("spina ventosa")
*22. Tuberous sclerosis
*23. Wilson's disease

* May be multiple.

*Reference:*
1. Jones SN, Stoker DJ: Radiology at your fingertips; lesions of the terminal phalanx. Clin Radiol 1988; 39:478-485

## Gamut B-132

## DACTYLITIS*

**COMMON**
1. Pyogenic osteomyelitis (esp. salmonella)
2. Sickle cell anemia: hand-foot S. (infarction with or without osteomyelitis)
3. Tuberculosis (spina ventosa)

**UNCOMMON**
1. Atypical mycobacteria infection; BCG immunization
2. Chronic granulomatous disease of childhood
3. Fungus disease$_g$ (eg, mycetoma, sporotrichosis)
4. Leprosy
5. [Neoplasm (eg, leukemia, metastasis, Ewing's sarcoma, angioma)]
6. Pancreatic fat necrosis (with elevated lipase)
7. Phalangeal microgeodic S.
8. Radiation necrosis
9. Sarcoidosis
10. Smallpox (eradicated by 1980)
11. Syphilis, yaws
12. Thermal injury (eg, frostbite, burn)
13. Tuberous sclerosis

* Varying degrees of bone destruction and expansion, periosteal reaction, and soft tissue swelling involving one or more bones of the hands and/or feet.

*References:*
1. Poznanski K, Beighton P: Gamut Index of Skeletal Dysplasias. Berlin: Springer-Verlag, 1984, pp 607-636
2. Swischuk LE: Differential Diagnosis in Pediatric Radiology. Baltimore: Williams & Wilkins, 1984, p 260

## Gamut B-133

## CLUBBING OF THE FINGERS OR TOES

### COMMON
1. Alveolar capillary block (eg, pulmonary interstitial fibrosis - sarcoidosis, scleroderma, pneumoconiosis)
2. Bronchogenic carcinoma
3. Cirrhosis of liver
4. Congenital heart disease (esp. tetralogy$_g$, pulmonary stenosis, PDA, VSD)
5. Pulmonary hypertrophic osteoarthropathy (See D-98)

### UNCOMMON
1. Acromegaly
2. Bird-headed dwarfism (Seckel S.)
3. Colitis, chronic (eg, ulcerative, Crohn's, amebic, tuberculous)
4. Cystic fibrosis (mucoviscidosis)
5. Familial idiopathic osteoarthropathy (Currarino)
6. Hajdu-Cheney S. (osteolysis)
7. [Hyperparathyroidism]
8. Idiopathic
9. Immotile cilia S.
10. Larsen S.
11. [Metastases to fingers]
12. Myxedema; hyperthyroidism; thyroid acropachy
13. Osler-Weber-Rendu S.
14. Pachydermoperiostosis
15. POEMS S.
16. Polycythemia
17. Sprue

18. Subacute bacterial endocarditis
19. Urinary tract infection, chronic

*References:*
1. Greenfield GB: Radiology of Bone Diseases. (ed 5) Philadelphia: Lippincott, 1990
2. Taybi H, Lachman RS: Radiology of Syndromes, Metabolic Disorders, and Skeletal Displasias. (ed 3) Chicago: Year Book Medical Publ, 1990, p 868

## Gamut B-134

# SYMPHALANGISM (FUSION OF PHALANGES IN A DIGIT)

## COMMON

1. Isolated anomaly (esp. PIP joints of fingers - "Shrewsbury mark," and DIP joints of toes)

## UNCOMMON

1. Acrocephalosyndactyly S. (Apert, others)
2. Brachydactyly B and C
3. Carpal-tarsal coalition
4. Cushing symphalangism
5. Diastrophic dysplasia
6. Hand-foot-genital S.
7. Multiple synostosis S.
8. Oculo-dento-osseous dysplasia
9. Popliteal pterygium S.
10. Short rib-polydactyly S., type I
11. Symphalangism-surdity S. (WL symphalangism-brachydactyly S.)

*References:*
1. Poznanski AK: The Hand in Radiologic Diagnosis. (ed 2) Philadelphia: W.B. Saunders, 1984, p 917

2. Poznanski AK: Foot manifestations of the congenital malformation syndromes. Semin Roentgenol 1970;5:354-366
3. Swischuk LE: Differential Diagnosis in Pediatric Radiology. Baltimore: Williams & Wilkins, 1984, pp 255-256
4. Taybi H, Lachman RS: Radiology of Syndromes, Metabolic Disorders, and Skeletal Dysplasias. (ed 3) Chicago: Year Book Medical Publ, 1990, p 876

## Gamut B-135

## CONTRACTURE OF A DIGIT

1. Ainhum
2. Arthrogryposis multiplex congenita (amyoplasia)
3. Burn
4. Camptodactyly
5. Congenital contractural arachnodactyly
6. Congenital or acquired ring contraction, annular band
7. Dupuytren's contracture
8. Volkmann's ischemic contracture

*Reference:*

1. Greenfield GB: Radiology of Bone Diseases. (ed 5) Philadelphia: Lippincott, 1990

# CAMPTODACTYLY (FLEXION DEFORMITY OF ONE OR MORE DIGITS)

## ACQUIRED

*1. Arthritis (esp. rheumatoid)
*2. Burn; frostbite
*3. Contracture
 4. Digital fibroma
*5. Infection
 6. Neoplasm
*7. Trauma

## CONGENITAL

 1. Aarskog S.
 2. Adducted thumb S.
 3. Arthrogryposis multiplex congenita; distal arthrogryposis
 4. Camptobrachydactyly
 5. Camptodactyly-ankylosis-pulmonary hypoplasia S.
 6. Cerebrohepatorenal S. (Zellweger S.)
 7. Fetal alcohol S.
 8. Focal dermal hypoplasia (Goltz S.)
 9. Goodman camptodactyly S., A and B
 10. Gordon S.
 11. Grebe S.
*12. Holt-Oram S.
 13. Idiopathic hypercalcemia (Williams S.)
 14. Isolated absence or hypoplasia of a phalanx
 15. Lenz microphthalmia S.
*16. Marfan S.; congenital contractural arachnodactyly
 17. Meckel S.
 18. Monosomy 21 S.
*19. Nail-patella S. (osteo-onychodysplasia)
*20. Oculo-dento-osseous dysplasia

---

\*21. Orofaciodigital S. I
22. Pectoral aplasia-syndactyly S. (Poland S.)
23. Pena-Shokeir S. I and II
24. Popliteal pterygium S.
25. Roberts S.
26. Trisomy 8 S.
\*27. Trisomy 13 S.
28. Trisomy 18 S.
29. Weaver-Smith S.
30. Whistling face S. (Freeman-Sheldon S.)

\* Common.

### References:

1. Poznanski AK: The Hand in Radiologic Diagnosis. (ed 2) Philadelphia: W.B. Saunders, 1984, p 916
2. Swischuk LE: Differential Diagnosis in Pediatric Radiology. Baltimore: Williams & Wilkins, 1984, pp 254-255
3. Taybi H, Lachman RS: Radiology of Syndromes, Metabolic Disorders, and Skeletal Dysplasias. (ed 3) Chicago: Year Book Medical Publ, 1990, pp 866-867

**Gamut B-137**

# SYNDACTYLY
## (SOFT TISSUE AND/OR BONY UNION BETWEEN ADJACENT DIGITS)

### COMMON
1. Acrocephalopolysyndactyly, all types
2. Acrocephalosyndactyly, all types
3. Cornelia de Lange S.
4. Isolated anomaly
5. Oculo-dento-osseous dysplasia

### UNCOMMON
1. Aarskog S.
2. Arthrogryposis

3. Basal cell nevus S. (Gorlin S.)
4. Bloom S.
5. Brachydactyly A-2 and B
6. Chondrodysplasia punctata (Conradi's disease)
7. Chondroectodermal dysplasia (Ellis-van Creveld S.)
8. Cloverleaf skull S.
9. Cryptophthalmos-syndactyly S. (Fraser S.)
10. EEC S.
11. Epidermolysis bullosa
12. Fanconi S. (pancytopenia-dysmelia S.)
13. Fetal aminopterin S.
14. Fetal hydantoin S.
15. Focal dermal hypoplasia (Goltz S.)
16. Greig cephalopolysyndactyly S.
17. Holt-Oram S.
18. Hypoglossia-hypodactyly S.
19. Incontinentia pigmenti S.
20. Laurence-Moon-Biedl S.
21. Myositis (fibrodysplasia) ossificans progressiva
22. Oculo-mandibulo-facial S. (Hallermann-Streiff S.)
23. Orofaciodigital S.
24. Osteogenesis imperfecta tarda
25. Otopalatodigital S.
26. Pectoral aplasia-syndactyly S. (Poland S.)
27. Pierre Robin S.
28. Popliteal pterygium S.
29. Prader-Willi S.
30. Pseudothalidomide S.
31. Roberts S.
32. Rubinstein-Taybi S.
33. Sclerosteosis
34. Short rib-polydactyly S., type 1
35. Silver-Russell S.
36. Smith-Lemli-Opitz S.
37. Thrombocytopenia-absent radius (TAR) S.
38. Tricho-rhino-phalangeal dysplasia
39. Triploidy
40. Trisomy 13 S.
41. Trisomy 18 S.
42. Trisomy 21 S. (Down S.) (toes)

NOTE: There are over 20 other minor congenital syndromes with syndactyly that are listed in the books by Poznanski and Taybi.

### References:

1. Jones KL: Smith's Recognizable Patterns of Human Malformation. Philadelphia: W.B. Saunders, 1988
2. Poznanski AK: The Hand in Radiologic Diagnosis. (ed 2) Philadelphia: W.B. Saunders, 1984, p 914
3. Taybi H, Lachman RS: Radiology of Syndromes, Metabolic Disorders, and Skeletal Dysplasias. (ed 3) Chicago: Year Book Medical Publ, 1990, p 876

## Gamut B-138

## POLYDACTYLY

### COMMON

1. Acrocephalopolysyndactyly
2. Bardet-Biedl S.; Laurence-Moon-Biedl S.; Biemond S. II
3. Chondroectodermal dysplasia (Ellis-van Creveld S.)
4. Fanconi S. (pancytopenia-dysmelia S.)
5. Isolated anomaly

### UNCOMMON

1. Acrorenal S.
2. Asphyxiating thoracic dysplasia (Jeune S.)
3. Blackfan-Diamond S.
4. Bloom S.
5. C S.
6. Chondrodysplasia punctata (Conradi's disease)
7. Dubowitz S.
8. Focal dermal hypoplasia (Goltz S.)
9. Grebe S. (toes)
10. Greig cephalopolysyndactyly S.
11. Holt-Oram S.
12. Lacrimo-auriculo-dento-digital S. (LADD S.)

13. Lissencephaly S.
14. McKusick-Kaufman S. (hereditary hydrometrocolpos)
15. Meckel S.
16. Mesomelic dysplasia (Werner type)
17. Möbius S.
18. Myositis (fibrodysplasia) ossificans progressiva
19. Orofaciodigital S. II (Mohr S.)
20. Pectoral aplasia-syndactyly S. (Poland S.)
21. Prune-belly S. (Eagle-Barrett S.)
22. Rieger S.
23. Rubinstein-Taybi S.
24. Short rib-polydactyly S., types 1, 2, 3
25. Silver-Russell S.
26. Smith-Lemli-Opitz S.
27. Stickler S. (arthro-ophthalmopathy)
28. Trisomy 13 S.
29. Trisomy 21 S. (Down S.)
30. VATER association

*References:*
1. Edeiken J, Dalinka M, Karasick D: Edeiken's Roentgen Diagnosis of Diseases of Bone. (ed 4) Baltimore: Williams & Wilkins, 1989
2. Jones KL: Smith's Recognizable Patterns of Human Malformation. Philadelphia: W.B. Saunders, 1988
3. Poznanski AK: Foot manifestations of the congenital malformation syndromes. Semin Roentgenol 1970;5:354-366
4. Poznanski AK: The Hand in Radiologic Diagnosis. (ed 2) Philadelphia: W.B. Saunders, 1984, pp 266-278
5. Swischuk LE: Differential Diagnosis in Pediatric Radiology. Baltimore: Williams & Wilkins, 1984, p 255
6. Taybi H, Lachman RS: Radiology of Syndromes, Metabolic Disorders, and Skeletal Dysplasias. (ed 3) Chicago: Year Book Medical Publ, 1990, p 875

B. Bone

# MACRODACTYLY

1. Enchondromatosis (Ollier's disease); Maffucci S.
2. Hemangioma
3. Idiopathic
4. Klippel-Trenaunay-Weber S.
5. Lymphangioma
6. Macrodystrophia lipomatosa
7. Melorheostosis
8. Neurofibromatosis
9. Plexiform neuroma
10. Proteus S.

*Reference:*
1. Taybi H, Lachman RS: Radiology of Syndromes, Metabolic Disorders, and Skeletal Dysplasias. (ed 3) Chicago: Year Book Medical Publ, 1990, p 873

# ARACHNODACTYLY (LONG FINGERS)

**COMMON**
1. Marfan S.

**UNCOMMON**
1. Basal cell nevus S. (Gorlin)
2. Congenital contractural arachnodactyly
3. Ehlers-Danlos S.
4. Frontometaphyseal dysplasia
5. Goodman camptodactyly S. B
6. Homocystinuria
7. Ichthyosis syndromes
8. Marden-Walker S.

9. Multiple endocrine neoplasia, type III (multiple neuroma S.)
10. Myotonic dystrophy
11. Rieger S.
12. Sotos S.
13. Stickler S. (arthro-ophthalmopathy)
14. XYY S.

*References:*
1. Poznanski AK: The Hand in Radiologic Diagnosis. (ed 2) Philadelphia: W.B. Saunders, 1984, p 918
2. Taybi H, Lachman RS: Radiology of Syndromes, Metabolic Disorders, and Skeletal Dysplasias. (ed 3) Chicago: Year Book Medical Publ, 1990, p 864

## Gamut B-141

## BRACHYDACTYLY (LOCALIZED)

### COMMON
1. Acro-osteolysis (eg, congenital, leprosy) (See B-127)
2. Congenital syndromes with short hands and feet (esp. chondrodysplasias, mucopolysaccharidoses$_g$) (See B-145)
3. Congenital syndromes with short metacarpals or metatarsals (See B-144)
4. Congenital syndromes with short phalanges (See B-123 to B-125)
5. Idiopathic
6. Osteomyelitis, dactylitis (eg, bacterial, tuberculous, yaws, smallpox)
7. Pseudohypoparathyroidism, pseudopseudohypoparathyroidism
8. Sickle cell anemia (hand-foot S.)
9. Trauma (eg, thermal, electrical, epiphyseal cartilage injury, fracture)

**UNCOMMON**
1. Arthritis (esp. juvenile rheumatoid)
2. Basal cell nevus S. (Gorlin S.)
3. Cone-shaped epiphyses (See B-29)
4. Enchondromatosis (Ollier's disease)
5. Epiphyseal dysostosis or dysplasia
6. Familial brachydactylies
7. Kashin-Beck disease (in Manchuria and Russia)
8. Myositis (fibrodysplasia) ossificans progressiva
9. Turner S.

*References:*
1. Greenfield GB: Radiology of Bone Diseases. (ed 5) Philadelphia: Lippincott, 1990
2. Poznanski AK: The Hand in Radiologic Diagnosis. (ed 2) Philadelphia: W.B. Saunders, 1984
3. Taybi H, Lachman RS: Radiology of Syndromes, Metabolic Disorders, and Skeletal Dysplasias. (ed 3) Chicago: Year Book Medical Publ, 1990, pp 864-865

## Gamut B-142

# CONGENITAL SYNDROMES WITH GENERALIZED BRACHYDACTYLY

**COMMON**
1. Achondroplasia
2. Chondroectodermal dysplasia (Ellis-van Creveld S.)
3. Mucopolysaccharidoses (eg, Hurler, Morquio, Maroteaux-Lamy)
4. Pseudohypoparathyroidism, pseudopseudohypoparathyroidism

**UNCOMMON**
1. Aarskog S.
2. Achondrogenesis
3. Acrocephalopolysyndactyly
4. Acrocephalosyndactyly
5. Acrodysostosis

6. Acromesomelic dysplasia
7. Asphyxiating thoracic dysplasia
8. Ateleosteogenesis
9. Campomelic dysplasia
10. Diastrophic dysplasia
11. Grebe chondrodysplasia
12. Hypochondroplasia
13. Hypophosphatasia
14. Metaphyseal chondrodysplasia (McKusick)
15. Metatropic dysplasia
16. Orofaciodigital S. I
17. Prader-Willi S.
18. Pseudoachondroplasia
19. Pseudoleprechaunism (Patterson S.)
20. Rothmund-Thomson S.
21. Thanatophoric dysplasia
22. Tricho-rhino-phalangeal dysplasia
23. Trisomy 21 S. (Down S.)
24. Weill-Marchesani S.
25. XXXXX S.

*References:*

1. Jones KL: Smith's Recognizable Patterns of Human Malformation. Philadelphia: W.B. Saunders, 1988
2. Poznanski AK: The Hand in Radiologic Diagnosis. (ed 2) Philadelphia: W.B. Saunders, 1984, p 244
3. Taybi H, Lachman RS: Radiology of Syndromes, Metabolic Disorders, and Skeletal Dysplasias. (ed 3) Chicago: Year Book Medical Publ, 1990, pp 864-865

## Gamut B-143

## SHORT METACARPALS OR METATARSALS (EXCLUDING GENERALIZED SHORTENING)

### COMMON
1. Arthritis (eg, juvenile rheumatoid, septic)
2. Congenital syndromes (See B-144)

3. Idiopathic, isolated anomaly
4. Infarction (eg, sickle cell anemia)
5. Osteomyelitis (eg, bacterial, yaws, smallpox)
6. Trauma (eg, thermal, electrical, epiphyseal cartilage injury, fracture)

## UNCOMMON
1. Hypoparathyroidism
2. Hypothyroidism, cretinism
3. Myotonic dystrophy
4. Radiation or radium injury

### References:
1. Edeiken J, Dalinka M, Karasick D.: Edeiken's Roentgen Diagnosis of Diseases of Bone. (ed 4) Baltimore: Williams & Wilkins, 1989
2. Greenfield GB: Radiology of Bone Diseases. (ed 5) Philadelphia: Lippincott, 1990

## Subgamut B-143A

# SHORT FOURTH METACARPAL*

## COMMON
1. Idiopathic
2. Osteomyelitis (esp. bacterial, yaws)
3. Pseudohypoparathyroidism, pseudopseudohypoparathyroidism
4. Trauma
5. Turner S. (gonadal dysgenesis)

## UNCOMMON
1. Basal cell nevus S. (Gorlin)
2. Dyschondrosteosis
3. Juvenile rheumatoid arthritis

4. Multiple epiphyseal dysplasia (Fairbank)
5. Sickle cell anemia with infarction

* Positive metacarpal sign: a line tangential to the heads of the fourth and fifth metacarpals passes through (rather than distal to) the head of the third metacarpal.

*Reference:*
1. Burgener FA, Kormano M: Differential Diagnosis in Conventional Radiology. New York: Thieme Medical Publ, 1991, p 267

## Gamut B-144

## CONGENITAL SYNDROMES WITH SHORT METACARPALS OR METATARSALS

### COMMON
1. Basal cell nevus S. (Gorlin)
2. Chondrodysplasia punctata (Conradi's disease)
*3. Cornelia de Lange S. (1st metacarpal)
*4. Diastrophic dysplasia (hitchhiker thumb)
5. Enchondromatosis (Ollier's disease)
*6. Holt-Oram S.
7. Hypothyroidism, cretinism
8. Mucopolysaccharidoses (eg, Hurler, Hunter); mucolipidosis II (I-cell disease)
*9. Myositis (fibrodysplasia) ossificans progressiva (thumb and great toe)
10. Pseudohypoparathyroidism, pseudopseudohypoparathyroidism
11. Turner S. (4th metacarpal)

### UNCOMMON
1. Acrofacial dysostosis (Nager S.)
2. Acromesomelic dysplasia

   3.  Aplasia cutis congenita (absent metacarpals)
   4.  Biemond S. I (4th metacarpal)
   5.  Brachydactyly A-1, C*, E
   6.  C syndrome
   7.  Camptobrachydactly
   8.  Cat's cry S. (5th metacarpal)
  *9.  Cephaloskeletal dysplasia (Taybi-Linder S)
 *10.  Chromosome 18 q- S.
  11.  Cockayne S.
  12.  Coffin-Siris S.
  13.  Cohen S.
  14.  Dyggve-Melchior-Clausen S.
  15.  Dyschondrosteosis (4th metacarpal)
 *16.  Dyssegmental dysplasia
  17.  Epiphyseal dysostosis
 *18.  Fanconi S. (pancytopenia-dysmelia S.)
  19.  Fetal alcohol S.
  20.  Grebe S.
 *21.  Hand-foot-genital S.
  22.  Ichthyosis syndromes
 *23.  Juberg-Hayward S.
  24.  Larsen S.
  25.  Megaepiphyseal dwarfism
  26.  Multiple cartilaginous exostoses
  27.  Multiple epiphyseal dysplasia (Fairbank)
  28.  Osteoglophonic dwarfism
  29.  Otopalatodigital S.
  30.  Pallister-Hall S. (4th metacarpal)
  31.  Poland S.
 *32.  Radial hypoplasia syndromes
  33.  Robinow S.
  34.  Rothmund-Thomson S.
 *35.  Rubinstein-Taybi S. (thumb and great toe)
  36.  Short rib-polydactyly S., types 1, 2, and 3
  37.  Silver-Russell S. (5th metacarpal)
  38.  Sjögren-Larsson S.
  39.  Spondyloepiphyseal dysplasia
 *40.  Symphalangism-brachydactyly S.
  41.  Thanatophoric dysplasia
  42.  Tricho-rhino-phalangeal dysplasia

*43. Trisomy 9p S.
*44. Trisomy 18 S.
*45. VATER association
46. Weaver S.
47. Weill-Marchesani S.

* Short first metacarpal primarily.

*References:*
1. Kozlowksi K, Beighton P: Gamut Index of Skeletal Dysplasias. Berlin: Springer-Verlag, 1984, pp 72-73
2. Poznanski AK: The Hand in Radiologic Diagnosis. (ed 2) Philadelphia: W.B. Saunders, 1984, pp 908-909
3. Swischuk LE: Differential Diagnosis in Pediatric Radiology. Baltimore: Williams & Wilkins, 1984, pp 247-250
4. Taybi H, Lachman RS: Radiology of Syndromes, Metabolic Disorders, and Skeletal Dysplasias. (ed 3) Chicago: Year Book Medical Publ, 1990, p 874

## Gamut B-145

# CONGENITAL SYNDROMES WITH SHORT HANDS AND FEET (ACROMELIA)

**COMMON**
1. Achondroplasia
2. Enchondromatosis (Ollier's disease)
3. Mucopolysaccharidoses (eg, Hurler, Hunter, Morquio)
4. Pseudohypoparathyroidism, pseudopseudohypoparathyroidism

**UNCOMMON**
1. Aarskog S.
2. Achondrogenesis
3. Acrodysostosis (peripheral dysostosis)
4. Acromesomelic dysplasia

B. Bone

5. Asphyxiating thoracic dysplasia
6. Cephaloskeletal dysplasia (Taybi-Linder S.)
7. Chondroectodermal dysplasia (Ellis-van Creveld S.)
8. Cockayne S.
9. Diastrophic dysplasia
10. Hand-foot-genital S.
11. Hypochondroplasia
12. Hypopituitarism
13. [Isolated anomaly]
14. Léri's pleonosteosis
15. Metaphyseal chondrodysplasias
16. Metatropic dysplasia
17. Mucolipidoses$_g$
18. Multiple cartilaginous exostoses
19. Multiple epiphyseal dysplasia (Fairbank)
20. Noonan S.
21. Orofaciodigital S.
22. Prader-Willi S.
23. Progeria
24. Pseudoachondroplasia
25. Short rib-polydactyly S.
26. Smith-Lemli-Opitz S.
27. Spondylo-epi-metaphyseal dysplasia
28. Spondylometaphyseal dysplasia
29. Thanatophoric dysplasia
30. Tricho-rhino-phalangeal dysplasia
31. Trisomy 21 S. (Down S.)
32. Weill-Marchesani S.

*References:*
1. Felson B (ed): Dwarfs and Other Little People. Semin Roentgenol 1973;8:257
2. Greenfield GB: Radiology of Bone Diseases. (ed 5) Philadelphia: Lippincott, 1990
3. Kozlowski K, Beighton P: Gamut Index of Skeletal Dysplasias. Berlin: Springer-Verlag, 1984, p 72
4. Taybi H, Lachman RS: Radiology of Syndromes, Metabolic Disorders, and Skeletal Dysplasias. (ed 3) Chicago: Year Book Medical Publ, 1990, p 872

## ACQUIRED DISEASES CAUSING SHORT HANDS AND FEET

1. Acro-osteolysis (See B-127)
2. Hypopituitarism
3. Leprosy
4. Lipoid dermatoarthritis
5. Osteomyelitis, severe (eg, bacterial, yaws, smallpox)
6. Rheumatoid arthritis, arthritis mutilans
7. Sickle cell anemia (hand-foot S.)
8. Trauma; surgery; ritual (eg, Chinese bound feet)

### Gamut B-147

## SPADE HAND (SMALL, SQUARE HAND WITH SHORTENING OF ALL BONES)

**COMMON**
1. Achondroplasia
2. Hypochondroplasia
3. Mucopolysaccharidoses

**UNCOMMON**
1. Achondrogenesis
2. Acrodysostosis (peripheral dysostosis)
3. Asphyxiating thoracic dysplasia
4. Cephaloskeletal dysplasia (Taybi-Linder S.)
5. Diastrophic dysplasia
6. Metaphyseal chondrodysplasias (esp. Jansen)
7. Metatropic dysplasia
8. Orofaciodigital S.
9. Pleonosteosis (Léri)
10. Pseudoachondroplasia

11. Short rib-polydactyly S.
12. Thanatophoric dysplasia

*References:*
1. Swischuk LE: Differential Diagnosis in Pediatric Radiology. Baltimore: Williams & Wilkins, 1984, p 254
2. Taybi H, Lachman RS: Radiology of Syndromes, Metabolic Disorders, and Skeletal Dysplasias. (ed 3) Chicago: Year Book Medical Publ, 1990, p 872

## Gamut B-148

## CONTRACTED HAND (CLAW-HAND)

### Acquired

1. Arthritis (esp. rheumatoid)
2. Burn, electrical injury
3. Diabetes
4. Dupuytren contracture
5. Epidermolysis bullosa
6. Frostbite
7. Leprosy
8. Neoplasm
9. Neurologic disorder
10. Reflex sympathetic dystrophy, Sudeck's atrophy
11. Trauma

### Congenital

1. Arthrogryposis
2. Chondrodysplasia punctata (Conradi's disease)
3. Congenital contractural arachnodactyly
4. Diastrophic dysplasia
5. Distal arthrogryposis (Gordon S.)
6. EEC S.
7. Freeman-Sheldon S. (whistling face S.)

8. Larsen S.
9. Léri's pleonosteosis
10. Monosomy 21 S.
11. Mucopolysaccharidoses; $GM_1$ gangliosidosis
12. Myotonic dystrophy
13. Pena-Shokeir S. I
14. Trisomy 13 S.
15. Trisomy 18 S.
16. Ulnar drift S. (digitotalar dysmorphism)

*Reference:*
1. Poznanski AK: The Hand in Radiologic Diagnosis. (ed 2) Philadelphia: W.B. Saunders, 1984, p 916

## Gamut B-149

## LARGE HANDS FOR AGE

### COMMON

1. Acromegaly; pituitary gigantism
2. Cerebral gigantism (Sotos S.)
3. Hyperthyroidism, active or treated (eg, thyroid acropachy)
4. Marfan S.
5. Precocious puberty

### UNCOMMON

1. Beckwith-Wiedemann S.
2. Coffin-Lowry S.
3. Frontometaphyseal dysplasia
4. Lipoatrophic diabetes (total lipodystrophy)
5. Pachydermoperiostosis
6. Patterson S. (pseudoleprechaunism)
7. Stickler S. (arthro-ophthalmopathy)

*References:*
1. Poznanski AK: The Hand in Radiologic Diagnosis. (ed 2) Philadelphia: W.B. Saunders, 1984, p 918
2. Taybi H, Lachman RS: Radiology of Syndromes, Metabolic Disorders, and Skeletal Dysplasias. (ed 3) Chicago: Year Book Medical Publ, 1990, p 872

### Gamut B-150

## ASYMMETRY IN SIZE OF HAND BONES (See Gamuts B-13 to B-15)

## Acquired

### SMALL BONES OF ONE HAND
1. Acro-osteolysis (See B-127)
2. Ainhum
3. Arrest of epiphyseal growth
   a. Fracture
   b. Juvenile rheumatoid arthritis
   c. Osteomyelitis (eg, septic, yaws, smallpox)
   d. Radiation injury
   e. Surgery
   f. Thermal injury (eg, burn, frostbite)
   g. Wringer injury
4. Paralysis

### LARGE BONES OF ONE HAND
1. Bone neoplasm
2. Hyperemia
   a. Hemangioma, arteriovenous fistula
   b. Infection
   c. Juvenile rheumatoid arthritis
3. Paget's disease

# Congenital

## GENERAL ASYMMETRY
1. Beckwith-Wiedemann S.
2. Hemiatrophy
3. Hemihypertrophy (See B-14)
4. Silver-Russell S.
5. Wilms' tumor

## SMALL BONES OF ONE HAND
1. Amniotic bands
2. Aplasia, hypoplasia
3. Chondrodysplasia punctata (Conradi's disease)
4. Poland S.
5. Warfarin embryopathy

## LARGE BONES OF ONE HAND
1. Enchondromatosis; Maffucci S.
2. Fibrous dysplasia
3. Hemangioma, arteriovenous fistula
4. Klippel-Trenaunay-Weber S.
5. Lymphangiectasia
6. Macrodactyly
7. Macrodystrophia lipomatosa
8. Melorheostosis
9. Neurofibromatosis

*Reference:*
1. Poznanski AK: The Hand in Radiologic Diagnosis. (ed 2) Philadelphia: W.B. Saunders, 1984, p 917

## GENERALIZED FAILURE OF MODELING OR TUBULATION IN THE HAND (WIDE OR THICK BONES) (See Gamuts B-11, B-12)

### Acquired

1. Anemia$_g$ (esp. thalassemia, sickle cell anemia)
2. Fluorosis
3. Fracture, healed
4. Infarction (eg, hand-foot S.)
5. Infection, osteomyelitis
6. Neoplasm
7. Rickets (healing); biliary disease in infancy
8. Subperiosteal hemorrhage (eg, hemophilia, osteogenesis imperfecta with trauma)

### Congenital

1. Achondrogenesis
2. Craniodiaphyseal dysplasia
3. Craniometaphyseal dysplasia
4. Enchondromatosis (Ollier's disease)
5. Engelmann's disease (diaphyseal dysplasia)
6. Fibrous dysplasia
7. Hyperphosphatasia
8. Melorheostosis
9. Metaphyseal dysplasia (Pyle's disease)
10. Mucolipidoses$_g$; fucosidosis, mannosidosis, GM$_1$ gangliosidosis
11. Niemann-Pick disease
12. Oculo-dento-osseous dysplasia
13. Osteopetrosis
14. Sclerosteosis
15. Singleton-Merten S.

*Reference:*
1. Poznanski AK: The Hand in Radiologic Diagnosis. (ed 2) Philadelphia: W.B. Saunders, 1984, p 901

## Gamut B-152

# ABNORMAL TAPERING OF SHORT TUBULAR BONES OF THE HANDS AND FEET

### PROXIMAL TAPERING
1. Cornelia de Lange S.
2. Mucopolysaccharidoses (eg, Hurler, Hunter, Morquio); mucolipidoses

### DISTAL TAPERING
1. Acro-osteolysis (See B-127)
2. Diabetes
3. Epidermolysis bullosa
4. Hyperparathyroidism
5. Leprosy; other neurotrophic diseases
6. Raynaud's disease
7. Scleroderma
8. Thermal injury (eg, burn, frostbite)

*Reference:*
1. Greenfield GB: Radiology of Bone Diseases. (ed 5) Philadelphia: Lippincott, 1990

## Gamut B-153

# NEUROTROPHIC BONE CHANGES (POINTED OR SPINDLED BONES) IN THE HANDS OR FEET

## COMMON

1. [Amputation (congenital, traumatic, or surgical)]
2. Arteriosclerosis obliterans; Raynaud's disease; Buerger's disease
3. Diabetes
4. Leprosy
5. Psoriatic arthritis
6. Rheumatoid arthritis
7. Scleroderma, dermatomyositis
8. Septic arthritis (pyarthrosis)
9. Spinal cord trauma or disease (eg, pernicious anemia, syringomyelia, spina bifida, meningomyelocele, neoplasm)
10. Thermal injury (eg, burn, frostbite, electrical)
11. Trophic ulcer of soft tissue with underlying destruction

## UNCOMMON

1. Acrodystrophic neuropathy
2. [Acro-osteolysis (See B-127)]
3. [Ainhum]
4. Amyloid neuropathy
5. Charcot-Marie-Tooth S.
6. [Clubbing of fingers]
7. Congenital indifference to pain
8. Congenital pseudarthrosis
9. Ergot intoxication
10. Hicks S. (familial sensory neural radiculopathy)
11. Idiopathic
12. Malnutrition (alcoholism or nutritional neuropathy)
13. Peripheral nerve injury
14. Porphyria

15. [Pyknodysostosis]
16. Riley-Day S. (familial dysautonomia)
17. Tabes dorsalis
18. Trench foot

*References:*
1. Gondos B: The pointed tubular bone. Radiology 1972; 105: 541-545
2. Greenfield GB: Radiology of Bone Diseases. (ed 5) Philadelphia: Lippincott, 1990
3. Hodgson JR, Pugh DG, Young HH: Roentgenologic aspect of certain lesions of bone: neurotrophic or infectious? Radiology 1948;50:65-70
4. Kozlowski K, Beighton P: Gamut Index of Skeletal Dysplasias. Berlin: Springer-Verlag, 1984, pp 76-77

## Gamut B-154

# WELL-DEFINED SOLITARY OR MULTIPLE LUCENT DEFECTS IN BONES OF THE HANDS, WRISTS, FEET, OR ANKLES

## COMMON
1. Bone cyst, developmental cyst
2. Enchondroma
3. Gout
4. Osteoarthritis
5. Posttraumatic (eg, avascular necrosis with cystic radiolucency following scaphoid or lunate fracture)
6. Rheumatoid arthritis; juvenile rheumatoid arthritis

## UNCOMMON
1. Amyloidosis
2. Aneurysmal bone cyst
3. Chondroblastoma
4. Chondromyxoid fibroma

5. Driller's disease (carpals)
6. Enchondromatosis (Ollier's disease)
7. Epidermoid inclusion cyst (distal phalanx)
8. Fibromatosis
9. Fibrous dysplasia
10. Ganglion (esp. intraosseous)
11. Giant cell reparative granuloma
12. Giant cell tumor
13. Glomus tumor (distal phalanx)
14. Granuloma (eg, foreign body, palm thorn)
15. Hemangioma; Maffucci S.
16. Hemochromatosis
17. Hemophilic pseudotumor
18. Histiocytosis $X_g$
19. Kienböck disease (lunate necrosis)
20. Lipoma (esp. calcaneus)
21. Metastasis
22. Microgeodic S.
23. Mucopolysaccharidosis I-S (Scheie)
24. Multiple myeloma
25. Nonossifying fibroma
26. Osteoid osteoma
27. Osteomyelitis, cystic (eg, tuberculous, atypical mycobacterial, fungal, partially treated bacterial infection)
28. Sarcoidosis
29. Sickle cell disease (hand-foot S.)
30. Sinus histiocytosis
31. Subungual keratoma (distal phalanx)
32. Tuberous sclerosis
33. [Vascular channels, esp. phalanges]
34. Villonodular synovitis
35. Xanthomatosis

*Reference:*

1. Poznanski AK: The Hand in Radiologic Diagnosis. (ed 2) Philadelphia: W.B. Saunders, 1984, p 919

# SCLEROTIC FOCUS IN BONES OF THE HANDS OR FEET

## NORMAL VARIANT
*1. Bone island; enostoma

## CONGENITAL DISORDER
1. Enchondromatosis
2. Fibrous dysplasia
3. Gardner S.
4. Melorheostosis
5. Multiple cartilaginous exostoses
6. Osteopathia striata
7. Osteopoikilosis
8. Tuberous sclerosis

## INFLAMMATORY
*1. Osteomyelitis, chronic; mycetoma
2. Syphilis
3. Yaws

## NEOPLASTIC
*1. Enchondroma
2. Nonossifying fibroma, healing
3. Osteoblastic metastasis
4. Osteoblastoma
5. Osteoid osteoma
6. Sarcoma (eg, osteosarcoma, chondrosarcoma, Ewing's)

## TRAUMATIC
*1. Healing fracture

## OTHER
*1. Avascular necrosis (eg, steroid therapy, trauma to scaphoid or lunate)
2. Infarct (eg, sickle cell disease)
3. Paget's disease

* Common.

*Reference:*
1. Poznanski AK: The Hand in Radiologic Diagnosis. (ed 2) Philadelphia: W.B. Saunders, 1984, p 899

## Gamut B-156

# TROPICAL DISEASES INVOLVING THE HANDS AND FEET

## COMMON
1. Filariasis (elephantiasis)
2. Leprosy
3. Sickle cell dactylitis (hand-foot S.)
4. Tuberculosis
5. Yaws, syphilis

## UNCOMMON
1. Ainhum
2. Guinea worm infection (dracunculiasis)
3. Kaposi sarcoma
4. Loiasis
5. Mycetoma (Madura foot); fungus diseases$_g$
6. Smallpox (residual deformities)
7. Tropical ulcer (usually tibia)

*Reference:*
1. Reeder MM, Palmer PES: The Radiology of Tropical Diseases, with Epidemiological, Pathological and Clinical Correlation. Baltimore: Williams & Wilkins, 1981

# CONGENITAL CONDITIONS ASSOCIATED WITH CLUBFOOT OR OTHER FOOT DEFORMITY

## COMMON
1. Faulty intrauterine positioning
*2. Neurologic or neuromuscular disease (eg, myotonic dystrophy, meningomyelocele, spina bifida)

## UNCOMMON
1. Aminopterin fetopathy (varus)
2. Arthrogryposis multiplex congenita
3. Bloom S.
4. Cerebrohepatorenal S. (Zellweger S.)
5. Chondrodysplasia punctata (Conradi's disease)
6. Chondroectodermal dysplasia (Ellis-van Creveld S.) (valgus)
7. Chromosome 4p S. (Wolf S.)
8. Chromosome 18q S.
9. Cornelia de Lange S.
10. Diastrophic dysplasia
11. Ehlers-Danlos S.
12. Homocystinuria (pes planus or cavus, everted feet)
13. Larsen S.
14. Marfan S. (long great toes, hammer toes)
15. Mietens-Weber S. (pes valgus planus)
16. Mucopolysaccharidoses$_g$ (eg, Hurler, Hunter, Morquio) (pes planus or cavus; misshapen tarsals)
17. Nail-patella S. (osteo-onychodysplasia)
18. Neurofibromatosis
19. Otopalatodigital S. (tarsal fusion)
20. Popliteal pterygium S.
21. Potter S. (renal agenesis)
22. Smith-Lemli-Opitz S.
23. Thrombocytopenia-absent radius (TAR) S.
*24. Trisomy 13 S.
*25. Trisomy 18 S.

26. Weaver-Smith S.
27. Whistling face S. (Freeman-Sheldon S.)
28. XXXXX S.
29. XXXXY S.

\* May have vertical talus.

### References:
1. Jones KL: Smith's Recognizable Patterns of Human Malformation. Philadelphia: W.B. Saunders, 1988
2. Poznanski AK: Foot manifestations of the congenital malformation syndromes. Semin Roentgenol 1970;5:354-366

---

## Gamut B-158

# CONGENITAL SYNDROMES WITH ACCESSORY CARPAL OR TARSAL OSSICLES

1. Anatomic variant
\*2. Brachydactyly A-1
\*3. Chondroectodermal dysplasia (Ellis-van Creveld S.)
\*4. Diastrophic dysplasia
5. [Dysplasia epiphysealis hemimelica (Trevor's disease)]
6. Grebe S.
7. Hand-foot-genital S.
8. Hollister S.
9. Holt-Oram S.
\*10. Larsen S.
\*11. Otopalatodigital S.
\*12. Stickler S. (arthro-ophthalmopathy)
13. Ulnar dimelia

\* Distal carpal row.

### References:
1. Kozlowski K, Beighton P: Gamut Index of Skeletal Dysplasias. Berlin: Springer-Verlag, 1984, pp 74-75

---

2. Poznanski AK: The Hand in Radiologic Diagnosis. (ed 2) Philadelphia: W.B. Saunders, 1984, pp 196-201

## Gamut B-159

# CONGENITAL SYNDROMES WITH SMALL CARPALS

## COMMON

1. Arthrogryposis
2. Chondrodysplasia punctata (Conradi's disease)
3. Morquio S.
*4. Multiple epiphyseal dysplasia (Fairbank)
5. Spondyloepiphyseal dysplasia

## UNCOMMON

1. Aarskog S.
2. Bird-headed dwarfism (Seckel S.)
3. Dyggve-Melchior-Clausen S.
*4. Farber S.
5. Frontometaphyseal dysplasia
6. Fucosidosis
7. Gordon S.
8. Kniest dysplasia
*9. Lipoid proteinosis
10. Metatropic dysplasia
*11. Osteoglophonic dwarfism
*12. Osteolysis (carpal-tarsal)
*13. Parastremmatic dwarfism
14. Spondylometaphyseal dysplasia
*15. Winchester S.

* With erosions or irregular margins.

### Reference:

1. Poznanski AK: The Hand in Radiologic Diagnosis. (ed 2) Philadelphia: W.B. Saunders, 1984, p 902

B. Bone

## Gamut B-160

# FRAGMENTED, IRREGULAR, OR SCLEROTIC CARPAL OR TARSAL BONES

### COMMON
1. Arthritis (esp. rheumatoid, pyogenic, gouty)
2. Aseptic necrosis (esp. scaphoid)
3. Infection (eg, mycetoma, osteomyelitis)
4. Normal variant (tarsals)
5. Trauma, postoperative changes

### UNCOMMON
1. Chondrodysplasia punctata (Conradi's disease)
2. Congenital bipartite bone
3. Morquio S.
4. Multiple epiphyseal dysplasia (Fairbank)
5. Spondyloepiphyseal dysplasia
6. Winchester S.

*Reference:*
1. Swischuk LE: Differential Diagnosis in Pediatric Radiology. Baltimore: Williams & Wilkins, 1984, pp 261-263

## Gamut B-161

# CARPAL OR TARSAL FUSION

### COMMON
1. Arthritis (esp. rheumatoid, juvenile chronic, pyogenic, fungal)
2. Arthrogryposis multiplex congenita

3. Normal variant, isolated anomaly (esp. triquetrum-lunate, talus-calcaneus, capitate-hamate, trapezium-trapezoid or navicular) as in Yoruba tribe of Nigeria
4. Traumatic; surgical

## UNCOMMON
1. Acrocephalopolysyndactyly (Carpenter S.)
2. Acrocephalosyndactyly (Apert S.)
3. Acromegaly
4. Baller-Gerold S.
5. Chondroectodermal dysplasia (Ellis-van Creveld S.) (capitate-hamate)
6. Chromosomal abnormalities
7. Cleft hand or foot
8. Craniofacial dysostosis (Crouzon S.) (calcaneus-cuboid)
9. Diastrophic dysplasia
10. Dyschondrosteosis; Madelung's deformity
11. EEC S.
12. F S.
13. Fetal alcohol S.
14. Frontometaphyseal dysplasia
15. Hand-foot-genital S.
16. Holt-Oram S.
17. Keratoderma palmaris et plantaris familiaris (tylosis)
18. Kniest dysplasia
19. LEOPARD S. (Lentiginosis S.)
20. Mesomelic dysplasia (Nievergelt type)
21. Multiple synostosis S.
22. Osteomyelitis
23. Otopalatodigital S. (capitate-hamate)
24. Reflex sympathetic dystrophy
25. Rothmund-Thomson S.
26. Scleroderma; dermatomyositis
27. Symphalangism-surdity S.
28. Thalidomide embryopathy
29. Turner S.

*References:*
1. Cope JR: Carpal coalition. Clin Radiol 1974;25:261-266
2. Kozlowski K, Beighton P: Gamut Index of Skeletal Dysplasias. Berlin: Springer-Verlag, 1984, p 74
3. Poznanski AK: Foot manifestations of the congenital malformation syndromes. Semin Roentgenol 1970;5:354-366
4. Poznanski AK: The Hand in Radiologic Diagnosis. (ed 2) Philadelphia: W.B. Saunders, 1984, pp 201-207
5. Taybi H, Lachman RS: Radiology of Syndromes, Metabolic Disorders, and Skeletal Dysplasias. (ed 3) Chicago: Year Book Medical Publ, 1990

## Gamut B-162

## CONGENITAL SYNDROMES ASSOCIATED WITH AN ABNORMAL CARPAL ANGLE*

### DECREASED ANGLE (LESS THAN 124°)
1. Dyschondrosteosis; Madelung's deformity
2. Hurler S.
3. Mesomelic dysplasia (Langer type)
4. Morquio S.
5. Multiple cartilaginous exostoses
6. Turner S.

### INCREASED ANGLE (GREATER THAN 139°)
1. Arthrogryposis
2. Cerebral gigantism (Sotos S.)
3. Chondroectodermal dysplasia (Ellis-van Creveld S.)
4. Cleidocranial dysplasia
5. Frontometaphyseal dysplasia
6. Larsen S.
7. Marfan S.
8. Multiple epiphyseal dysplasia (Fairbank)
9. Otopalatodigital S.
10. Pfeiffer-like S.

11. Stickler S. (arthro-ophthalmopathy)
12. Tricho-rhino-phalangeal dysplasia

* Normal carpal angle is 131.5° ( + or - 7.2°).

*References:*
1. Poznanski AK: The Hand in Radiologic Diagnosis. (ed 2) Philadelphia: W.B. Saunders, 1984, pp 193-195
2. Swischuk LE: Differential Diagnosis in Pediatric Radiology. Baltimore: Williams & Wilkins, 1984, p 260

## Gamut B-163

## CARPAL ANOMALIES SEEN IN COMMON CONGENITAL SYNDROMES*

| | Os Centrale (one or more) | Extra Distal Carpals | Os Triangulare | Irregular Carpal Margins | Abnormally Shaped Scaphoid | Absent or Hypoplastic Scaphoid | Scaphoid Fused to Other Carpals | Abnormally Shaped Capitate | Absent or Hypoplastic Capitate | Some Carpal Fusion | Decreased Carpal Angle | Increased Carpal Angle | Diminution in Size of the Carpus |
|---|---|---|---|---|---|---|---|---|---|---|---|---|---|
| Arthrogryposis | | | O | | O | | O | O | | X | | X | X |
| Diastrophic dysplasia | | X | | X | O | | O | O | | O | | O | X |
| Dyschondrosteosis | | | | | | | | | | O | X | | |
| Ellis-van Creveld S. | | X | | | | | | | | X | | | |
| Epiphyseal dysplasia | | | | X | O | | | X | X | | | X | X |
| Fanconi's anemia | | | | | X | X | | | | | | | |
| Hand-foot-genital S. | X | | O | | X | | X | | | X | | | |
| Holt-Oram S. | X | | | | X | O | X | O | | O | | | |
| Homocystinuria | | | | | | | | X | | | | | |
| Otopalatodigital S. | O | O | | | O | | O | X | | O | | | O |
| Symphalangism | | | | | | | O | | | X | | | |
| Turner S. | | | | | | | | | | O | X | | O |

(Modified from Poznanski AK, Holt JF; AJR 1971;112:443-459)

* X = commonly present; O = occasionally present

# HYPOPLASIA OR APLASIA OF THE RADIUS[+] AND/OR THUMB

## COMMON

*1. Cornelia de Lange S.
2. Fanconi S. (pancytopenia-dysmelia S.)
3. Holt-Oram S.
*4. Isolated anomaly
*5. Phocomelia (eg, thalidomide embryopathy)
6. Thrombocytopenia-absent radius (TAR) S.

## UNCOMMON

1. Acrofacial dysostosis (Nager)
2. Baller-Gerold S. (craniosynostosis-radial dysplasia or aplasia)
3. Bird-headed dwarfism (Seckel S.)
4. Blackfan-Diamond S.
5. Craniosynostosis-radial dysplasia
6. Duane/radial dysplasia S.
7. Dyschondrosteosis
8. Ectodermal dysplasia
*9. Ives-Houston S.
10. Juberg-Hayward S.
11. Lacrimo-auriculo-dento-digital S. (LADD S.)
12. Mesomelic dysplasia
13. Pena-Shokeir S.
14. Poland S.
*15. Pseudothalidomide S.
16. Ring D chromosome S.
*17. Roberts S.
18. Rothmund-Thomson S.
19. Trisomy 13 S.
20. Trisomy 18 S.
21. VATER association

* May have ulnar hypoplasia as well.
+ Radial hypoplasia may be seen with certain congenital heart diseases; renal anomalies; esophageal, duodenal, or anal atresia; rib anomalies; Klippel-Feil S.; kyphoscoliosis; and hypoplasia or spina bifida of the lumbosacral spine.

*References:*
1. Edeiken J, Dalinka M, Karasick D: Edeiken's Roentgen Diagnosis of Diseases of Bone. (ed 4) Baltimore: Williams & Wilkins, 1989
2. Jones KL: Smith's Recognizable Patterns of Human Malformation. Philadelphia: W.B. Saunders, 1988
3. Kozlowski K, Beighton P: Gamut Index of Skeletal Dysplasias. Berlin: Springer-Verlag, 1984, p 65
4. Poznanski AK: The Hand in Radiologic Diagnosis. (ed 2) Philadelphia: W.B. Saunders, 1984, pp 244-248, 911
5. Swischuk LE: Differential Diagnosis in Pediatric Radiology. Baltimore: Williams & Wilkins, 1984, pp 187-188

## Gamut B-165

## DISORDERS ASSOCIATED WITH MADELUNG DEFORMITY[*]

1. Dyschondrosteosis (Léri-Weill disease)
2. Enchondromatosis (Ollier's disease); Maffucci S.
3. Hurler S. (tilt of distal radius and ulna towards each other)
4. LEOPARD S. (Lentiginosis S.)
5. Multiple cartilaginous exostoses (diaphyseal aclasis)
6. Trauma in childhood (pseudo-Madelung deformity)
7. Turner S.

[*] Premature fusion of ulnar aspect of distal radial epiphysis resulting in (1) ulnar and volar angulation of distal radial articular surface, (2) decreased carpal angle, and (3) dorsal subluxation of distal ulna.

*References:*
1. Kozlowski K, Beighton P: Gamut Index of Skeletal Dysplasias. Berlin: Springer-Verlag, 1984, p 65
2. Poznanski AK: The Hand in Radiologic Diagnosis. (ed 2) Philadelphia: W.B. Saunders, 1984, p 904
3. Taybi H, Lachman RS: Radiology of Syndromes, Metabolic Disorders, and Skeletal Dysplasias. (ed 3) Chicago: Year Book Medical Publ, 1990, p 874

## Gamut B-166

# RADIOULNAR SYNOSTOSIS

**COMMON**
1. Ehlers-Danlos S.
2. Holt-Oram S.
3. Idiopathic, isolated anomaly
4. Multiple cartilaginous exostoses (distal forearm)
5. Trauma (interosseous ligament ossification)

**UNCOMMON**
1. Acrocephalosyndactyly, Pfeiffer type
2. Cloverleaf skull S.
3. Femoral-facial S.
4. Fetal alcohol S.
5. Infantile cortical hyperostosis (Caffey's disease)
6. Klinefelter S. (XXY S.); XXXY S.
7. Lacrimo-auriculo-dento-digital S. (LADD S.)
8. Mesomelic dysplasia (Nievergelt type)
9. Multiple synostosis S.
10. Nager acrofacial dysostosis
11. Thalidomide embryopathy
12. Thanatophoric dysplasia
13. Trisomy 18 S.
14. XXXXX S.; XXXXY S.

*References:*
1. Kozlowski K, Beighton P: Gamut Index of Skeletal Dysplasias. Berlin: Springer-Verlag, 1984, pp 64-65
2. Taybi H, Lachman RS: Radiology of Syndromes, Metabolic Disorders, and Skeletal Dysplasias. (ed 3) Chicago: Year Book Medical Publ, 1990, p 877

## Gamut B-167

# DEFORMITY OF THE FOREARM

**COMMON**
1. Fracture of radial shaft with dislocation of distal ulna
2. Generalized bone growth disturbance (eg, under-constriction or overconstriction of diametaphyses) (See B-10, B-11)
3. Monteggia fracture (fracture of ulnar shaft with dislocation of radial head)
4. Proximal radioulnar dislocation (incl. "nursemaid's elbow")

**UNCOMMON**
1. Congenital radioulnar synostosis (See B-166)
2. Enchondromatosis (Ollier's disease) with shortened ulna
3. Hypoplasia or aplasia of radius or ulna (See B-164)
4. Isolated anomaly
5. Madelung's deformity (See B-165)
6. Multiple cartilaginous exostoses (diaphyseal aclasis) with short ulna, curved radius, and often radial head dislocation
7. Osteogenesis imperfecta (bowed radius and ulna)

*Reference:*
1. Burgener FA, Kormano M: Differential Diagnosis in Conventional Radiology. New York: Thieme Medical Publ, 1991, pp 254-255

# CONGENITAL SYNDROMES WITH ELBOW ANOMALY (INCLUDING RADIAL HEAD HYPOPLASIA, PROXIMAL RADIOULNAR DISLOCATION, CUBITUS VALGUS)

**COMMON**

1. Larsen S.
*2. Multiple cartilaginous exostoses
*3. Nail-patella S. (osteo-onychodysplasia)
+*4. Noonan S.
*5. Otopalatodigital S.
+6. Turner S.

**UNCOMMON**

1. Acromesomelic dysplasia
2. Aminopterin fetopathy
*3. Bird-headed dwarfism (Seckel S.)
*4. Campomelic dysplasia
5. Cerebro-costo-mandibular S.
+6. Cerebrohepatorenal S. (Zellweger S.)
7. Chondroectodermal dysplasia (Ellis-van Creveld S.)
8. Chromosomal abnormalities (18p-S., 20p S.)
9. Cleidocranial dysplasia
10. Cloverleaf skull
*11. Coffin-Siris S.
*12. Cornelia de Lange S.
*13. Craniofacial dysostosis (Crouzon S.)
14. Cutis laxa
15. Diastrophic dysplasia
+*16. Dyschondrosteosis
17. Enchondromatosis (Ollier's disease)
*18. Familial idiopathic acro-osteolysis
*19. Fanconi S. (pancytopenia-dysmelia S.)
20. Frontometaphyseal dysplasia
21. Holt-Oram S.

22. Idiopathic; isolated anomaly
*23. Klinefelter S. (XXY S.)
*24. Mesomelic dysplasia (Nievergelt type)
25. Metaphyseal dysplasia (Pyle's disease)
*26. Mietens-Weber S.
27. Multiple synostosis S.
28. Neurofibromatosis
29. Oculo-dento-osseous S.
+30. Pleonosteosis (Léri)
*31. Spondylo-epi-metaphyseal dysplasia with joint laxity
32. Thrombocytopenia-absent radius (TAR) S.
33. Trisomy 8 S.
+34. Trisomy 22 S.
*35. XXXXY S.; XXXXX S.

* Proximal radioulnar dislocation.
+ Increased carrying angle (cubitus valgus).

*References:*

1. Greenfield GB: Radiology of Bone Diseases. (ed 5) Philadelphia: Lippincott, 1990
2. Jones KL: Smith's Recognizable Patterns of Human Malformation. Philadelphia: W.B. Saunders, 1988
3. Kozlowski K, Beighton P: Gamut Index of Skeletal Dysplasias. Berlin: Springer-Verlag, 1984, p 66
4. Taybi H, Lachman RS: Radiology of Syndromes, Metabolic Disorders, and Skeletal Dysplasias. (ed 3) Chicago: Year Book Medical Publ, 1990, p 870

## Gamut B-169

# DISPLACED ELBOW FAT PAD

**COMMON**
1. Infection, synovitis
2. Rheumatoid arthritis
3. Trauma with hemorrhage

**UNCOMMON**

1. Gout
2. Hemophilia
3. Leukemia
4. Metastasis
5. Neuropathic joint
6. Osteoarthritis
7. Osteochondritis dissecans
8. Osteoid osteoma
9. Pseudogout (CPPD crystal deposition disease)
10. Synovial osteochondromatosis
11. Synovial sarcoma
12. Villonodular synovitis

*Reference:*

1. Murphy WA, Siegel MJ: Elbow fat pads with new signs and extended differential diagnosis. Radiology 1977;124:659-665

## Gamut B-170

# GROOVED DEFECT, EROSION, OR DEFORMITY OF THE HUMERAL HEAD

**COMMON**

*1. Arthritis (esp. rheumatoid, ankylosing spondylitis, gout, infectious)
*2. Avascular necrosis (esp. steroid therapy, sicklemia)
*3. Chronic dislocation (Hill-Sachs defect)
*4. Fracture (esp. of greater tuberosity)

**UNCOMMON**

*1. Arteriovenous fistula, traumatic
*2. Glenohumeral dysplasia
*3. Hemophilia
4. [Humerus varus]
*5. Multicentric reticulohistiocytosis (lipoid dermatoarthritis)

---

*6. Periarthrosis humeroscapularis
*7. Pigmented villonodular synovitis
 8. Rickets
*9. Rotator cuff tear with atrophy and upward
    subluxation
10. Syringomyelia (neurotrophic joint)
*11. Tuberculosis

\* Grooved defect or erosion of humeral head.

### References:
1. Hill HA, Sachs MD: The grooved defect of the humeral head.
   Radiology 1940;35:690-700
2. Burgener FA, Kormano M: Differential Diagnosis in Conventional Radiology. (ed 2) New York: Thieme Medical Publ,
   1991, p 252

## Gamut B-171

# CONGENITAL SYNDROMES WITH ABNORMAL SCAPULA (USUALLY HYPOPLASIA)

### COMMON
1. Cleidocranial dysplasia
2. Isolated anomaly
3. Mucopolysaccharidoses (eg, Hurler S., Maroteaux-Lamy S.)
4. Nail-patella S. (osteo-onychodysplasia)
5. Sprengel's deformity; Klippel-Feil S.

### UNCOMMON
1. Achondrogenesis
2. Achondroplasia (flat inferior angle)
3. Basal cell nevus S. (Gorlin S.)
4. Campomelic dysplasia
5. CHILD S. (ichthyosis-limb reduction S.)

6. Dyggve-Melchior-Clausen S.
7. Dyssegmental dyslasia
8. Fetal varicella S.
9. Hallermann-Streiff S.
10. Holt-Oram S.
11. Kinky-hair S. (Menkes S.)
12. LEOPARD S. (lentiginosis S.)
13. Mucolipidosis II; fucosidosis
14. Poland S.
15. Proteus S.
16. Scapuloiliac dysostosis (Kosenow-Sinios)
17. Short rib-polydactyly S.
18. Thanatophoric dysplasia
19. Thrombocytopenia-absent radius S. (TAR S.)

*References:*

1. Kozlowski K, Beighton P: Gamut Index of Skeletal Dysplasias. Berlin: Springer-Verlag, 1984, p 54
2. Taybi H, Lachman RS: Radiology of Syndromes, Metabolic Disorders, and Skeletal Dysplasias. (ed 3) Chicago: Year Book Medical Publ, 1990, p 883

---

## Gamut B-172

# LESION OF THE SCAPULA IN AN INFANT OR CHILD

**COMMON**

*1. Benign bone tumor (esp. osteochondroma; also enchondroma, hemangioma, lymphangioma, aneurysmal bone cyst)
2. Fracture

**UNCOMMON**

1. Arthritis involving glenohumeral joint (incl. neurotrophic due to syringomyelia)

---

2. Bone cyst
3. Brachial plexus injury (winged scapula)
4. Congenital syndromes with hypoplasia (See B-171)
5. Erb's paralysis
*6. Fibrous dysplasia
*7. Histiocytosis $X_g$
*8. Infantile cortical hyperostosis (Caffey's disease)
9. Leukemia, lymphoma$_g$
*10. Metastasis
*11. Osteomyelitis
*12. Sarcoma (esp. Ewing's)
13. Sprengel's deformity

\* May cause enlargement or expansion of scapula.

### Reference:
1. Swischuk LE: Differential Diagnosis in Pediatric Radiology. Baltimore: Williams & Wilkins, 1984, pp 269-270

---

## Gamut B-173

# LESION OF THE CLAVICLE IN AN INFANT OR CHILD

### COMMON
1. Osteomyelitis
2. Trauma (fracture, dislocation, battered child S.)

### UNCOMMON
1. Achondroplasia
2. Benign bone neoplasm
3. Congenital hypoplasia or absence (eg, cleidocranial dysplasia, pyknodysostosis) (See B-174)
4. Endosteal hyperostosis (van Buchem, Worth)
5. Fibrous dysplasia; other fibrocystic lesion
6. Handlebar (hypoplastic, squat) clavicle (See B-174A)

---

B. Bone                                                    237

7. Histiocytosis $X_g$
8. Hyperparathyroidism (esp. secondary)
9. Infantile cortical hyperostosis (Caffey's disease)
10. Leukemia, lymphoma$_g$
11. Malignant bone neoplasm (esp. osteosarcoma, Ewing's sarcoma)
12. Metaphyseal dysplasia (Pyle's disease)
13. Metastasis
14. Mucopolysaccharidoses (eg, Hurler S.)
15. Oculo-dento-osseous dysplasia (expansion of clavicles)
16. Osteodysplasty (Melnick-Needles S.)
17. Osteogenesis imperfecta
18. Osteopetrosis
19. Progeria
20. Pseudarthrosis, congenital or traumatic
21. Rheumatoid arthritis, juvenile
22. Syphilis
23. Tuberculosis

---

**Gamut B-174**

## APLASTIC, HYPOPLASTIC, OR THIN CLAVICLE

**COMMON**

1. Cleidocranial dysplasia
2. Holt-Oram S.
3. Osteodysplasty (Melnick-Needles S.)
*4. Progeria (thin clavicle)
5. Pyknodysostosis

**UNCOMMON**

1. Birth trauma to brachial plexus (unilateral)
2. CHILD S.
*3. Cockayne S. (thin clavicle)

---

4. Coffin-Siris S.
5. Congenital clavicular pseudarthrosis
6. Focal dermal hypoplasia (Goltz S.)
7. Fucosidosis
*8. Larsen S. (thin clavicle)
9. Scapuloiliac dysostosis
10. Spondyloepiphyseal dysplasia (delayed ossification)
*11. Trisomy 13 S. (thin clavicle)
*12. Trisomy 18 S. (thin clavicle)
*13. Turner S. (thin clavicle laterally)

* Thin or slender clavicle.

*References:*
1. Jones KL; Smith's Recognizable Patterns of Human Malformation. Philadelphia: W.B. Saunders, 1988
2. Kozlowski K, Beighton P: Gamut Index of Skeletal Dysplasias. Berlin: Springer-Verlag, 1984, pp 53-54
3. Taybi H, Lachman RS: Radiology of Syndromes, Metabolic Disorders, and Skeletal Dysplasias. (ed 3) Chicago: Year Book Medical Publ, 1990, p 881

## Subgamut B-174A

## HANDLEBAR (HYPOPLASTIC, SQUAT) CLAVICLE

1. Asphyxiating thoracic dysplasia (Jeune S.)
2. Diastrophic dysplasia
3. Holt-Oram S.
4. Hurler S. (short, thick clavicle)
5. [Normal variant (improper positioning of chest)]
6. Thrombocytopenia-absent radius (TAR) S.
7. Trisomy 18 S.

*Reference:*
1. Swischuk LE: Differential Diagnosis in Pediatric Radiology. Baltimore: Williams & Wilkins, 1984, p 266

# BROAD, THICKENED, OR ENLARGED CLAVICLE
## (See Gamut B-176)

## COMMON

1. Neoplasm, benign (eg, cartilaginous tumor, osteoma) or malignant (eg, osteosarcoma, Ewing's sarcoma, metastasis, myeloma)
2. [Normal variant or improper positioning of chest, esp. in a child]
3. Osteomyelitis, chronic productive (incl. salmonella, syphilis)
4. Paget's disease
5. Posttraumatic (healed fracture with callus)

## UNCOMMON

1. Copper deficiency (Menkes S.)
2. Distal osteosclerosis
3. Endosteal hyperostosis (van Buchem, Worth)
4. Fibrous dysplasia
5. Histiocytosis $X_g$ (esp. healed)
6. Holt-Oram S.
7. Hyperphosphatasia
8. Infantile cortical hyperostosis (Caffey's disease)
9. Lymphoma$_g$
10. Metaphyseal dysplasia (Pyle's disease)
11. Mucolipidoses; fucosidosis
12. Mucopolysaccharidoses (esp. Hurler S.)
13. Oculo-dento-osseous dysplasia
14. Osteodysplasty (Melnick-Needles S.)
15. Winchester S.

*Reference:*

1. Taybi H, Lachman RS: Radiology of Syndromes, Metabolic Disorders, and Skeletal Dysplasias. (ed 3) Chicago: Year Book Medical Publ, 1990, p 881

## Gamut B-176

# SCLEROSIS AND/OR PERIOSTEAL REACTION INVOLVING THE CLAVICLE

**COMMON**

*1. Arthritis of sternoclavicular or acromioclavicular joint (eg, osteoarthritis, septic arthritis)
 2. Bone sarcoma (eg, osteosarcoma, Ewing's)
 3. Fracture with callus
 4. Metastasis (esp. osteoblastic)
 5. Osteomyelitis (incl. salmonella, syphilis, sclerosing osteomyelitis)
 6. Paget's disease

**UNCOMMON**

 *1. Avascular necrosis (Friedreich's disease)
 *2. Condensing osteitis of clavicle
  3. Endosteal hyperostosis (van Buchem, Worth)
  4. Histiocytosis $X_g$
  5. Hypertrophic osteoarthropathy
  6. Hypervitaminosis A
  7. Infantile cortical hyperostosis (Caffey's disease)
  8. Leukemia, lymphoma$_g$ (esp. Hodgkin's)
  9. Osteoid osteoma
 10. Osteoma
 *11. Sternocostoclavicular hyperostosis
 *12. Tietze S.

\* Involves sternal end of clavicle.

*Reference:*

 1. Appell RG, et al: Condensing osteitis of the clavicle in childhood: A rare sclerotic bone lesion. Pediatr Radiol 1983; 13:301-306

## Gamut B-177

# EROSION, DESTRUCTION, PENCILING, OR DEFECT OF THE OUTER END OF THE CLAVICLE

**COMMON**
*1. Hyperparathyroidism, primary or secondary
 2. Metastasis
 3. Myeloma
*4. Osteomyelitis (esp. pyogenic, tuberculous)
*5. Posttraumatic osteolysis (eg, weight lifter)
*6. Rheumatoid arthritis
 7. Rickets
 8. Surgical procedure

**UNCOMMON**
 1. Amyloidosis
 2. Congenital syndromes with hypoplasia of the clavicle (eg, cleidocranial dyplasia) (See B-174)
 3. Gout
 4. Histiocytosis $X_g$ (eosinophilic granuloma)
 5. Lymphoma$_g$ (esp. Hodgkin's disease)
 6. Multicentric reticulohistiocytosis (lipoid dermatoarthritis)
 7. Neurogenic osteolysis
 8. Primary bone neoplasm (eg, Ewing's sarcoma)
*9. Progeria
 10. Pyknodysostosis
 11. Reiter S.
 12. Sarcoidosis
*13. Scleroderma

* Penciled or pointed distal end of clavicle.

*References:*
 1. Greenfield GB: Radiology of Bone Diseases. (ed 5) Philadelphia: Lippincott, 1990
 2. Greenway GD, Danzig LA, Resnick D, et al: The painful shoulder. Med Radiogr Photog 1982;58:22-67
 3. Jacobson HG, Siegelman SS: RSNA Refresher Course Syllabus

## Gamut B-178

## TIBIOTALAR TILT

## Congenital

1. Dysplasia epiphysealis hemimelica (Trevor's disease)
2. Endosteal hyperostosis (van Buchem)
3. Metaphyseal chondrodysplasia
4. Multiple epiphyseal dysplasia (Fairbank)
5. Nail-patella S. (osteo-onychodysplasia)
6. Spondyloepiphyseal dysplasia

## Developmental

**COMMON**
1. Fibrous dysplasia
2. Neurofibromatosis

**UNCOMMON**
1. Enchondromatosis (Ollier's disease)
2. Multiple cartilaginous exostoses

## Acquired

**COMMON**
1. Blount's disease
2. Fracture (eg, Salter III or IV fracture of distal tibia; fractured femur with abnormal stress)
3. [Pseudotibiotalar tilt (flexing knee and externally rotating foot during radiography)]
4. Rheumatoid arthritis (esp. juvenile)

**UNCOMMON**
1. Avascular necrosis (eg, with chronic renal failure)
2. Bleeding disorder$_g$ with chronic hemarthrosis (esp. hemophilia, leukemia)

3. Cretinism, adult
4. Femoral bowing
5. Hypoparathyroidism
6. Hypophosphatasia
7. Osteomyelitis of tibia, chronic (incl. syphilis, yaws, tropical ulcer)
8. Poliomyelitis
9. Rickets
10. Sickle cell disease

*Reference:*
1. Griffiths H, Wandtke J: Tibiotalar tilt - A new slant. Skeletal Radiol 1981;6:193-197

## **Gamut B-179**

## **ISOLATED TIBIAL BOWING**

### **COMMON**
1. Blount's disease (tibia vara)
2. Osteomyelitis (esp. syphilis-saber shin; yaws-boomerang tibia; tropical ulcer)
3. Paget's disease
4. Physiological (idiopathic) anterior or posterior tibial bowing
5. Trauma (eg, epiphyseal injury, malunited fracture)

### **UNCOMMON**
1. Absence or hypoplasia of fibula (See B-181)
2. Elongation of fibula (See B-180)
3. Fibrous dysplasia
4. Klippel-Trenaunay-Weber S. or limb hypertrophy (See B-14)
5. Neurofibromatosis (usually lateral bowing)
6. Rickets

*Reference:*

1. Kozlowski K, Beighton P: Gamut Index of Skeletal Dysplasias. Berlin: Springer-Verlag, 1984, p 67

## Gamut B-180

# ELONGATION OF FIBULA

1. Achondroplasia
2. Hypochondroplasia
3. Mesomelic dysplasia
4. Metaphyseal chondrodysplasia (McKusick)
5. Muscular disorder$_g$
6. Pseudoachondroplasia
7. Spondylo-epi-metaphyseal dysplasia

*Reference:*

1. Kozlowski K, Beighton P: Gamut Index of Skeletal Dysplasias. Berlin: Springer-Verlag, 1984, p 67

## Gamut B-181

# HYPOPLASIA OF FIBULA[*]

1. Bird-headed dwarfism (Seckel S.)
2. Campomelic dysplasia
3. Chondroectodermal dysplasia (Ellis-van Creveld S.)
4. Chromosomal abnormalities
5. de la Chapelle dysplasia

[*] Usually seen with tibial hypoplasia, but predominant fibular changes may be seen in above dysplasias. There are at least eight other rare syndromes listed in Taybi's text.

*References:*
1. Kozlowski K, Beighton P: Gamut Index of Skeletal Dysplasias. Berlin: Springer-Verlag, 1984, p 68
2. Taybi H, Lachman RS: Radiology of Syndromes, Metabolic Disorders, and Skeletal Dysplasias. (ed 3) Chicago: Year Book Medical Publ, 1990, p 872

## Gamut B-182

# CONGENITAL SYNDROMES WITH ABSENT, HYPOPLASTIC, DYSPLASTIC, BIPARTITE, OR DISLOCATED PATELLA

**COMMON**

1. Nail-patella S. (osteo-onychodysplasia) (absent or hypoplastic)

**UNCOMMON**

1. Acrocephalopolysyndactyly (Carpenter S.) (dislocated)
2. Arthrogryposis
3. Cerebrohepatorenal S. (calcific flecks in patella)
4. Diastrophic dysplasia (dislocated, hypoplastic, or multipartite)
5. Familial absence of patella; Seckel's bird-headed dwarfism (absent)
6. Kuskokwim S. (hypoplastic)
7. Mesomelic dysplasia (Werner type)
8. Multiple epiphyseal dysplasia (dislocated or bipartite)
9. Neurofibromatosis (absent)
10. Popliteal pterygium S. (absent or bipartite)
11. Rubinstein-Taybi S. (dislocated)
12. Spondylo-epi-metaphyseal dysplasia
13. Spondyloepiphyseal dysplasia

14. Stickler S. (arthro-ophthalmopathy) (dislocated)
15. Trisomy 8 S.

*References:*
1. Jones KL: Smith's Recognizable Patterns of Human Malformation. Philadelphia: W.B. Saunders, 1988
2. Kozlowski K, Beighton P: Gamut Index of Skeletal Dysplasias. Berlin: Springer-Verlag, 1984, p 67
3. Taybi H, Lachman RS: Radiology of Syndromes, Metabolic Disorders, and Skeletal Dysplasias. (ed 3) Chicago: Year Book Medical Publ, 1990, pp 874-875

## Gamut B-183

# ABNORMAL POSITION OF THE PATELLA (PATELLA ALTA OR BAJA)

### PATELLA ALTA (HIGH PATELLA)
1. Chondromalacia of patella
2. Neuromuscular disorders$_g$ (eg, poliomyelitis, cerebral palsy)
3. Osgood-Schlatter's disease
4. Osteomyelitis of femur; arthritis with joint effusion
5. Rupture of patellar ligament
6. Sinding-Larsen disease (avascular necrosis of inferior ossification center of patella)
7. Subluxation, recurrent

### PATELLA BAJA OR PROFUNDA (LOW PATELLA)
1. Achondroplasia; other bone dysplasias
2. Paresis of quadriceps muscle (eg, poliomyelitis)
3. Rheumatoid arthritis, juvenile
4. Rupture of quadriceps tendon
5. Surgical transposition of tibial tuberosity

*Reference:*
1. Burgener FA, Kormano M: Differential Diagnosis in Conventional Radiology. New York: Thieme Medical Publ, 1991, pp 229-230

## Gamut B-184

# LYTIC PATELLAR LESION

## COMMON

1. Chondroblastoma
2. Chondromalacia
3. Cystic osteomyelitis; Brodie's abscess; tuberculosis
4. Enchondroma
5. Giant cell tumor

## UNCOMMON

1. Aneurysmal bone cyst
2. Bone cyst
3. Brown tumor of hyperparathyroidism
4. Dorsal defect of patella ´
5. Gout
6. Hemangioma
7. Histiocytosis $X_g$
8. Metastasis
9. Myeloma
10. Osteoblastoma
11. Osteochondritis dissecans

*Reference:*
1. Goergen TG, Resnick D, Greenway G, et al: Dorsal defect of the patella (DDP): A characteristic radiographic lesion. Radiology 1979;130:333-336

## Gamut B-185

# ENLARGEMENT OF THE DISTAL FEMORAL INTERCONDYLAR NOTCH

**COMMON**
1. Hemophilia

**UNCOMMON**
1. Juvenile chronic arthritis
2. Psoriatic arthritis
3. Rheumatoid arthritis (esp. juvenile)
4. Tuberculous arthritis

## Gamut B-186

# ENLARGED MEDIAL FEMORAL CONDYLE

1. Blount's disease (tibia vara)
2. Chondrodystrophies
3. Cornelia de Lange S.
4. Dyschondrosteosis
5. Posttraumatic
6. Prader-Willi S.
7. Turner S.
8. Vitamin D-resistant rickets

*Reference:*

1. Swischuk LE: Differential Diagnosis in Pediatric Radiology. Baltimore: Williams & Wilkins, 1984, p 218

## Gamut B-187

# BRIGHT INTRAMEDULLARY SIGNAL ON T2-WEIGHTED IMAGE OF THE KNEE WITH INTACT CORTEX

1. Bone bruise (contusion, trabecular fracture)
2. Leukemia
3. Lymphoma
4. Metastasis
5. Osteosarcoma
6. Regrowth of hematopoietic marrow

*Reference:*
1. Crues JV, et al: Chapter 63, In: Stark DD, Bradley WG (eds): Magnetic Resonance Imaging. (ed 2) St. Louis: CV Mosby, 1992

## Gamut B-188

# HIGH INTRAMEDULLARY SIGNAL ON T2-WEIGHTED IMAGE OF THE KNEE WITH DISRUPTED CORTEX

1. Osteochondritis dessicans (chronic recurrent trauma)
2. Posttraumatic osteonecrosis
3. Spontaneous osteonecrosis
4. Type II bone contusion

*Reference:*
1. Crues JV, et al: Chapter 63, In: Stark DD, Bradley WG (eds): Magnetic Resonance Imaging. (ed 2) St. Louis: CV Mosby, 1992

## Gamut B-189

# GENU VARUM (BOW LEGS)

**COMMON**
1. Idiopathic; physiologic prenatal bowing; tibial torsion in infants
*2. Osteoarthritis, primary or secondary (may be associated with medial displacement of femur–genu laxum)
3. Rickets, all causes
*4. Tibia vara (Blount's disease)
*5. Trauma (fracture of medial condyle of femur or tibia)

**UNCOMMON**
1. Achondroplasia, pseudoachondroplasia
2. Campomelic dysplasia
*3. Dysplasia epiphysealis hemimelica (Trevor's disease)
*4. Epiphyseal-metaphyseal injury (trauma, infection, radiation, hypervitaminosis A)
5. Femoral anteversion
6. Hyperparathyroidism
7. Hyperphosphatasia
8. Hypochondroplasia
*9. Localized neoplasm (eg, osteochondroma, juxta-articular chondroma of lateral aspect of knee)
10. Metaphyseal chondrodysplasia (esp. Schmid type)
11. Spondylo-epi-metaphyseal dysplasia
12. Spondyloepiphyseal dysplasia congenita
13. Thanatophoric dysplasia
14. Turner S.

* Usually or always unilateral.

*References:*
1. Burgener FA, Kormano M: Differential Diagnosis in Conventional Radiology. (ed 2) New York: Thieme Medical Publ, 1991, p 262

2. Kozlowski K, Beighton P: Gamut Index of Skeletal Dysplasias. Berlin: Springer-Verlag, 1984, p 66
3. Silverman FN (ed): Caffey's Pediatric X-ray Diagnosis. (ed 8) Chicago: Year Book Medical Publ, 1985, vol 1, pp 812-813
4. Swischuk LE: Differential Diagnosis in Pediatric Radiology. Baltimore: Williams & Wilkins, 1984, pp 180-182
5. Taybi H, Lachman RS: Radiology of Syndromes, Metabolic Disorders, and Skeletal Dysplasias. (ed 3) Chicago: Year Book Medical Publ, 1990, p 872

## Gamut B-190

## GENU VALGUM (KNOCK-KNEES)

### COMMON
*1. Arthritis (eg, juvenile rheumatoid arthritis; secondary osteoarthritis involving lateral compartment of knee, such as rupture of lateral meniscus or severe rheumatoid arthritis)
2. Flatfeet
3. Physiologic
4. Regional muscular weakness from neurologic or neuromuscular disease$_g$

### UNCOMMON
1. Achondroplasia
2. Acrocephalopolysyndactyly (Carpenter S.)
3. Chondroectodermal dysplasia (Ellis-van Creveld S.)
4. Dyschondrosteosis
*5. Dysplasia epiphysealis hemimelica (Trevor's disease)
6. Engelmann's disease (diaphyseal dysplasia)
*7. Epiphyseal-metaphyseal injury (trauma, infection, radiation)
8. Hajdu-Cheney S. (osteolysis)
9. Hypophosphatasia

B. Bone

*10. Localized neoplasm (eg, osteochondroma,
      juxta-articular chondroma of medial aspect of knee)
11. Metaphyseal chondrodysplasia
12. Metaphyseal dysplasia (Pyle's disease)
13. Mucopolysaccharidoses (eg, Hurler, Morquio)
14. Multiple epiphyseal dysplasia (Fairbank)
15. Nail-patella S. (osteo-onychodysplasia)
16. Parastremmatic dwarfism
17. Rickets (with hypotonia)
18. Spondyloepiphyseal dysplasia

* Usually or always unilateral.

### References:

1. Swischuk LE: Differential Diagnosis in Pediatric Radiology.
   Baltimore: Williams & Wilkins, 1984, pp 180-182
2. Taybi H, Lachman RS: Radiology of Syndromes, Metabolic
   Disorders, and Skeletal Dysplasias. (ed 3) Chicago: Year
   Book Medical Publ, 1990, p 872

### Gamut B-191

## COXA VARA (UNILATERAL OR BILATERAL)

### COMMON
1. Avascular necrosis of femoral head (eg, steroid therapy, sickle cell anemia, collagen disease$_g$, Gaucher's
   disease, radiation) (See B-51)
2. Idiopathic (primary) coxa vara of childhood
3. Legg-Perthes disease (late)
4. Malunited fracture of femoral neck (incl.
   epiphyseal-metaphyseal fracture; battered child S.)
5. Paget's disease
6. Rickets; osteomalacia
7. Slipped capital femoral epiphysis (late) (See B-194)

## UNCOMMON

1. Congenital syndromes (See B-191A)
2. Femoral neck lesion, other (eg, osteomyelitis)
3. Fibrous dysplasia
4. Hyperparathyroidism (esp. secondary–renal osteodystrophy)
5. Hypothyroidism (slipped epiphysis)
6. Rheumatoid arthritis

*Reference:*
1. Swischuk LE: Differential Diagnosis in Pediatric Radiology. Baltimore: Williams & Wilkins, 1984, pp 183-186

### Subgamut B-191A

## CONGENITAL SYNDROMES WITH COXA VARA

### COMMON

1. Achondroplasia
2. Fibrous dysplasia
3. Multiple epiphyseal dysplasia (Fairbank)
4. Osteogenesis imperfecta
5. Spondyloepiphyseal dysplasia (congenita or tarda)

### UNCOMMON

1. Arthrogryposis
2. Cleidocranial dysplasia
3. Congenital coxa vara (femoral neck defect; hypoplasia of proximal femur)
4. Cretinism, hypothyroidism
5. Diastrophic dysplasia
6. Dyggve-Melchior-Clausen S.; Smith-McCort S.
7. Enchondromatosis (Ollier's disease)
8. Femoral-facial S.
9. Frontometaphyseal dysplasia
10. Hyperphosphatasia

11. Hypophosphatasia
12. Kniest dysplasia
13. Metaphyseal chondrodysplasia (Schmid)
14. Metatropic dysplasia
15. Meyer dysplasia of femoral head
16. Morquio S.
17. Osteodysplasty (Melnick-Needles S.)
18. Osteopetrosis
19. Pseudoachondroplasia
20. Pseudohypoparathyroidism,
    pseudopseudohypoparathyroidism
21. Schwartz-Jampel S.
22. Shwachman S.
23. Spondylo-epi-metaphyseal dysplasia
24. Spondylometaphyseal dysplasia (Kozlowski)

*References:*
1. Kozlowski K, Beighton P: Gamut Index of Skeletal Dysplasias. Berlin: Springer-Verlag, 1984, pp 58-59
2. Swischuk LE: Differential Diagnosis in Pediatric Radiology. Baltimore: Williams & Wilkins, 1984, pp 183-186
3. Taybi H, Lachman RS: Radiology of Syndromes, Metabolic Disorders, and Skeletal Dysplasias (ed 3) Chicago: Year Book Medical Publ, 1990, pp 869-870

## Gamut B-192

## COXA VALGA

**COMMON**
1. Chronic leg injury
2. Congenital dislocation of hip (untreated)
3. Paralytic disorder, neuromuscular disorder$_g$, chronic muscle hypotonia (eg, meningomyelocele, cerebral palsy, muscular dystrophy, poliomyelitis)
4. Rheumatoid arthritis (incl. juvenile)

**UNCOMMON**
1. Acrocephalopolysyndactyly (Carpenter S.)
2. Arthrogryposis
3. Cleidocranial dysplasia
4. Coffin-Lowry S.
5. Dyschondrosteosis
6. Dysplasia epiphysealis hemimelica (Trevor's disease)
7. Frontometaphyseal dysplasia
8. Hypoplasia or agenesis of sacrum; caudal regression S.
9. Metaphyseal dysplasia (Pyle's disease)
10. Mucopolysaccharidoses (eg, Hurler, Hunter, Morquio); fucosidosis; mannosidosis
11. Osteodysplasty (Melnick-Needles S.)
12. Otopalatodigital S.
13. Prader-Willi S.
14. Progeria
15. Pseudohypoparathyroidism
16. Pyknodysostosis
17. Schwartz-Jampel S.
18. Stickler S.(arthro-ophthalmopathy)
19. Turner S. (gonadal dysgenesis)
20. XXXXY S.

*References:*
1. Swischuk LE: Differential Diagnosis in Pediatric Radiology. Baltimore: Williams & Wilkins, 1984, pp 183-186
2. Taybi H, Lachman RS: Radiology of Syndromes, Metabolic Disorders, and Skeletal Dysplasias. (ed 3) Chicago: Year Book Medical Publ, 1990, p 869

B. Bone

# FRAGMENTED OR IRREGULAR FEMORAL HEAD

## COMMON

1. Arthritis, advanced (eg, rheumatoid, purulent, degenerative, posttraumatic, gouty, neurotrophic)
2. Avascular necrosis, all causes (See B-51)
3. Congenital dislocation of the hip, after treatment
4. Legg-Perthes disease (osteochondrosis of femoral epiphysis)
5. Occlusive vascular disease; thromboembolic disease
6. Sickle cell anemia
7. Steroid therapy, Cushing S.
8. Traumatic dislocation; fracture of femoral neck; surgical or manipulative trauma

## UNCOMMON

1. Achondroplasia
2. Adrenogenital S.
3. Chondrodysplasia punctata (Conradi's disease)
4. Cretinism, hypothyroidism
5. Diabetes
6. Diastrophic dysplasia
7. Dysplasia epiphysealis hemimelica (Trevor's disease)
8. Elsbach dysplasia (bilateral hereditary microepiphyseal dysplasia)
9. Enchondromatosis (Ollier's disease)
10. Gaucher's disease
11. Hemophilia, Christmas disease
12. Hereditary arthro-ophthalmopathy (Stickler S.)
13. Infection
14. Leukemia
15. Meyer dysplasia of femoral head
16. Mucopolysaccharidoses (esp. Hurler, Hunter, Morquio); pseudo-Hurler polydystrophy
17. Multiple epiphyseal dysplasia (Fairbank)

18. Osteochondritis dissecans
19. Osteochondromuscular dystrophy (Schwartz-Jampel S.)
20. Pancreatitis, acute or chronic; alcoholism
21. Renal osteodystrophy; postrenal transplantation
22. Rickets, all types
23. Sarcoidosis
24. Slipped capital femoral epiphysis (late)
25. Spondyloepiphyseal dysplasia
26. Tricho-rhino-phalangeal dysplasia
27. Winchester S.

*References:*
1. Greenfield GB: Radiology of Bone Diseases. (ed 5) Philadelphia: Lippincott, 1990
2. Kozlowski K, Beighton P: Gamut Index of Skeletal Dysplasias. Berlin: Springer-Verlag, 1984, pp 57-58
3. Swischuk LE: Differential Diagnosis in Pediatric Radiology. Baltimore: Williams & Wilkins, 1984, pp 212-214

## Subgamut B-193A

## FEMORAL HEAD DYSPLASIA

1. Elsbach dysplasia (bilateral hereditary microepiphyseal dysplasia)
2. Legg-Perthes disease
3. Meyer dysplasia
4. Multiple epiphyseal dysplasia (Fairbank)
5. Subchondral dysplasia (osteochondritis dissecans)

## Gamut B-194

# SLIPPED CAPITAL FEMORAL EPIPHYSIS

**COMMON**
1. Idiopathic (age 9-17)
2. Renal osteodystrophy
3. Trauma

**UNCOMMON**
1. Congenital coxa vara
2. Gaucher's disease
3. Gigantism (hyperpituitarism); rapid growth spurt; growth hormone therapy; pituitary tumor
4. Hemophilia
5. Hyperparathyroidism
6. Hypothyroidism
7. Metaphyseal chondrodysplasia
8. Obesity; mechanical stress
9. Pseudohypoparathyroidism, pseudopseudohypoparathyroidism
10. Radiation therapy
11. Rickets; poor nutrition
12. Scurvy
13. Steroid therapy; Cushing S.
14. Syphilis
15. Trisomy 21 S. (Down's S.)

*References:*
1. Greenfield GB: Radiology of Bone Diseases. (ed 5) Philadelphia: Lippincott, 1990
2. Steinbach HL, Young DA: The roentgen appearance of pseudohypoparathyroidism (PH) and pseudo-pseudohypoparathyroidism (PPH). AJR 1966;97:49-66
3. Taybi H, Lachman RS: Radiology of Syndromes, Metabolic Disorders, and Skeletal Dysplasias. (ed 3) Chicago: Year Book Medical Publ, 1990, pp 871-872

## Gamut B-195

# LOCAL COMPLICATIONS OF TOTAL HIP REPLACEMENT

**COMMON**
1. Aseptic loosening; subsidence
2. Dislocation
3. Hematoma
4. Heterotopic bone formation (myositis ossificans)
5. Phlebitis

**UNCOMMON**
1. Foreign body (granulomatous) reaction; excessive granulation tissue
2. Fracture of femur or pelvis
3. Fracture of prosthesis or cement
4. Greater trochanteric bursitis or separation; nonunion of osteotomy
5. Infection
6. Lucent line (fibrous tissue-not loosening)
7. Malpositioning of prosthesis; ectopic placement of cement
8. Osteolysis, local
9. Protrusion of either femoral or acetabular components
10. Vascular or neurologic impairment secondary to surgical complications or migration of prosthesis or cement

*References:*
1. Errico TJ, Fetto JF, Waugh TR: Heterotopic ossification: Incidence and relation to trochanteric osteotomy in 100 total hip arthroplasties. Clin Orthop 1984;190:138-141
2. Gaskill MF: Local complications of total hip replacements. Semin Roentgenol 1986;21:3-4
3. Heist KP: Complications of total hip replacement. J Am Osteopath Assoc 1981;80:356-365

# RADIOGRAPHIC FINDINGS SUGGESTING LOOSENING AND/OR INFECTION OF TOTAL HIP PROSTHESES

## PLAIN FILM FINDINGS

1. Bone destruction
2. Cement-bone lucency widening of 2 mm or more
3. Development or widening of metal-cement lucency
4. Migration of prosthetic components
5. Motion of components demonstrable on stress views or fluoroscopy

## ARTHROGRAPHIC FINDINGS

1. Extension of contrast material between cement and bone or between prosthesis and bone
2. Filling of irregular para-articular cavities or fistulous tracts indicating infection

## SCINTIGRAPHIC FINDINGS

1. Diffuse uptake, especially around both components, suggests infection
2. Focal uptake around femoral component (seen in septic or aseptic loosening)
3. Increased activity in acetabular and/or femoral shaft regions after 6 to 10 months postoperatively
4. Increased gallium uptake in comparison to bone agent uptake suggests infection, but is insensitive

*Reference:*

1. Weissman BN: Total joint replacement: Fixation of prosthetic components. Syllabus for the Categorical Course on Diagnostic Techniques in the Musculoskeletal System. American College of Radiology, 1986, pp 119-131

## Gamut B-196

# PROTRUSIO ACETABULI, UNILATERAL OR BILATERAL

## COMMON

1. Degenerative joint disease, primary (osteoarthritis) or secondary (incl. hemophilia, hemochromatosis)
2. Normal variant (children age 4-12)
3. Osteomalacia, rickets
4. Paget's disease
5. Primary or idiopathic (Otto pelvis) (eg, coxa vara with retroversion of femoral neck)
6. Renal osteodystrophy
7. Rheumatoid arthritis (incl. juvenile)
8. Trauma (acetabular fracture with medial dislocation of hip)

## UNCOMMON

1. Arthritis, other (eg, ankylosing spondylitis, juvenile chronic arthritis, gout, psoriatic)
2. Fibrous dysplasia
3. Hydatid disease
4. Hyperparathyroidism
5. Hyperphosphatasia
6. Infectious arthritis (eg, pyogenic, tuberculous)
7. Marfan S.
8. Mucopolysaccharidoses (esp. Morquio S.)
9. Neoplasm involving acetabulum, primary or meta-static, with medial dislocation of hip
10. Ochronosis (alkaptonuria)
11. Osteogenesis imperfecta tarda
12. Osteoporosis
13. Postsurgical (eg, medial dislocation of femoral head prosthesis following total hip replacement)
14. Radiation therapy (esp. in a child)
15. Stickler S. (arthro-ophthalmopathy)
16. Turner S.

*References:*
1. Kuhlman JE et al: Acetabular protrusion in the Marfan syndrome. Radiology 1987;164:415-417
2. McEwen C, Poppel MH, Poker N, Jacobson HG: Protrusio acetabuli in rheumatoid arthritis. Radiology 1956;66:33-40
3. Murray RO, Jacobson HG, Stoker DJ: The Radiology of Skeletal Disorders. (ed 3) London: Churchill Livingstone, 1990
4. Taybi H, Lachman RS: Radiology of Syndromes, Metabolic Disorders, and Skeletal Dysplasias. (ed 3) Chicago: Year Book Medical Publ, 1990, p 879

## Gamut B-197

# CONGENITAL SYNDROMES WITH AN ABNORMAL PELVIS
## (See Gamuts B-198 to B-200)

**COMMON**
1. Achondroplasia (small trident pelvis, short sacroiliac notches)
2. Mucopolysaccharidoses (eg, Hurler, Morquio) (flared iliac wings, steep acetabular roofs, narrow pelvic inlet, coxa valga)
3. Trisomy 21 S. (Down S.) (hypoplastic, flared iliac wings, decreased acetabular and iliac angles, ischial tapering)

**UNCOMMON**
1. Achondrogenesis (sacral, pubic, ischial bones not ossified, flat acetabula)
2. Asphyxiating thoracic dysplasia (Jeune S.) (flared ilia, trident pelvis)
3. Campomelic dysplasia (narrow pelvis with poor ossification)
4. Caudal hypoplasia or aplasia (narrow pelvis with absence or hypoplasia of sacrum)
5. Chondrodysplasia punctata (Conradi's disease) (trapezoid ilium)

---

6. Chondroectodermal dysplasia (Ellis-van Creveld S.) (trident pelvis)
7. Cleidocranial dysplasia (wide pubic symphysis)
8. Cockayne S. (small square pelvis)
9. Diastrophic dysplasia (short thick iliac bones)
10. Hypochondroplasia (small pelvis)
11. Kniest dysplasia (trefoil-shaped pelvis, coxa vara)
12. Marfan S. (wide pelvic cavity, vertical ilia)
13. Metaphyseal chondrodysplasias (abnormal acetabula)
14. Metatropic dysplasia (small iliac height and sacro-sciatic notches)
15. Nail-patella S. (osteo-onychodysplasia) (iliac horns)
16. Osteodysplasty (Melnick-Needles S.) (narrow pelvis with flared iliac wings, flat acetabula and tapered ischia)
17. Osteogenesis imperfecta tarda (protrusio acetabuli)
18. Osteopetrosis (alternating bands of increased density)
19. Rubinstein-Taybi S. (flared ilia, small iliac index)
20. Spondyloepiphyseal dysplasia (squared ilia, delayed pubic and femoral head ossification)
21. Thanatophoric dysplasia (squared ilia with small sacrosciatic notches, trident pelvis)
22. Trisomy 18 S. (small "antimongoloid" pelvis with vertical ilia, steep acetabular angles)
23. Tuberous sclerosis (patchy sclerotic densities)

## Gamut B-198

# TYPES OF ABNORMAL PELVIC CONFIGURATION IN AN INFANT OR CHILD

## SHORT SACROILIAC NOTCHES

1. Achondroplasia
2. Metatropic dysplasia

3. Short rib-polydactyly S., type 1 (Saldino-Noonan)
4. Thanatophoric dysplasia

## CRENATED ILIAC CRESTS
1. Dyggve-Melchior-Clausen S.
2. Parastremmatic dwarfism
3. Smith-McCort S.

## RETARDED PELVIC OSSIFICATION
1. Achondrogenesis
2. Campomelic dysplasia
3. Cleidocranial dysplasia

## NARROW PELVIS
1. Campomelic dysplasia
2. Morquio S.
3. Osteodysplasty (Melnick-Needles S.)

## ILIAC HORNS
1. Nail-patella S. (osteo-onychodysplasia)

## DECREASED ACETABULAR ANGLE (See B-199)
1. Achondroplasia
2. Arthrogryposis
3. Hypothyroidism, cretinism
4. Trisomy 21 S. (Down S.)

## TRIDENT PELVIS (TRIRADIATE ACETABULUM)
1. Achondroplasia
2. Asphyxiating thoracic dysplasia (Jeune S.)
3. Chondroectodermal dysplasia (Ellis-van Creveld S.)
4. Thanatophoric dysplasia

*Reference:*
1. Kozlowski K, Beighton P: Gamut Index of Skeletal Dysplasias. Berlin: Springer-Verlag, 1984, pp 56-57

# CONGENITAL SYNDROMES WITH FLAT OR DECREASED ACETABULAR ANGLE

## TYPE A PELVIS (SMALL, SQUARE ILIAC WINGS AND IRREGULAR ACETABULAR ROOFS)

1. Achondrogenesis, types I and II
*2. Achondroplasia
3. Asphyxiating thoracic dysplasia (Jeune S.)
4. Caudal regression S.
5. Cephaloskeletal dysplasia (Taybi-Linder S.)
6. Chondrodysplasia punctata (rhizomelic form)
7. Chondroectodermal dysplasia (Ellis-van Creveld S.)
8. Dyggve-Melchior-Clausen S.
9. Dyssegmental dysplasia
10. Hypochondroplasia
11. Kniest dysplasia
12. Metaphyseal chondrodysplasias (advanced)
13. Metatropic dysplasia
14. Morquio S.
15. Short rib-polydactyly S. (Saldino-Noonan type)
16. Spondyloepiphyseal dysplasia congenita
17. Thanatophoric dysplasia

## TYPE B PELVIS (ILIAC WINGS OUTWARDLY FLARED AND LESS SQUARE)

1. Acrocephalopolysyndactyly (Carpenter S.)
2. Acrocephalosyndactyly (Waardenburg)
3. Aminopterin fetopathy
*4. Arthrogryposis
5. Bladder exstrophy
6. Cleidocranial dysplasia
7. Cockayne S.
8. Cornelia de Lange S.
9. Hypophosphatasia
*10. Hypothyroidism, cretinism

11. Metaphyseal chondrodysplasias (mild)
12. Mucopolysaccharidoses; mucolipidoses
13. Nail-patella S. (osteo-onychodysplasia)
14. Osteodysplasty (Melnick-Needles S.)
15. Osteogenesis imperfecta
16. Popliteal pterygium S.
17. Prune-belly S. (Eagle-Barrett S.)
18. Rubinstein-Taybi S.
19. Sacral agenesis
20. Trisomy 13 S.
*21. Trisomy 21 S. (Down S.)

\* Common.

*References:*
1. Swischuk LE: Differential Diagnosis in Pediatric Radiology. Baltimore: Williams & Wilkins, 1984, pp 272-273
2. Taybi H, Lachman RS: Radiology of Syndromes, Metabolic Disorders, and Skeletal Dysplasias. (ed 3) Chicago: Year Book Medical Publ, 1990, p 878

**Gamut B-200**

## CONGENITAL SYNDROMES WITH DELAYED OR DEFECTIVE PUBIC OSSIFICATION

**COMMON**
1. Chondrodystrophies (See B-1)
2. Cleidocranial dysplasia
3. Ehlers-Danlos S.
4. Prune-belly S. (Eagle-Barrett S.)
5. Spondyloepiphyseal dysplasia congenita

**UNCOMMON**
1. Achondrogenesis
2. Campomelic dysplasia

3. Chondrodysplasia punctata (Conradi's disease)
4. Chromosome 4p- S. (Wolf S.)
5. Cryptophthalmia S.
6. Dyggve-Melchior-Clausen S.
7. Focal dermal hypoplasia (Goltz S.)
8. Hypophosphatasia, severe
9. Larsen S.
10. Sjögren-Larsson S.
11. Taybi-Linder S.
12. Trisomy 9p+ S.

*References:*
1. Swischuk LE: Differential Diagnosis in Pediatric Radiology. Baltimore: Williams & Wilkins, 1984, pp 273-276
2. Taybi H, Lachman RS: Radiology of Syndromes, Metabolic Disorders, and Skeletal Dysplasias. (ed 3) Chicago: Year Book Medical Publ, 1990, p 879

## Gamut B-201

## WIDENING OF THE PUBIC SYMPHYSIS

**COMMON**
1. Osteitis pubis, early (after pelvic surgery, parturition)
2. Pregnancy
3. Traumatic dislocation

**UNCOMMON**
1. Ankylosing spondylitis; rheumatoid arthritis (early)
2. Congenital anorectal, genital, or urinary tract malformation; anal atresia; caudal regression S.
3. Congenital syndromes (esp. cleidocranial dysplasia) (See B-200)
4. Diastasis recti
5. Epispadias, hypospadias
6. Exstrophy of the bladder

7. Hyperparathyroidism
8. Hypothyroidism
9. Idiopathic
10. Malignant neoplasm, primary or metastatic, lymphoma$_g$, multiple myeloma
11. Osteomyelitis (eg, pyogenic, tuberculous)
12. Osteonecrosis pubis (chronic stress in young athletes)
13. Paraplegia with neurogenic bone resorption (incl. syringomyelia)
14. Pubic hypoplasia

*References:*
1. Muecke EC, Currarino G: Congenital widening of the pubic symphysis. AJR 1968;103:179-185
2. Swischuk LE: Differential Diagnosis in Pediatric Radiology. Baltimore: Williams & Wilkins, 1984, pp 273-276

## Gamut B-202

# BRIDGING OR FUSION OF THE PUBIC SYMPHYSIS

## COMMON

1. Ankylosing spondylitis (late)
2. Degenerative changes; osteoarthrosis
3. Idiopathic
4. Infection, healed (eg, tuberculous or pyogenic osteomyelitis)
5. Osteitis pubis, healed
6. Posttraumatic; postparturition
7. Rheumatoid arthritis (late)

## UNCOMMON

1. Fluorosis
2. Myositis ossificans (pseudomarsupial bones)

3. Ochronosis (alkaptonuria)
4. Postradiation therapy
5. Surgical fusion

*References:*

1. Forrester DM, Brown JC, Nesson JW: The Radiology of Joint Disease. (ed 3) Philadelphia: W.B. Saunders, 1987
2. Resnick D, Niwayama G: Diagnosis of Bone and Joint Disorders. (ed 2) Philadelphia: W.B. Saunders, 1988
3. Schwarz G, Schwarz GS: Noninfectious symphysial bridging and pseudomarsupial bones. AJR 1966;97:687-692

## Gamut B-203

# CONGENITAL SYNDROMES WITH ELEVEN PAIRS OF RIBS

## COMMON

1. [Normal variant]
2. Trisomy 21 S. (Down S.)

## UNCOMMON

1. Asphyxiating thoracic dyplasia (Jeune S.)
2. Atelosteogenesis
3. Campomelic dysplasia
4. Cleidocranial dysplasia
5. Short rib-polydactyly S.
6. Trisomy 18 S.

*Reference:*

1. Taybi H, Lachman RS: Radiology of Syndromes, Metabolic Disorders, and Skeletal Dysplasias. (ed 3) Chicago: Year Book Medical Publ, 1990, p 882

## Gamut B-204

# THIN, RIBBON-LIKE, OR TWISTED RIBS

**COMMON**
1. Idiopathic; congenital hypoplasia; cervical rib
2. Myotonic dystrophy; myotubular myopathy; hypotonia; Werdnig-Hoffmann disease
*3. Neurofibromatosis
4. Osteoporosis, severe
*5. Regenerated rib (after resection)

**UNCOMMON**
1. Achondrogenesis, types I and II
2. Aminopterin fetopathy
3. Angiomatosis (Gorham's disease)
*4. Basal cell nevus S. (Gorlin S.)
5. Campomelic dysplasia
6. Cockayne S.
7. Contractural arachnodactyly
8. Hallermann-Streiff S.
9. Hyperparathyroidism
10. Larsen S.
11. Metaphyseal chondrodysplasia (Jansen)
12. Morquio S. (posterior portion)
*13. Osteodysplasty (Melnick-Needles S.)
14. Osteogenesis imperfecta
15. Paraplegia; poliomyelitis
16. Progeria
17. Rheumatoid arthritis
18. Scleroderma
*19. Spondylocostal dysostosis
*20. Spondylothoracic dysplasia
21. 3-M S.
22. Trisomy 13 S.
23. Trisomy 18 S.
24. Trisomy 21 S. (Down S.)
25. Turner S.

* Ribs may be twisted.

*References:*
1. Greenfield GB: Radiology of Bone Diseases. (ed 5) Philadelphia: Lippincott, 1990
2. Kozlowski K, Beighton P: Gamut Index of Skeletal Dysplasias. Berlin: Springer-Verlag, 1984, pp 51-52
3. Murray RO, Jacobson HG, Stoker DJ: The Radiology of Skeletal Disorders. (ed 3) London: Churchill Livingstone, 1990
4. Swischuk LE: Differential Diagnosis in Pediatric Radiology. Baltimore: Williams & Wilkins, 1984, p 284
5. Taybi H, Lachman RS: Radiology of Syndromes, Metabolic Disorders, and Skeletal Dysplasias. (ed 3) Chicago: Year Book Medical Publ, 1990, p 882

## Gamut B-205

## WIDE OR THICKENED RIBS

**COMMON**
1. Achondroplasia
2. Acromegaly
3. Anemia$_g$ (esp. thalassemia, sickle cell disease)
4. Fibrous dysplasia
5. Fluorosis
6. Mucopolysaccharidoses
7. Normal variant
8. Paget's disease
9. Posttraumatic (healed fractures with callus)
10. Rickets (rosary)

**UNCOMMON**
1. Basal cell nevus S. (Gorlin)
2. Craniodiaphyseal dysplasia
3. Dysosteosclerosis
4. Endosteal hyperostosis (van Buchem, Worth)
5. Erdheim-Chester disease
6. Fucosidosis, mannosidosis, GM$_1$ gangliosidosis
7. Gaucher's disease, Niemann-Pick disease

8. Hyperphosphatasia
9. Hypochondroplasia
10. Infantile cortical hyperostosis (Caffey's disease)
11. Melorheostosis
12. Metaphyseal chondrodysplasia (Schmid)
13. Metaphyseal dysplasia (Pyle's disease)
14. Mucolipidosis II, III
15. Oculo-dento-osseous dysplasia
16. Osteogenesis imperfecta congenita (thick bone type)
17. Osteomyelitis, healed; actinomycosis
18. Osteopetrosis
19. Pachydermoperiostosis
20. Polycythemia
21. Proteus S.
22. Pseudoachondroplasia
23. Scurvy
24. Trisomy 8 S.
25. Tuberous sclerosis
26. Weill-Marchesani S.

*References:*
1. Greenfield GB: Radiology of Bone Diseases. (ed 5) Philadelphia: Lippincott, 1990
2. Taybi H, Lachman RS: Radiology of Syndromes, Metabolic Disorders, and Skeletal Dysplasias. (ed 3) Chicago: Year Book Medical Publ, 1990, p 883

## Gamut B-206

## SHORT RIBS*

**COMMON**
1. Achondroplasia
2. [Rickets, all types]

**UNCOMMON**
1. Achondrogenesis, types I and II
2. Asphyxiating thoracic dysplasia (Jeune S.)

3. Campomelic dysplasia
4. Cerebro-costo-mandibular S.
5. Chondroectodermal dysplasia (Ellis-van Creveld S.)
6. Cleidocranial dysplasia
7. Dyssegmental dysplasia
8. Enchondromatosis (Ollier's disease)
9. Fibrochondrogenesis; hypochondrogenesis
10. Hypophosphatasia
11. Immune deficiency (severe combined) and adenosine deaminase deficiency
12. Mandibuloacral dysplasia
13. Metatropic dysplasia
14. Mucopolysaccharidoses (esp. Morquio S.)
15. Osteodysplasty (Melnick-Needles S.)
16. Osteogenesis imperfecta
17. Pseudoachondroplasia
18. Short rib-polydactyly S., types 1, 2, and 3
19. Spondylocostal dysostosis
20. Spondyloepiphyseal dysplasia congenita
21. Thanatophoric dysplasia

\* Usually associated with small thorax.

*References:*
1. Campbell JB: Personal communication
2. Greenfield GB: Radiology of Bone Diseases. (ed 5) Philadelphia: Lippincott, 1990
3. Kozlowski K, Beighton P: Gamut Index of Skeletal Dysplasias. Berlin: Springer-Verlag, 1984, pp 50-51
4. Taybi H, Lachman RS: Radiology of Syndromes, Metabolic Disorders, and Skeletal Dysplasias. (ed 3) Chicago: Year Book Medical Publ, 1990, p 882

# MULTIPLE SYMMETRICAL ANTERIOR RIB ENLARGEMENT, FLARING, OR CUPPING

## COMMON

1. Achondroplasia
2. Normal variant
3. Rickets, all types (See B-46)
4. Scurvy

## UNCOMMON

1. Asphyxiating thoracic dysplasia; other narrow thorax-short rib syndromes
2. Farber lipogranulomatosis
3. Hypophosphatasia
4. Infantile nutritional copper deficiency; kinky-hair S. (Menkes S.)
5. Leukemia (chloromas)
6. Metaphyseal chondrodysplasias (Jansen, McKusick, Schmid types); Shwachman S.
7. Short rib-polydactyly S.
8. Spondylometaphyseal dysplasia
9. Thalassemia
10. Thanatophoric dysplasia

*References:*

1. Austin JHM: Chloroma; report of a patient with unusual rib lesions. Radiology 1969; 93:671-672
2. Kozlowski K, Beighton P: Gamut Index of Skeletal Dysplasias. Berlin: Springer-Verlag, 1984, p 53
3. Taybi H, Lachman RS: Radiology of Syndromes, Metabolic Disorders, and Skeletal Dysplasias. (ed 3) Chicago: Year Book Medical Publ, 1990, p 882

## Gamut B-208

# CLASSIFICATION OF RIB NOTCHING

## Arterial

1. High aortic obstruction
   a. Coarctation of aorta
2. Low aortic obstruction
   a. Aortic thrombosis
3. Subclavian obstruction
   a. Blalock-Taussig procedure (unilateral)
   b. Pulseless disease (eg, Takayasu's arteritis); advanced arteriosclerosis
4. Pulmonary oligemia
   a. Absent pulmonary artery (unilateral)
   b. Ebstein's anomaly
   c. Emphysema
   d. Pseudotruncus arteriosus
   e. Pulmonary valvular stenosis or atresia
   f. Tetralogy of Fallot$_g$

## Venous

1. Obstruction of superior vena cava, innominate or subclavian vein

## Arteriovenous

1. A-V fistula of chest wall (intercostal artery-vein)
2. Pulmonary A-V fistula

## Neurogenic

1. Intercostal neurofibroma or neurilemoma
2. Neurofibromatosis
3. Bulbar poliomyelitis; quadriplegia

## Osseous

1. Hyperparathyroidism
2. Osteodysplasty (Melnick-Needles S.)
3. Thalassemia

## Miscellaneous

1. Idiopathic; normal variant
2. Indwelling catheter

*References:*
1. Boone ML, Swenson BE, Felson B: Rib notching: Its many causes. Am J Roentgenol 1964;91:1075-1088
2. Felson B, Weinstein AW, Spitz HB: Principles of Chest Roentgenology: A Programmed Text. Philadelphia: W.B. Saunders, 1965, p 197

### Gamut B-209

# RESORPTION OR NOTCHING OF THE SUPERIOR RIB MARGINS

## COMMON
1. Collagen disease$_g$ (eg, rheumatoid arthritis, sclero-derma, lupus)
2. Hyperparathyroidism
3. Localized pressure effect (eg, thoracic drainage tube, rib retractor, intercostal neurofibroma, multiple cartilaginous exostoses)

## UNCOMMON
1. Coarctation of thoracic aorta (superior and inferior margins)
2. Idiopathic
3. Intercostal muscle atrophy in restrictive lung disease

4. Marfan S.
5. Neurofibromatosis
6. Osteogenesis imperfecta
7. Poliomyelitis, paralysis
8. Radiation therapy
9. Sjögren S.

*References:*
1. Eisenberg RL: Clinical Imaging: An Atlas of Differential Diagnosis. Rockville, MD: Aspen Publishers, 1988, pp 704-707
2. Greenfield GB: Radiology of Bone Diseases. (ed 5) Philadelphia: Lippincott, 1990
3. Sargent EN, Turner AF, Jacobson G: Superior marginal rib defects. AJR 1969;106:491-505

## Gamut B-210

## RIB LESION IN A CHILD

### Congenital

*1. Achondroplasia
*2. Bifid rib, supernumerary rib, synostosis
*3. Cervical rib
*4. Coarctation of aorta (rib notching)
*5. Hypoplasia or absence
  6. Mucopolysaccharidoses (eg, Hurler, Morquio)
  7. Neurofibromatosis
  8. Osteochondrodysplasias, other (See B-1)
  9. Osteopetrosis
*10. Thalassemia, sickle cell anemia

### Inflammation

1. Infantile cortical hyperostosis (Caffey's disease)
2. Granulomatous disease of childhood

3. Hydatid disease
*4. Osteomyelitis (eg, bacterial, tuberculous, fungal)

# Neoplasm

1. Angioma
2. Chondromyxoid fibroma
*3. Enchondroma
4. Hamartoma
5. Leukemia, lymphoma$_g$
6. Metastasis (esp. neuroblastoma)
7. Neurofibroma
8. Osteoblastoma
9. Osteochondroma
10. Osteoma
11. Sarcoma (eg, Ewing's, osteosarcoma)

# Miscellaneous

*1. Fibrocystic lesion (cyst, nonossifying fibroma, fibrous dysplasia)
2. Histiocytosis X$_g$
*3. Rib notching, other causes (See B-208)
*4. Rickets, all types (See B-46)
5. Scurvy
*6. Trauma (eg, fracture, callus, regenerated rib)

* Common.

## Gamut B-211

# SHORT LESION OF A RIB
# (LESS THAN 6 CM)
# (See Gamut B-212)

**COMMON**

1. Bone cyst
2. Brown tumor of hyperparathyroidism
3. Enchondroma
4. Fibrous dysplasia
5. Fracture, callus
6. Histiocytosis $X_g$ (esp. eosinophilic granuloma)
7. Metastasis
8. Osteochondroma, exostosis
9. Osteomyelitis (eg, bacterial, tuberculous, fungal)
10. Plasmacytoma, multiple myeloma

**UNCOMMON**

1. Angioma, arteriovenous fistula
2. Chondroblastoma
3. Chondromyxoid fibroma
4. Gaucher's disease
5. Giant cell tumor
6. Hamartoma
7. Lipoma
8. Lymphoma$_g$ (esp. Hodgkin's)
9. Nonossifying fibroma
10. Osteoblastoma
11. Osteoid osteoma
12. Osteoma
13. Sarcoma (eg, Ewing's, osteosarcoma, chondrosarcoma)

## Gamut B-212

# LONG LESION OF A RIB
## (OVER 6 CM - USUALLY EXPANSILE)
### (See Gamut B-211)

**COMMON**
1. Fibrous dysplasia
2. [Fused or bifid rib]
3. Metastasis (esp. breast, prostate, lung, kidney, neuroblastoma)
4. Osteomyelitis (eg, bacterial, tuberculous, fungal)
5. Plasmacytoma, multiple myeloma
6. Sarcoma (eg, osteosarcoma, chondrosarcoma, Ewing's)
7. [Surgical removal; regeneration]

**UNCOMMON**
1. Aneurysmal bone cyst
2. Bone cyst
3. Chondromyxoid fibroma
4. Gaucher's disease
5. Histiocytosis $X_g$
6. Hydatid cyst
7. Melorheostosis
8. Paget's disease

*Reference:*
1. Omell GH, Anderson LS, Bramson RT: Chest wall tumors. Radiol Clin North Am 1973;11:197-214

# MULTIPLE EXPANDING RIB LESIONS

## COMMON
1. Anemia$_g$ (eg, thalassemia, sickle cell)
2. Metastases
3. Multiple myeloma

## UNCOMMON
1. Angiomas
2. Brown tumors of hyperparathyroidism
3. Enchondromatosis (Ollier's disease)
4. Endosteal hyperostosis (van Buchem, Worth)
5. Engelmann's disease (diaphyseal dysplasia)
6. Fibrous dysplasia
7. Gaucher's disease
8. Histiocytosis X$_g$
9. Hydatid disease
10. Hypophosphatasia
11. Infantile cortical hyperostosis (Caffey's disease)
12. Leukemia (chloromas)
13. Mucopolysaccharidoses (esp. Hurler, Morquio)
14. Multiple cartilaginous exostoses (diaphyseal aclasis)
15. Osteogenesis imperfecta
16. Pachydermoperiostosis
17. Paget's disease
18. Rickets (rosary)
19. Scurvy

# CONGENITAL STERNAL ABNORMALITY

## HYPERSEGMENTATION
1. Trisomy 21 S. (Down S.)

## UNDERSEGMENTATION (OFTEN WITH HYPOPLASIA AND PREMATURE FUSION)
1. Campomelic dysplasia
2. Cornelia de Lange S.
3. Noonan S.
4. Trisomy 18 S.

## PECTUS CARINATUM (PIGEON BREAST)

1. Congenital heart disease (esp. cyanotic)
2. Isolated finding
3. Morquio S.
4. Noonan S.
5. Spondyloepiphyseal dysplasia congenita
6. Undersegmentation, hypoplasia (see above)

## PECTUS EXCAVATUM
1. Congenital bowing of tibia
2. Congenital heart disease
3. Ehlers-Danlos S.
4. Homocystinuria
5. Idiopathic; isolated finding
6. Marfan S.
7. Mitral valve prolapse S.
8. Newborn with respiratory distress
9. Osteogenesis imperfecta

*Reference:*
1. Swischuk LE: Differential Diagnosis in Pediatric Radiology. Baltimore: Williams & Wilkins, 1984, p 278

---

## Gamut B-215

# EROSION, SCLEROSIS, AND/OR FUSION OF THE STERNOMANUBRIAL SYNCHONDROSIS OR STERNOCLAVICULAR JOINTS

### COMMON
1. Ankylosing spondylitis
2. Degenerative arthritis
3. Posttraumatic, postsurgical
4. Psoriatic arthritis
5. Rheumatoid arthritis

### UNCOMMON
1. Congenital fusion anomaly
2. Enteropathic arthritis
3. Fluorosis
4. Infection (pyogenic, tuberculous)
5. Reiter S.
6. Relapsing polychondritis

*Reference:*

1. Burgener FA, Kormano M: Differential Diagnosis in Conventional Radiology. (ed 2) New York: Thieme Medical Publ, 1991, p 224

B. Bone

# C

# Calvarium (Skull)

## ABNORMAL SIZE OR SHAPE

## ABNORMAL DENSITY OR THICKNESS

| C-12 | Diffuse or Widespread Increased Density, Sclerosis, or Thickening of the Calvarium |
|------|-----------|
| C-12A | Congenital Conditions with Increased Density or Thickening of the Skull |
| C-13 | Localized Increased Density, Sclerosis, or Thickening of the Base of Skull (See Gamut C-14) |
| C-14 | Generalized Increased Density, Sclerosis, or Thickening of the Base of the Skull (See Gamut C-13) |
| C-15 | Thinning of the Skull, Localized or Generalized |

## DESTRUCTION

| C-16 | Diffuse or Widespread Demineralization or Destruction of the Skull (Including "Salt and Pepper" Skull) |
|------|-----------|
| C-17 | Erosion of the Inner Table of the Skull |
| C-18 | Button Sequestrum of the Skull |
| C-19 | Solitary Osteolytic Skull Lesion (See Gamut C-20) |
| C-20 | Radiolucent Lesion or Bone Defect in the Skull, Solitary or Multiple (See Gamut C-19) |

## SELLA TURCICA

| C-21 | Enlarged, Eroded, or Destroyed Sella Turcica (Including Intrasellar or Parasellar Mass on CT or MRI) |
|------|-----------|
| C-22 | Small Sella Turcica |
| C-23 | Abnormal Sellar Configuration |

## MISCELLANEOUS

| C-24 | Normal Skull Variants That May Simulate a Fracture |
|------|-----------|
| C-25 | Multiple Wormian (Sutural) Bones |

C

## Gamut C-1

# PREMATURE CRANIOSYNOSTOSIS (CRANIOSTENOSIS)

**COMMON**
1. Congenital syndromes (See C-1B)
*2. Decreased intracranial pressure (brain atrophy, shunted hydrocephalus - "contracting skull")
3. Primary (idiopathic) craniosynostosis (See C-1A)

**UNCOMMON**
*1. Anemia$_g$ (eg, sickle cell, thalassemia, iron deficiency)
*2. Cretinism, hypothyroidism (treated)
*3. Hyperthyroidism
*4. Hypervitaminosis D
5. Microcephaly (failure of brain growth)
*6. Polycythemia vera
*7. Rickets (hypophosphatemic, treated; vitamin D resistant)

*Secondary synostosis.

*References:*
1. Cohen MM Jr: Genetic perspective on craniosynostosis and syndromes with craniosynostosis. Neurosurgery 1977;47: 886
2. David DJ, Poswillo D, Simpson D: The Craniosynostoses. Berlin: Springer-Verlag, 1982
3. Duggan CA, Keever EB, Gay BB Jr: Secondary craniosynostosis. AJR 1970;109:277-293
4. Jones KL: Smith's Recognizable Patterns of Human Malformation. (ed 3) Philadelphia: W.B. Saunders, 1988
5. Newton TH, Potts DG: Radiology of the Skull and Brain. St. Louis: C.V. Mosby, 1971, vol 1, book 1, pp 222-228
6. Swischuk LE: Differential Diagnosis in Pediatric Radiology. Baltimore: Williams & Wilkins, 1984, p 350
7. Taybi H, Lachman RS: Radiology of Syndromes, Metabolic Disorders, and Skeletal Dysplasias. (ed 3) Chicago: Year Book Medical Publ, 1990, p 852

# CLASSIFICATION OF PRIMARY (IDIOPATHIC) PREMATURE CRANIOSYNOSTOSIS

1. **Brachycephaly** (short, wide, slightly high head with "harlequin" orbits) - bilateral coronal sutures
2. **Microcephaly** (small round head) - all sutures (universal craniosynostosis)
3. **Oxycephaly** (tall, wide, short head) or **turricephaly** (tower-shaped, pointed head with overgrowth of bregma and flat, underdeveloped lower posterior fossa) - bilateral lambdoid and coronal sutures
4. **Plagiocephaly** (oblique asymmetrical head) - unilateral coronal suture (with flattening of ipsilateral frontoparietal region, elevation of ipsilateral sphenoid wing, and unilateral "harlequin" orbit) and/or lambdoid suture
5. **Scaphocephaly** (boat head) or **dolichocephaly** (long, narrow, slightly high head) - sagittal suture
6. **Trigonocephaly** (triangular head; narrow in front, broad behind with hypotelorism) - metopic suture
7. **Triphyllocephaly (cloverleaf skull or kleeblattschädel)** - trilobular skull with frontal and temporal bulges - intrauterine premature closure of sagittal, coronal, and lambdoid sutures

*References:*
1. Newton TH, Potts DG: Radiology of the Skull and Brain. St. Louis: C.V. Mosby, 1971, vol 1, book 1, p 222
2. Silverman FN (ed): Caffey's Pediatric X-ray Diagnosis. (ed 8) Chicago: Year Book Medical Publ, 1985, pp 36-43
3. Swischuk LE: Differential Diagnosis in Pediatric Radiology. Baltimore: Williams & Wilkins, 1984, p 331
4. Swischuk LE: Imaging of the Newborn, Infant, and Young Child. (ed 3) Baltimore: Williams & Wilkins, 1989, pp 906-913

## Subgamut C-1B

# CONGENITAL SYNDROMES WITH PREMATURE CRANIOSYNOSTOSIS

**COMMON**
1. Achondroplasia (base of skull)
2. Acrocephalopolysyndactyly (Carpenter and other types)
3. Acrocephalosyndactyly (Apert and other types)
4. Asphyxiating thoracic dysplasia
5. Chondrodysplasia punctata (Conradi's disease)
6. Cloverleaf skull (kleeblattschädel)
7. Craniofacial dysostosis (Crouzon S.)
8. Hypophosphatasia (late)
9. Mucopolysaccharidoses (eg, Hurler S.; Maroteaux-Lamy S.); mucolipidosis III; fucosidosis
10. Rubella S.
11. Thanatophoric dysplasia
12. Trisomy 21 S. (Down S.)

**UNCOMMON**
1. Acrocraniofacial dysostosis
2. Adducted thumb S. (Christian S.)
3. Adrenogenital S.
4. Aminopterin fetopathy
5. Baller-Gerold S.
6. Bird-headed dwarfism (Seckel S.)
7. C S.
8. Chromosomal syndromes (5p-, 7q+, 13)
9. Craniotelencephalic dysplasia
10. Fetal hydantoin S.
11. Fetal trimethadione S.
12. Idiopathic hypercalcemia (Williams S.)
13. Meckel S.
14. Metaphyseal chondrodysplasia (Jansen)
15. Oculo-mandibulo-facial S. (Hallermann-Streiff S.)
16. Osteoglophonic dysplasia
17. Trisomy 18 S.

*References:*
1. Cohen MM Jr: Genetic perspective on craniosynostosis and syndromes with craniosynostosis. Neurosurgery 1977;47: 886
2. David DJ, Poswillo D, Simpson D: The Craniosynostoses. Berlin: Springer-Verlag, 1982
3. Jones KL: Smith's Recognizable Patterns of Human Malformation. Philadelphia:W.B. Saunders, 1988
4. Newton TH, Potts DG: Radiology of the Skull and Brain. St. Louis: C.V. Mosby, 1971, vol 1, book 1, pp 222-228
5. Swischuk LE: Differential Diagnosis in Pediatric Radiology. Baltimore:Williams & Wilkins, 1984, p 350
6. Taybi H, Lachman RS: Radiology of Syndromes, Metabolic Disorders, and Skeletal Dysplasias. (ed 3) Chicago:Year Book Medical Publ, 1990, p 852

## Gamut C-2

## MICROCEPHALY (MICROCRANIA)

**COMMON**
1. Cerebral atrophy; perinatal brain damage from hypoxia
2. Craniosynostosis, total
3. Encephalocele
4. Idiopathic small brain (micrencephaly)
5. Prenatal irradiation or infection (eg, toxoplasmosis, rubella, cytomegalovirus, herpes, syphilis)

**UNCOMMON**
1. Adducted thumb S.
2. Aminopterin fetopathy
3. Beckwith-Wiedemann S.
4. Bird-headed dwarfism (Seckel S.)
5. C S.
6. Cephaloskeletal dysplasia (Taybi-Linder S.)
7. Cerebro-oculo-facial-skeletal S.
8. Chondrodysplasia punctata (Conradi's disease)
9. Chromosome syndromes [eg, 4p-, 5p-(cat cry S.), 18q-,22]
10. Cockayne S.

11. Coffin-Siris S.
12. Cornelia de Lange S.
13. Deprivation dwarfism
14. Dubowitz S.
15. Dyggve-Melchior-Clausen S.
16. Familial
17. Fanconi anemia
18. Fetal alcohol S.
19. Fetal hydantoin S.
20. Fetal trimethadione S.
21. Goltz S.
22. "Happy puppet" S.
23. Holoprosencephaly (arhinencephaly)
24. Homocystinuria
25. Incontinentia pigmenti
26. Johanson-Blizzard S.
27. Kinky-hair S. (Menkes S.)
28. Langer-Giedion S.
29. Lenz microphthalmia S.
30. Lesch-Nyhan S.
31. Lissencephaly S.
32. Meckel S.
33. Noonan S.
34. [Normal variant]
35. Prader-Willi S.
36. Riley-Day S.
37. Rubinstein-Taybi S.
38. Smith-Lemli-Opitz S.
39. Trisomy 13 S.
40. Trisomy 18 S.
41. Trisomy 21 S. (Down S.)

*References:*
1. Felson B (ed): Dwarfs and other little people. Semin Roentgenol 1973:8:133-263
2. Newton TH, Potts DG: Radiology of the Skull and Brain. St. Louis: C.V. Mosby, 1971, vol 1, book 1, pp 151-152
3. Jones KL: Smith's Recognizable Patterns of Human Malformation. Philadelphia: W.B. Saunders, 1988
4. Taybi H, Lachman RS: Radiology of Syndromes, Metabolic Disorders, and Skeletal Dysplasias. (ed 3) Chicago: Year Book Medical Publ, 1990, p 854

## Gamut C-3

# MACROCEPHALY (MACROCRANIA)

**COMMON**
1. [Calvarial thickening (eg, congenital anemias$_g$)]
*2. Congenital syndromes  (See C-3A)
*3. Craniostenosis
4. Hydrocephalus
*5. Subdural hematoma

**UNCOMMON**
1. Aneurysm of vein of Galen
2. Aqueduct stenosis
3. Arnold-Chiari malformation
4. Choroid plexus papilloma
*5. Expansion of middle fossa
6. Hydranencephaly
7. Infection causing hydrocephalus (eg, meningitis, toxoplasmosis)
8. Megalencephaly
9. Porencephaly
10. Posterior fossa cyst (eg, dermoid, teratoma, Dandy-Walker S.)
*11. Tumor or subarachnoid cyst adjacent to calvarium

*May be asymmetrical.

*References:*
1. Harwood-Nash DC, Fitz CR: Large heads and ventricles in infants. Radiol Clin North Am 1975;13:119-224
2. Newton TH, Potts DG: Radiology of the Skull and Brain. St. Louis: C.V. Mosby, 1971, vol 1, book 1, pp 144-151
3. Scotti LN, Maravilla K, Hardman DR: The enlarging head - angiographic evaluation of megacephaly. American Roentgen Ray Society Scientific Exhibit, Atlanta, 1975
4. Swischuk LE: Differential Diagnosis in Pediatric Radiology. Baltimore: Williams & Wilkins, 1984, pp 329-330

## Subgamut C-3A

# CONGENITAL SYNDROMES WITH MACROCEPHALY*

## COMMON
1. Achondroplasia, hypochondroplasia
2. Hydrocephalus
3. Hyperostosis diseases (eg, osteopetrosis, craniometaphyseal dysplasia, Camurati-Engelmann disease, pyknodysostosis, hyperphosphatasia)
4. Mucopolysaccharidoses$_g$ (incl. Hurler, Hunter, Morquio, Maroteaux-Lamy); GM$_1$ gangliosidosis
5. Neurofibromatosis

## UNCOMMON
1. Achondrogenesis, hypochondrogenesis
2. Beckwith-Wiedemann S.
3. Campomelic dysplasia
4. Cerebral gigantism (Sotos S.)
5. Cerebrohepatorenal S. (Zellweger S.)
6. Cleidocranial dysplasia
7. Cranioectodermal dysplasia
8. Dandy-Walker S.
9. Familial megalencephaly; megalencephaly syndromes
10. Greig cephalopolysyndactyly S.
11. Hypomelanosis of Ito
12. Klippel-Trenaunay-Weber S.
13. Kniest dysplasia
14. Marfan S.
15. Noonan S.
16. Osteogenesis imperfecta
17. Pituitary gigantism or dwarfism
18. Proteus S.
19. Riley-Smith S.
20. Robinow S.
21. Schwarz-Lélek S.
22. [Silver-Russell S.]

23. Spondyloepiphyseal dysplasia congenita (lethal)
24. Tay-Sachs disease
25. Thanatophoric dysplasia
26. Tuberous sclerosis

\* Many dwarfs have relative macrocephaly.

*References:*

1. DeMyer W: Megalencephaly in children: clinical syndromes, genetic patterns, and differential diagnoses from other causes of megalocephaly. Neurology 1972;22:634-643
2. Holt JF, Kuhns LR: Macrocranium and macrocephaly in neurofibromatosis. Skeletal Radiol 1976;1:25-28
3. Jones KL: Smith's Recognizable Patterns of Human Malformation. Philadelphia: W.B. Saunders, 1988
4. Swischuk LE: Differential Diagnosis in Pediatric Radiology. Baltimore: Williams & Wilkins, 1984, p 329
5. Taybi H, Lachman RS: Radiology of Syndromes, Metabolic Disorders, and Skeletal Dysplasias. (ed 3) Chicago: Year Book Medical Publ, 1990, pp 853-854

## Gamut C-4

# ABNORMAL CONTOUR OF THE CALVARIUM
## (See Gamuts C-1 to C-10)

**COMMON**

1. Achondroplasia, other congenital syndromes
2. Fibrous dysplasia, leontiasis ossea
3. Hemiatrophy of brain (eg, Sturge-Weber S.; Dyke-Davidoff-Masson S.); localized cerebral atrophy
4. Hydrocephalus
5. Paget's disease (eg, tam-o'-shanter skull) (See C-4A)
6. Postoperative
7. Postural flattening, usually occipital (eg, cerebral palsy); postural asymmetry from scoliosis
8. Premature craniosynostosis (See C-1, C-1A)
9. Trauma (incl. obstetrical)

**UNCOMMON**
1. Arachnoid cyst
2. Craniolacunia
3. Craniofacial dysostosis (Crouzon S.)
4. Craniopagus twins
5. Dandy-Walker S.
6. Encephalocele
7. Hyperphosphatasia
8. Hypertelorism; cranium bifidum
9. Microcephaly
10. Neoplasm
11. Neurofibromatosis
12. Porencephalic cyst; cerebral cyst
13. Rickets, healed, with bossing
14. Silver-Russell S.
15. Subdural hematoma, chronic; hygroma

## Subgamut C-4A

# TAM-O'-SHANTER SKULL (THICKENING OF THE SKULL VAULT WITH BASILAR INVAGINATION)

**COMMON**
1. Paget's disease

**UNCOMMON**
1. Fibrous dysplasia
2. Hypophosphatasia
3. Neurofibromatosis
4. Osteogenesis imperfecta
5. Osteomalacia, rickets

## Gamut C-5

# UNILATERAL SMALL CRANIUM

**COMMON**
1. Cerebral hemiatrophy (eg, Dyke-Davidoff-Masson S.; Sturge-Weber S.)
2. Normal (slight)
3. Trauma (depressed skull fracture)
4. Unilateral lambdoid or coronal craniosynostosis

**UNCOMMON**
1. Head positioning in infancy (postural flattening)
2. Radiation therapy
3. Silver-Russell S. (congenital hemiatrophy)

## Gamut C-6

# BIPARIETAL BOSSING

1. Bilateral coronal synostosis, isolated or with Crouzon S.
2. Bilateral subdural hematoma, chronic
3. Cleidocranial dysplasia
4. Cloverleaf skull (kleeblattschädel)
5. Pyknodysostosis
6. Rickets, healed

*Reference:*
1. Swischuk LE: Differential Diagnosis in Pediatric Radiology. Baltimore: Williams & Wilkins, 1984, p 336

　　　　　　　　　　C. Calvarium (Skull)

## Gamut C-7

# LOCALIZED BULGE OF THE CALVARIUM OR SCALP

**COMMON**

1. Anemia, chronic$_g$ (eg, sickle cell, iron deficiency)
2. Cephalhematoma
3. Metastatic carcinoma or neuroblastoma
4. Myeloma

**UNCOMMON**

1. Arachnoid cyst with erosion
2. Dermoid cyst, intradiploic
3. Fibrous dysplasia
4. Histiocytosis X$_g$
5. Intracranial neoplasm (large) with erosion of calvarium
6. Leptomeningeal cyst
7. Meningioma
8. Paget's disease with secondary malignant neoplasm
9. Porencephalic cyst
10. Primary neoplasm of calvarium (eg, sarcoma, osteoma)
11. Scalp neoplasm or cyst
12. Subdural hematoma

*Reference:*
1. Swischuk LE: Differential Diagnosis in Pediatric Radiology. Baltimore: Williams & Wilkins, 1984, p 337

## Gamut C-8

# BASILAR INVAGINATION

**COMMON**

1. Arnold-Chiari malformation
2. Congenital craniovertebral anomaly
   a. Atlantoaxial dislocation with or without congenital separation of odontoid

---

    b. Atlanto-occipital fusion (assimilation)

    c. Klippel-Feil S.

    d. Stenosis of foramen magnum

    e. Unfused posterior arch of atlas

3. Osteogenesis imperfecta

4. Osteomalacia (See B-46); rickets

5. Paget's disease

## UNCOMMON

1. Achondroplasia
2. Aqueduct stenosis
3. Cleidocranial dysplasia
4. Craniofacial dysostosis (Crouzon S.)
5. Fibrous dysplasia
6. Hajdu-Cheney S. (idiopathic acro-osteolysis)
7. Histiocytosis $X_g$
8. Hydrocephalus, chronic
9. Hyperparathyroidism, primary or secondary (renal osteodystrophy)
10. Hypophosphatasia
11. Mucopolysaccharidoses (eg, Hurler, Morquio)
12. Occipital craniotomy in a child
13. Osteomyelitis (incl. syphilis, tuberculosis)
14. Osteopetrosis
15. Osteoporosis
16. Psoriatic arthritis
17. Pyknodysostosis
18. Rheumatoid arthritis; ankylosing spondylitis
19. Trauma, severe
20. Trisomy 21 S. (Down S.)

*References:*

1. Dolan KD: Cervicobasilar relationships. Radiol Clin North Am 1977;15:155-166
2. DuBoulay GH: Principles of X-ray Diagnosis of the Skull. (ed 2) London: Butterworths, 1980, pp 229-235
3. Epstein BS, Epstein JA: The association of cerebellar tonsillar herniation with basilar impression incident to Paget's disease. AJR 1969;107:535-542
4. Taybi H, Lachman RS: Radiology of Syndromes, Metabolic Disorders, and Skeletal Dysplasias. (ed 3) Chicago: Year Book Medical Publ, 1990, pp 851-852

# HYPOPLASIA OF THE BASE OF THE SKULL

**COMMON**
1. Achondroplasia
2. Cretinism
3. Trisomy 21 S. (Down S.)

**UNCOMMON**
1. Achondrogenesis
2. Acrocephalopolysyndactyly (Carpenter S.)
3. Acrocephalosyndactyly (Apert, Pfeiffer types)
4. Cranial dysplasia; cleidocranial dysplasia
5. Craniofacial dysostosis (Crouzon S.)
6. Oculo-mandibulo-facial S. (Hallermann-Streiff S.)
7. Orbital hypotelorism with arhinencephaly; trisomy 13 S.
8. Short rib-polydactyly S.
9. Thanatophoric dysplasia

*References:*
1. Dorst J: Personal communication
2. DuBoulay GH: Principles of X-ray Diagnosis of the Skull. (ed 2) London: Butterworths, 1980, pp 237-243

# FORAMEN MAGNUM ABNORMALITIES

## Enlargement

**COMMON**
1. Arnold-Chiari malformation
2. Cervical-occipital meningocele or encephalocele
3. Dandy-Walker cyst; other posterior fossa cysts

**UNCOMMON**
1. Neoplasm of posterior fossa or upper cervical spine
2. Syringobulbia

## Small or Irregular Foramen Magnum

1. Bilateral or unilateral occipitalization (fusion) of C1 to base of skull
2. Chondrodystrophies
   a. Achondroplasia
   b. Achondrogenesis
   c. Diastrophic dysplasia
   d. Metatropic dysplasia
   e. Thanatophoric dysplasia

*Reference:*
1. Swischuk LE: Differential Diagnosis in Pediatric Radiology. Baltimore:Williams & Wilkins, 1984, pp 359-361

## Gamut C-11

# LOCALIZED INCREASED DENSITY, SCLEROSIS, OR THICKENING OF THE CALVARIUM

**COMMON**
1. Anatomic variation (eg, sutural sclerosis; external occipital protuberance)
2. Anemia$_g$ (esp. sickle cell)
3. [Artifact; hair braid; overlying soft tissue tumor or sebaceous cyst]
4. Cephalhematoma; ossified subdural hematoma
5. Chronic osteomyelitis or adjacent cellulitis; tuberculosis; syphilis; mycetoma
6. [Depressed skull fracture]
7. Fibrous dysplasia

8. Hyperostosis frontalis interna
*9. Meningioma
*10. Metastasis, osteoblastic (eg, prostate, breast)
11. Osteoma
12. Paget's disease

**UNCOMMON**

1. Arteriovenous malformation of dura
2. Cerebral hemiatrophy; Davidoff-Dyke S.
3. [Dural calcification]
4. Frontometaphyseal dysplasia
*5. Hemangioma
6. Histiocytosis $X_g$, healing
7. Ischemic necrosis (eg, bone flap)
8. Lymphoma$_g$
9. Mastocytosis
10. Neurofibromatosis
11. Osteoblastoma
12. Osteochondroma
*13. Osteosarcoma
14. Radiation osteonecrosis; treated tumor (eg, brown tumor, lytic metastasis from breast)
15. Tuberous sclerosis

* Sunburst spiculations may be present.

*Reference:*

1. DuBoulay GH: Principles of X-ray Diagnosis of the Skull. (ed 2) London: Butterworths, 1980, pp 113-125

## Gamut C-12

### DIFFUSE OR WIDESPREAD INCREASED DENSITY, SCLEROSIS, OR THICKENING OF THE CALVARIUM

**COMMON**

1. Acromegaly
*2. Anemia$_g$ (sickle cell, thalassemia, iron deficiency, hereditary spherocytosis)

3. Cerebral atrophy in childhood (contracting skull)
4. Congenital syndromes; sclerosing bone dysplasias (See C-12A)
+5. Fibrous dysplasia, leontiasis ossea
6. Hydrocephalus, postshunting
7. Hyperostosis interna generalisata; Morgagni-Stewart-Morel S.
8. Hyperparathyroidism, primary or secondary, treated (renal osteodystrophy, esp. in patients on dialysis)
9. Normal, idiopathic
*10. Metastases, osteoblastic (eg, prostate, breast)
11. Myelosclerosis
12. Paget's disease ("cotton wool" appearance)

## UNCOMMON

1. AV malformation, large
2. Craniosynostosis (See C-1)
3. Cretinism, hypothyroidism (treated)
4. Cyanotic congenital heart disease, long standing
5. Dilantin therapy
6. Dystrophia myotonica
7. Fluorosis
8. Hemihypertrophy of cranium due to cerebral hemiatrophy (Dyke-Davidoff-Masson S.)
9. Homocystinuria
10. Hypervitaminosis D
11. Hypoparathyroidism
12. Increased intracranial pressure in adults, chronic (eg, from intermittent obstruction)
13. Infantile cortical hyperostosis (Caffey's disease)
*14. Leukemia, lymphoma$_g$
*15. Meningioma
16. Microcephaly
*17. Neuroblastoma metastases
18. Osteomyelitis, chronic; mycetoma
*19. Polycythemia (childhood)
20. Rickets, treated ("bossing"); vitamin D-resistant rickets
21. Syphilitic osteitis

\* May show vertical striations ("hair on end").

\+ May develop leontiasis ossea (lion-like facies) due to overgrowth of facial bones.

## References:

1. Anderson R, et al: Thickening of the skull in surgically treated hydrocephalus. AJR 1970;110:96-101
2. DuBoulay GH: Principles of X-ray Diagnosis of the Skull. (ed 2) London: Butterworths, 1980, pp 98-113
3. Griscom NT, Oh KS: The contracting skull; Inward growth of the inner table as a physiologic response to diminution of intracranial content in children. AJR 1970;110:106-110
4. Kattan KR: Calvarial thickening after Dilantin medication. AJR 1970;110:102-105
5. Swischuk LE: Differential Diagnosis in Pediatric Radiology. Baltimore: Williams & Wilkins, 1984, pp 338-341
6. Taybi H, Lachman RS: Radiology of Syndromes, Metabolic Disorders, and Skeletal Dysplasias. (ed 3) Chicago: Year Book Medical Publ, 1990
7. Teplick JG, Haskin ME: Roentgenologic Diagnosis. (ed 3) Philadelphia: W.B. Saunders, 1976

## Subgamut C-12A

# CONGENITAL CONDITIONS WITH INCREASED DENSITY OR THICKENING OF THE SKULL

## COMMON

+1. Craniometaphyseal dysplasia; metaphyseal dysplasia (Pyle's disease); frontometaphyseal dysplasia
2. Craniosynostosis (See C-1)
3. Cretinism, hypothyroidism
4. Cyanotic congenital heart disease, long standing
5. Endosteal hyperostosis (van Buchem S., Worth S.)
6. Engelmann's disease (diaphyseal dysplasia)
7. Fanconi anemia
+8. Fibrous dysplasia (leontiasis ossea) (incl. McCune-Albright S.)

9. Hemihypertrophy of cranium due to cerebral hemitrophy (Dyke-Davidoff-Masson S.)
10. Homocystinuria
+11. Hyperphosphatasia
12. Microcephaly
13. Mucopolysaccharidoses; $GM_1$ gangliosidosis
14. Osteopetrosis
15. Pachydermoperiostosis
16. Pseudohypoparathyroidism; pseudopseudohypoparathyroidism
17. Pyknodysostosis
18. Tuberous sclerosis

## UNCOMMON

1. Acrodysostosis
2. Adrenogenital S.
3. Cockayne S.
4. Craniodiaphyseal dysplasia
5. Distal osteosclerosis
6. Dysosteosclerosis
7. Idiopathic hypercalcemia (Williams S.)
8. Lawrence-Seip S.
9. Lenz-Majewski hyperostotic dwarfism
10. Marshall S.
11. Melorheostosis
12. Oculo-dento-osseous dysplasia
13. Osteodysplasty (Melnick-Needles S.)
14. Osteogenesis imperfecta tarda
15. Osteopathia striata
16. Otopalatodigital S.
17. Schwarz-Lélek S.
18. Sclerosteosis
19. Troell-Junet S.
20. Tubular stenosis (Kenny-Caffey S.)
21. Weill-Marchesani S.
22. XXXXY S.

+ May develop leontiasis ossea (lion-like facies) due to overgrowth of facial bones.

*References:*
1. Kozlowski K., Beighton P.: Gamut Index of Skeletal Dysplasias. Berlin: Springer-Verlag, 1984
2. Swischuk LE: Differential Diagnosis in Pediatric Radiology. Baltimore: Williams & Wilkins, 1984, pp 338-341
3. Taybi H, Lachman RS: Radiology of Syndromes, Metabolic Disorders, and Skeletal Dysplasias. (ed 3) Chicago: Year Book Medical Publ, 1990

## Gamut C-13

# LOCALIZED INCREASED DENSITY, SCLEROSIS, OR THICKENING OF THE BASE OF THE SKULL
## (See Gamut C-14)

**COMMON**
1. Fibrous dysplasia
2. Mastoiditis, chronic sclerotic
3. Meningioma

**UNCOMMON**
1. Chordoma (with calcification)
2. Lymphoepithelioma of nasopharynx or paranasal sinus
3. Lymphoma$_g$
4. Metastasis, osteoblastic
5. Nasopharyngeal infection, chronic (eg, tuberculosis)
6. Osteoma; chondroma
7. Petrositis or osteomyelitis, chronic
8. Radiation therapy for invasive carcinoma of ear, sphenoid sinus, or nasopharynx
9. Sarcoma (eg, osteosarcoma, chondrosarcoma, rhabdomyosarcoma)
10. Sphenoid sinusitis; mucocele

*References:*
1. Potter GD: Sclerosis of the base of the skull as a manifestation of nasopharyngeal carcinoma. Radiology 1970;94:35-38

2. Tsai FY, Lisella RS, Lee KF, et al: Osteosclerosis of base of skull as a manifestation of tumor invasion. AJR 1975;124: 256-264

## Gamut C-14

# GENERALIZED INCREASED DENSITY, SCLEROSIS, OR THICKENING OF THE BASE OF THE SKULL
### (See Gamut C-13)

**COMMON**
1. Fibrous dysplasia
2. Paget's disease

**UNCOMMON**
1. Anemia$_g$, primary (eg, thalassemia, sickle cell)
2. Cleidocranial dysplasia
3. Craniometaphyseal dysplasia
4. Cretinism
5. Engelmann's disease (diaphyseal dysplasia)
6. Fluorosis
7. Frontometaphyseal dysplasia
8. Hyperparathyroidism, primary or secondary (treated)
9. Hypervitaminosis D
10. Idiopathic hypercalcemia (Williams S.)
11. Melorheostosis
12. Meningioma
13. Metaphyseal chondrodysplasia (Jansen)
14. Metaphyseal dysplasia (Pyle's disease)
15. Neurofibromatosis
16. Osteodysplasty (Melnick-Needles S.)
17. Osteopathia striata
18. Osteopetrosis
19. Otopalatodigital S.
20. Pachydermoperiostosis

21. Pyknodysostosis
22. Ribbing's disease (hereditary multiple diaphyseal sclerosis)
23. Tricho-dento-osseous S.
24. Vitamin D-resistant rickets (healing)

*References:*

1. DuBoulay GH: Principles of X-ray Diagnosis of the Skull. (ed 2) London: Butterworths, 1980
2. Swischuk LE: Differential Diagnosis in Pediatric Radiology. Baltimore: Williams & Wilkins, 1984, p 344

## Gamut C-15

# THINNING OF THE SKULL, LOCALIZED OR GENERALIZED

## Localized

**COMMON**
1. Parietal thinning
2. Subdural hematoma, chronic

**UNCOMMON**
1. Congenital arachnoid cyst
2. Intracranial tumor, slow growing
3. Leptomeningeal cyst
4. Localized cerebral agenesis or atrophy
5. Localized temporal horn hydrocephalus
6. Necrosis of skull (eg, radiation therapy)
7. Neurofibromatosis
8. Porencephalic cyst

## Generalized

**COMMON**
1. Craniolacunia
2. Hydrocephalus, long standing

3. Normal (eg, prematurity)
4. Osteogenesis imperfecta

**UNCOMMON**
1. Aminopterin fetopathy
2. Cleidocranial dysplasia; cranial dysplasia
3. Hypophosphatasia
4. Increased intracranial pressure, other causes
5. Osteodysplasty (Melnick-Needles S.)
6. Progeria
7. Rickets
8. Trisomy 18 S.

*References:*
1. DuBoulay GH: Principles of X-ray Diagnosis of the Skull. (ed 2) London: Butterworths, 1980
2. Swischuk LE: Differential Diagnosis in Pediatric Radiology. Baltimore: Williams & Wilkins, 1984, pp 346-347

## Gamut C-16

# DIFFUSE OR WIDESPREAD DEMINERALIZATION OR DESTRUCTION OF THE SKULL (INCLUDING "SALT AND PEPPER" SKULL)

**COMMON**
*1. Hyperparathyroidism, primary or secondary
*2. Leukemia, lymphoma_g
*3. Metastatic carcinoma or neuroblastoma
*4. Multiple myeloma
*5. Osteomyelitis, diffuse
6. Osteoporosis (eg, senile, postmenopausal) (See B-44)

**UNCOMMON**
1. Anemia_g (eg, sickle cell, thalassemia)
2. Electric burn; thermal burn

3. Idiopathic
4. Meningioma or other meningeal neoplasm
5. Osteomalacia; rickets (See B-46)
6. Osteonecrosis
*7. Paget's disease (osteoporosis circumscripta)
8. Primary malignant neoplasm of skull (eg, Ewing's sarcoma)
9. Radiation necrosis; radium poisoning
10. Steroid therapy; Cushing S.
11. Syphilis

* May show mottled or "salt and pepper" destruction of calvarium.

## Gamut C-17

# EROSION OF THE INNER TABLE OF THE SKULL

**COMMON**

1. Metastasis
2. Osteomyelitis
3. Pacchionian granulation
4. Subdural hematoma, chronic

**UNCOMMON**

1. AV malformation of brain surface
2. Cisterna magna anomaly
3. Epidermoid
4. Glioma or cyst of superficial brain cortex (eg, oligodendroglioma, leptomeningeal cyst)
5. Hemangioma of skull
6. Histiocytosis $X_g$ (esp. eosinophilic granuloma)
7. Meningioma
8. Multiple myeloma
9. Neoplasm of dura, other (eg, sarcoma, melanoma)
10. Porencephaly
11. Sinus pericranii

## Gamut C-18

# BUTTON SEQUESTRUM OF THE SKULL[*]

**COMMON**
1. Eosinophilic granuloma
2. Metastatic carcinoma (esp. breast)
3. Osteomyelitis

**UNCOMMON**
1. [Burr hole or bone flap]
2. [Calvarial "doughnut", idiopathic]
3. Dermoid cyst
4. Epidermoid (primary cholesteatoma)
5. Fibrosing osteitis
6. [Hemangioma]
7. Meningioma
8. Multiple myeloma
9. Necrosis (eg, radiation therapy, radium poisoning, electric burn, electric shock therapy)
10. Paget's disease
11. Sarcoidosis
12. Syphilis
13. Tuberculosis

[*] Round radiolucent skull defect with central bony density or sequestrum.

*References:*
1. Newton TH, Potts DG: Radiology of the Skull and Brain. St. Louis: C.V. Mosby, 1971, p 759
2. Rosen IW, Nadel HI: Button sequestrum of the skull. Radiology 1969;92:969-971
3. Satin R, Usher MS, Goldenberg M: More causes of button sequestrum. J Can Assoc Radiol 1976;27:288-289
4. Sholkoff SD, Mainzer F: Button sequestrum revisited. Radiology 1971;100:649-652
5. Wells PO: Button sequestrum of eosinophilic granuloma of the skull. Radiology 1956;67:746-747

# SOLITARY OSTEOLYTIC SKULL LESION
## (See Gamut C-20)

**COMMON**

*1. Cholesteatoma (inflammatory)
*2. Epidermoid (primary cholesteatoma)
*3. Fibrous dysplasia
 4. Fracture (esp. depressed)
*5. Hemangioma
*6. Histiocytosis $X_g$ (esp. eosinophilic granuloma)
*7. Meningocele, encephalocele, cranium bifidum
 8. Metastasis
 9. Myeloma, plasmacytoma
10. Normal variant (eg, venous lake, enlarged emissary channel, inioindineal canal, pacchionian granulation, parietal foramen, parietal thinning)
*11. Osteomyelitis
12. Paget's disease (osteoporosis circumscripta)
*13. Surgical defect (eg, burr hole, craniotomy flap)

**UNCOMMON**

 1. Arachnoid cyst
 2. AV malformation
 3. Brown tumor of hyperparathyroidism
*4. Calvarial "doughnut", idiopathic
 5. Dermal sinus
 6. Dermoid cyst
 7. Ectopic glial tissue (occipital)
 8. Fibrosing osteitis
 9. Glomus jugulare tumor (base)
10. Hydatid cyst
11. Idiopathic
12. Intraosseous or chronic subdural hematoma
13. Leptomeningeal cyst
*14. Lymphoma$_g$
*15. Mucocele or neoplasm of paranasal sinus

\*16. Necrosis of skull (eg, radiation therapy, electrical or thermal burn)

\*17. Neoplasm of brain or dura with bone erosion (esp. meningioma)

18. Neoplasm or cyst of scalp (eg, carcinoma, rodent ulcer, neurofibroma, sebaceous cyst)

19. Neoplasm of skull, benign

20. Neurofibromatosis (eg, asterion or lambdoid suture defect, absent sphenoid wing)

\*21. Sarcoidosis

22. Sarcoma of bone

\*23. Syphilis

\*24. Tuberculosis, fungus disease_g

\* May have surrounding sclerosis.

### References:

1. DuBoulay GH; Principles of X-ray Diagnosis of the Skull. (ed 2) London: Butterworths, 1980, pp 57-94
2. Lane B: Erosions of the skull. Radiol Clin North Am 1974; 12:257-282
3. Taveras JM, Wood EH: Diagnostic Neuroradiology. (ed 2) Baltimore: Williams & Wilkins, vol 1, 1976

### Gamut C-20

# RADIOLUCENT LESION OR BONE DEFECT IN THE SKULL, SOLITARY OR MULTIPLE
## (See Gamut C-19)

## Congenital or Developmental Defect

1. Congenital arachnoid cyst

\*2. Congenital fibromatosis

\*3. [Craniolacunia (lacunar skull)]

4. Dermoid

5. Ectopic intradiploic glial tissue

6. Encephalocele, meningoencephalocele, dermal sinus, median cleft face S., cranium bifidum

---

7.  Epidermoid (primary cholesteatoma)
8.  Fibrous dysplasia (incl. cortical)
9.  Fontanelle
*10. Frontal fenestra
11.  Hemangioma or arteriovenous malformation of bone or scalp
12.  Inioindineal canal (emissary vein canal)
*13. Neurofibromatosis (eg, asterion or lambdoid suture defect, absent sphenoid wing)
*14. Pacchionian depression
*15. Parietal foramina
*16. Parietal thinning
*17. Venous lake or diploic channel
*18. Wide sutures (See C-27, C-28)

## Traumatic

*1. Burr hole; surgical defect; craniotomy
2.  Fibrosing osteitis
*3. Fracture, simple or depressed
4.  Hematoma (cephalhematoma, intradiploic, subdural); cephalhydrocele
5.  Leptomeningeal cyst

## Inflammatory

1.  Cholesteatoma
2.  Hydatid disease
3.  Mucocele of paranasal sinus
*4. Osteomyelitis, bacterial or fungal$_g$; abscess
*5. Sarcoidosis
*6. Syphilis, yaws
*7. Tuberculosis

## Neoplastic

1.  Aneurysmal bone cyst
2.  Chondroid lesion
3.  Chordoma of clivus
4.  Giant cell tumor (esp. complicating Paget's)

5. Glomus jugulare tumor
*6. Hemangioma, angiomatosis
7. Intracranial tumor with erosion
*8. Lymphoma$_g$, leukemia, chloroma
9. Malignant fibrous histiocytoma
10. Melanotic progonoma
11. Meningioma
*12. Metastasis (incl. neuroblastoma)
*13. Myeloma, plasmacytoma
14. Neoplasm of paranasal sinus or nasopharynx with erosion
15. Neurofibroma of bone or scalp
16. Sarcoma of bone (eg, Ewing's, osteosarcoma, chondrosarcoma, fibrosarcoma)
17. Skin or scalp tumor with invasion (eg, rodent ulcer)

# Miscellaneous

*1. Brown tumor of hyperparathyroidism
*2. Button sequestrum (See C-18)
3. Calvarial "doughnut", idiopathic
*4. Gaucher's disease; Niemann-Pick disease; Weber-Christian disease
5. Hemophilic pseudotumor
*6. Histiocytosis X$_g$
*7. Infantile cortical hyperostosis (Caffey's disease)
*8. Necrosis (eg, radiation therapy, electrical or thermal burn, postoperative bone flap necrosis)
9. Paget's disease (osteoporosis circumscripta)
*10. Parietal thinning, senile

*May be multiple.

*References:*
1. Du Boulay GH: Principles of X-ray Diagnosis of the Skull. (ed 2) London: Butterworths, 1980
2. Jacobson HG: Personal communication
3. Lane B: Erosions of the skull. Radiol Clin North Am 1974; 12:257-282
4. Lo Presti JM: Personal communication
5. Taveras JM, Wood EH: Diagnostic Neuroradiology. (ed 2) Baltimore: Williams & Wilkins, vol 1, 1976

# ENLARGED, ERODED, OR DESTROYED SELLA TURCICA (INCLUDING INTRASELLAR OR PARASELLAR MASS ON CT OR MRI)

## COMMON

1. Aneurysm or ectatic internal carotid artery (cavernous or suprasellar segment); carotid-cavernous fistula
2. Craniopharyngioma
3. Cretinism, hypothyroidism
4. Empty sella S.
5. Increased intracranial pressure, chronic (eg, obstructive hydrocephalus, dilated third ventricle, neoplasm, universal craniosynostosis)
6. Juxtasellar or suprasellar neoplasm, other (eg, meningioma, neurinoma of cranial nerves III to VI, optic chiasm glioma, epidermoid, dermoid, teratoma, hamartoma of tuber cinereum, hypothalamic glioma, germinoma, ectopic pinealoma)
7. [Osteoporosis; osteomalacia; hyperparathyroidism]
8. Pituitary adenoma (eg, chromophobe or eosinophilic adenoma, often with acromegaly or gigantism)

## UNCOMMON

1. Abscess, pituitary
2. Arachnoid cyst, suprasellar or intrasellar, congenital or acquired (eg, after intracranial bleeding, infection, or with storage disease)
3. Basilar (transsphenoid) encephalocele
4. Benign neoplasm of skull base (eg, ossifying fibroma, osteochondroma, osteoma, chondroma)
5. Chordoma
6. Frontal lobe neoplasm
7. Histiocytosis $X_g$ (often leading to diabetes insipidus)
8. Hypogonadism (incl. Turner S.)

9. Infundibular lesion (eg, metastasis, histiocytosis $X_g$, sarcoidosis)

10. Lymphoid hypophysitis (pituitary enlargement, usually with normal sella, in a postpartum woman with thyrotoxicosis)

11. Metastasis (esp. from lung or breast)

12. Mucocele of sphenoid sinus

13. Mucopolysaccharidoses (esp. Hurler S.); mucolipidosis

14. Neoplasm of sphenoid sinus or nasopharynx with local invasion (eg, carcinoma, angiofibroma, giant cell tumor)

15. Neurofibromatosis

16. Optic nerve neoplasm (eg, carcinoma, glioma, neurofibroma, meningioma)

17. Osteomyelitis, granuloma (eg, syphilis, tuberculosis, sarcoidosis, fungus disease$_g$)

18. Oxycephaly

19. Pituitary gland hypertrophy after adrenal ablation (Nelson S.) or with hypothyroidism

20. Pituitary neoplasm, other (eg, adenocarcinoma, carcinosarcoma, lymphoma$_g$, oncocytoma, prolactinoma, choristoma)

21. Postoperative change

22. Rathke cleft cyst

*References:*

1. Doyle FH: Radiology of the pituitary fossa. In: Lodge T, Steiner RE (eds): Recent Advances in Radiology. New York: Churchill Livingstone, 1979, vol 6, pp 121-143

2. DuBoulay GH: Principles of X-ray Diagnosis of the Skull. (ed 2) London: Butterworths, 1980

3. Kaufman B, Chamberlin WB Jr: The "empty" sella turcica. Acta Radiol 1970;13:413-425

4. Lee SH, Rao KC: Cranial Computed Tomography and MRI. (ed 2) New York: McGraw-Hill, 1987, pp 453-477

5. Newton TH, Potts DG: Radiology of the Skull and Brain. St. Louis: C.V. Mosby, 1971, vol 1, book 1, pp 372-402

6. Sage MR, Chan ESH, Reilly PL: The clinical and radiological features of the empty sella syndrome. Clin Radiol 1980; 31:513-519

7. Swischuk LE: Differential Diagnosis in Pediatric Radiology. Baltimore: Williams & Wilkins, 1984, pp 356-357

8. Taveras JM, Wood EH: Diagnostic Neuroradiology. (ed 2) Baltimore: Williams & Wilkins, 1976, vol 1, pp 65-89
9. Teasdale E, et al: The reliability of radiology in detecting prolactin-secreting pituitary microadenomas. Br J Radiol 1981;54:556-571
10. Tindall GT, Hoffman JC Jr: Evaluation of the abnormal sella turcica. Arch Intern Med 1980;140:1078-1083

## Gamut C-22

## SMALL SELLA TURCICA

### COMMON

1. Decreased intracranial pressure (eg, brain atrophy, successful shunt for hydrocephalus)
2. Hypopituitarism; growth hormone deficiency
3. Normal variant

### UNCOMMON

1. Cockayne S.
2. "Contracting skull" (postinflammatory or traumatic cerebral degeneration)
3. Cretinism, treated
4. Deprivation dwarfism
5. Fibrous dysplasia
6. Genetic (primordial) dwarfism
7. Microcephaly  (See C-2)
8. Myotonic dystrophy
9. Prader-Willi S.
10. Radiation therapy during childhood
11. Sheehan S. (postpartum pituitary necrosis)
12. Trisomy 21 S. (Down S.)
13. Vestigial or dysplastic sella

### References:

1. Newton TH, Potts DG: Radiology of the Skull and Brain. St. Louis: C.V. Mosby, 1971, vol 1, book 1, pp 371-372

2. Oh KS, Ledesma-Medina J, Bender TM: Practical Gamuts and Differential Diagnosis in Pediatric Radiology. Chicago: Year Book Medical Publ, 1982, p 8
3. Taybi H, Lachman RS: Radiology of Syndromes, Metabolic Disorders, and Skeletal Dysplasias. (ed 3) Chicago: Year Book Medical Publ, 1990, p 854

## Gamut C-23

# ABNORMAL SELLAR CONFIGURATION

## J-Shaped Sella Turcica

### COMMON
1. Hydrocephalus, mild arrested
2. Normal variant (5% of normal children)
3. Optic chiasm glioma

### UNCOMMON
1. Achondroplasia
2. Cretinism
3. Hurler S. (gargoylism)
4. Neurofibromatosis (sphenoid dysplasia)
5. Pituitary tumor extending anteriorly
6. Subarachnoid cyst (intrasellar)
7. Suprasellar tumor

## Elongated or Stretched Sella

1. Craniopharyngioma or other juxtasellar or suprasellar neoplasm (eg, meningioma)
2. Enlarging head (eg, storage diseases, chondro-dystrophies, hydrocephalus, megalencephaly)
3. Normal variant

## Omega or Scooped Sella

1. Normal (unilateral)
2. Optic chiasm tumor (glioma, neurofibroma)
3. Pituitary fossa tumor

## Dysplastic Sella

1. Neurofibromatosis

*Reference:*
1. Swischuk LE: Differential Diagnosis in Pediatric Radiology. Baltimore: Williams & Wilkins, 1984, pp 356-358

## Gamut C-24

# NORMAL SKULL VARIANTS THAT MAY SIMULATE A FRACTURE

1. Arterial groove (eg, meningeal vessels, middle temporal branch of superficial temporal artery, deep temporal branches of internal maxillary artery, supraorbital artery)
2. Artifact or soft tissue alteration (eg, skin laceration, skin fold, air trapped beneath skin, matted hair, hair braid, rubber band, tape, dressing, linen)
3. Emissary vein, venous lake, diploic channel, sinus groove
4. Fissure, synchondrosis, suture
   a. Cerebellar synchondrosis
   b. Coronal suture
   c. Innominate synchondrosis
   d. Interparietal suture
   e. Intersphenoid synchondrosis
   f. Lambdoid suture
   g. Lateral fissures of the foramen magnum
   h. Lateral interparietal fissure

  i. Lateral sphenoidal suture
  j. Median occipital fissure
  k. Mendosal suture
  l. Metopic suture
  m. Occipitomastoid suture
  n. Parietal fissure
  o. Parietomastoid suture
  p. Spheno-occipital synchondrosis
  q. Squamosal suture
  r. Transverse occipital suture
  s. Unfused planum sphenoidale
 5. Wormian (sutural) bone

### References:

1. Allen WE, Kier EL, Rothman SLG: Pitfalls in the evaluation of skull trauma. Radiol Clin North Am 1973;11:479-503
2. Keats TE: Atlas of Normal Roentgen Variants That May Simulate Disease. (ed 4) Chicago: Year Book Medical Publ, 1988
3. Swischuk LE: The normal pediatric skull: Variations and artifacts. Radiol Clin North Am 1972;10:277-290
4. Tomsick TA: Gamut: Normal skull variant that may simulate a fracture. Semin Roentgenol 1978;13:3

## Gamut C-25

# MULTIPLE WORMIAN (SUTURAL) BONES

## COMMON

1. Cleidocranial dysplasia
2. Cretinism, hypothyroidism
3. Hypophosphatasia
4. Normal; idiopathic
5. Osteogenesis imperfecta
6. Progeria
7. Pyknodysostosis

**UNCOMMON**
1. Aminopterin fetopathy
2. Cerebrohepatorenal S. (Zellweger S.)
3. Chondrodysplasia punctata (Conradi's disease)
4. Familial idiopathic osteoarthropathy (Currarino S.)
5. Hajdu-Cheney S. (idiopathic acro-osteolysis)
6. Hallermann-Streiff S.
7. Hydrocephalus, infantile
8. Kinky-hair S. (Menkes S.); copper deficiency
9. Metaphyseal chondrodysplasia (Jansen)
10. Osteopetrosis, infantile type; sclerosteosis
11. Pachydermoperiostosis
12. Prader-Willi S.
13. [Rickets]
14. Trisomy 21 S. (Down S.)

*References:*

1. Cremin B, Goodman H, Spranger J, et al: Wormian bones in osteogenesis imperfecta and other disorders. Skeletal Radiol 1982;8:35-38
2. Greenfield GB: Radiology of Bone Diseases. (ed 5) Philadelphia: Lippincott, 1990
3. Kozlowski K, Beighton P: Gamut Index of Skeletal Dysplasias. Berlin: Springer-Verlag, 1984, pp 35-36
4. Pryles CV, Khan AJ: Wormian bones. Am J Dis Child 1979;133:380-382
5. Taybi H, Lachman RS: Radiology of Syndromes, Metabolic Disorders, and Skeletal Dysplasias. (ed 3) Chicago: Year Book Medical Publ, 1990, p 855

## Gamut C-26

# DELAYED OR DEFECTIVE CRANIAL OSSIFICATION

## TRANSIENT
### (Spontaneous correction before 3 years of age)

1. Aminopterin fetopathy
2. Cerebrohepatorenal S. (Zellweger S.)

3. Congenital lacunar skull
4. Congenital scalp defect S.
5. Cutis laxa; Ehlers-Danlos S.
6. Hypophosphatasia
7. Kinky-hair S. (Menkes S.)
8. Metaphyseal chondrodysplasia (Jansen)
9. Mucopolysaccharidoses (eg, Hunter, Hurler)
10. Osteogenesis imperfecta
11. Rubinstein-Taybi S.
12. Silver-Russell S.
13. Trisomy 13 S.
14. Trisomy 18 S.
15. Trisomy 21 S. (Down S.)

## INTERMEDIATE
### (Spontaneous correction between 3 and 10 years)

1. Cretinism, hypothyroidism
2. Otopalatodigital S.
3. Pachydermoperiostosis
4. Progeria
5. Rickets

## PROTRACTED
### (Persistence beyond 10 years of age)

1. Cleidocranial dysplasia
2. Cranium bifidum occultum
3. Dermal sinus
4. Encephalocele
5. Frontonasal dysplasia
6. Hypertelorism with Sprengel's deformity
7. Oculo-mandibulo-facial S. (Hallermann-Streiff S.)
8. Parietal foramina; occipital foramina
9. Parietal thinning
10. Pyknodysostosis
11. Stanescu dysostosis
12. Tubular stenosis (Kenny-Caffey S.)

*Reference:*
1. Dorst JP: Personal communication

---

# DELAYED CLOSURE AND/OR INCOMPLETE OSSIFICATION OF SUTURES

## COMMON

1. Cleidocranial dysplasia
2. Cretinism, hypothyroidism
3. Hydrocephalus
4. Increased intracranial pressure (esp. brain neoplasm)
5. Infiltration of sutures (eg, metastatic neuroblastoma, leukemia)
6. Intrauterine growth failure or infection (eg, rubella S.)
7. Normal, prematurity
8. Osteogenesis imperfecta
9. Osteoporosis, severe
10. Rickets
11. Trisomy 21 S. (Down S.)


## UNCOMMON

1. Aminopterin fetopathy
2. Cerebrohepatorenal S. (Zellweger S.)
3. Cranium bifidum
4. Diencephalic S.
5. Familial idiopathic osteoarthropathy (Currarino S.)
6. Fetal primidone S.
7. Hajdu-Cheney S. (idiopathic acro-osteolysis)
8. Hallermann-Streiff S.
9. Hyperparathyroidism, primary infantile or secondary (renal osteodystrophy)
10. Hypoparathyroidism
11. Hypophosphatasia
12. Neurofibromatosis (bone defect along lambdoid suture)
13. Pachydermoperiostosis
14. Progeria
15. Prolonged parenteral hyperalimentation
16. Psychosocial (deprivation) dwarfism
17. Pyknodysostosis

18. Rubinstein-Taybi S.
19. Silver-Russell S.
20. Vitamin A deficiency or intoxication
21. Winchester S.

*References:*
1. Newton TH, Potts DG: Radiology of the Skull and Brain. St. Louis: C.V. Mosby, 1971, vol 1, book 1, pp 232-236
2. Taybi H, Lachman RS: Radiology of Syndromes, Metabolic Disorders, and Skeletal Dysplasias. (ed 3) Chicago: Year Book Medical Publ, 1990, pp 854-855

## Gamut C-28

# SEPARATION OR INFILTRATION OF SKULL SUTURES IN AN INFANT OR CHILD
## (See Gamut C-27)

### COMMON
1. Brain abscess, cerebritis
2. Brain neoplasm (eg, pinealoma, medulloblastoma)
3. Cerebral edema, hemorrhage, or contusion
4. Hydrocephalus
5. Incomplete ossification adjacent to sutures (See C-27)
6. Increased intracranial pressure, other causes
7. Lead poisoning, other encephalopathy
8. Leukemia, lymphoma$_g$
9. Meningitis, meningoencephalitis
10. Neuroblastoma, metastatic
11. Normal (esp. prematurity)
12. Subdural hematoma or hygroma

### UNCOMMON
1. Hydranencephaly
2. Hypervitaminosis A
3. Intracranial cyst

4. Megalencephaly
5. Pseudotumor cerebri
6. Rebound growth of brain and body after treatment for hypothyroidism or deprivation dwarfism

*References:*
1. Swischuk LE: Differential Diagnosis in Pediatric Radiology. Baltimore: Williams & Wilkins, 1984, pp 347-348
2. Swischuk LE: The growing skull. Semin Roentgenol 1974; 9:115-124

## Gamut C-29

# INCREASED SIZE OF THE VASCULAR GROOVES OF THE SKULL

## COMMON
1. AV malformation
2. Hemangioma of skull
3. Meningioma

## UNCOMMON
1. Collateral circulation (eg, thrombosis of a venous sinus, occlusion of internal carotid artery)
2. Fibrous dysplasia
3. Metastasis (eg, thyroid carcinoma, hypernephroma)
4. Pacchionian granulations
5. Paget's disease
6. Sarcoma or other malignant neoplasm of skull

## Gamut C-30

# "HAIR ON END" OR "SUNBURST" PATTERN IN THE SKULL

## Generalized ("Hair on End")

**COMMON**
1. Congenital hemolytic anemias$_g$ (eg, thalassemia, sickle cell disease, hereditary spherocytosis, elliptocytosis)

**UNCOMMON**
1. Congenital cyanotic heart disease with secondary polycythemia
2. Hypernephroma with increased erythropoiesis
3. Iron deficiency anemia, severe
4. Leukemia, lymphoma$_g$
5. Multiple myeloma
6. Polycythemia vera
7. Red cell enzyme deficiencies with secondary reticulocytosis (eg, pyruvate kinase, hexokinase, glucose-6-phosphate dehydrogenase)

## Localized ("Sunburst" Spiculations)

**COMMON**
1. Hemangioma
2. Meningioma
3. Metastasis (esp. neuroblastoma, prostate, breast)

**UNCOMMON**
1. Ewing's sarcoma
2. Osteosarcoma

*References:*
1. Greenfield GB: Radiology of Bone Diseases. (ed 5) Philadelphia: Lippincott, 1990

2. Kohler A, Zimmer EA: Borderlands of the Normal and Early Pathologic in Skeletal Radiology. New York: Grune & Stratton, 1968, p 202

3. Silverman FN: Caffey's Pediatric X-ray Diagnosis (ed 8) Chicago: Year Book Medical Publ, 1985, pp 79-85

4. Swischuk LE: Differential Diagnosis in Pediatric Radiology. Baltimore: Williams & Wilkins, 1984, pp 341-343

5. Wilson JD, et al: Harrison's Principles of Internal Medicine. (ed 12) New York: McGraw-Hill, 1991

# J

# Joints

J

## Gamut J-1

# CONGENITAL SYNDROMES WITH LIMITED JOINT MOBILITY

**COMMON**
1. Achondroplasia (elbow)
2. Arthrogryposis multiplex congenita
3. Bony exostoses or synostoses around a joint (See B-114 and B-115)
4. Mucopolysaccharidoses; $GM_1$ gangliosidosis

**UNCOMMON**
1. Acrocephalosyndactyly (Apert S.)
2. Cerebrohepatorenal S. (third and fifth fingers)
3. Chondrodysplasia punctata, severe (Conradi's disease)
4. Chondroectodermal dysplasia (Ellis-van Creveld S.)
5. Cockayne S.
6. Contractural arachnodactyly
7. Cornelia de Lange S. (elbow)
8. Diabetes, juvenile
9. Diastropic dysplasia
10. Dyschondrosteosis; Madelung's deformity (elbow, wrist)
11. Dysplasia epiphysealis hemimelica (Trevor's disease)
12. Familial dwarfism with stiff joints
13. Hereditary arthro-ophthalmopathy (Stickler S.)
14. Kniest dysplasia
15. Léri's pleonosteosis
16. Metaphyseal chondrodysplasias
17. Metatropic dysplasia
18. Mietens-Weber S. (knee)
19. Multiple cartilaginous exostoses
20. Multiple epiphyseal dysplasia (hip)
21. Myositis (fibrodysplasia) ossificans progressiva
22. Osteochondromuscular dystrophy (Schwartz-Jampel S.)
23. Otopalatodigital S. (elbow)

24. Parastremmatic dwarfism
25. Popliteal pterygium S.
26. Progeria
27. Spondyloepiphyseal dysplasia
28. Spondylometaphyseal dysplasia
29. Trisomy 13 S. (fingers)
30. Trisomy 18 S.
31. Weill-Marchesani S.
32. Winchester S.
33. XXXXY S.

*References:*
1. Jones KL: Smith's Recognizable Patterns of Human Malformation. Philadelphia: W.B. Saunders, 1988
2. Swischuk LE: Differential Diagnosis in Pediatric Radiology. Baltimore: Williams & Wilkins, 1984, p 288
3. Taybi H, Lachman RS: Radiology of Syndromes, Metabolic Disorders, and Skeletal Dysplasias. (ed 3) Chicago: Year Book Medical Publ, 1990, pp 868-869

## Gamut J-2

# CONGENITAL SYNDROMES WITH JOINT LAXITY OR HYPERMOBILITY

## COMMON
1. Marfan S.
2. Morquio S.
3. Trisomy 21 S. (Down S.)

## UNCOMMON
1. Bird-headed dwarfism (Seckel S.)
2. Braham-Lenz S.
3. Coffin-Siris S.
4. Cutis laxa-growth deficiency S.
5. Ehlers-Danlos S.
6. Focal dermal hypoplasia (Goltz S.)

7. Geroderma osteodysplastica
8. Hallermann-Streiff S.
9. Hereditary arthro-ophthalmopathy (Stickler S.)
10. Hypochondroplasia
11. Lenz-Majewski hyperostotic dwarfism
12. LEOPARD S. (lentiginosis S.)
13. Marfanoid hypermobility S.
14. Metaphyseal chondrodysplasia (McKusick)
15. Mucopolysaccharidoses
16. Nail-patella S. (osteo-onychodysplasia)
17. Oculo-cerebro-renal S. (Lowe S.)
18. Osteogenesis imperfecta, congenita and tarda
19. Osteolysis (Hajdu-Cheney S.)
20. Pseudoachondroplasia
21. Spondylo-epi-metaphyseal dysplasia with joint laxity
22. XXXXY S.

*References:*
1. Jones KL: Smith's Recognizable Patterns of Human Malformation. Philadelphia: W.B. Saunders, 1988.
2. Swischuk LE: Differential Diagnosis in Pediatric Radiology. Baltimore: Williams & Wilkins, 1984, p 288
3. Taybi H, Lachman RS: Radiology of Syndromes, Metabolic Disorders, and Skeletal Dysplasias (ed 3) Chicago: Year Book Medical Publ, 1990, p 873

## Gamut J-3

## CONGENITAL SYNDROMES WITH JOINT DISLOCATION OR SUBLUXATION (See Gamut J-2)

**COMMON**
1. Congenital dislocation of hip
2. Congenital dislocation of radial head

3. Dyschondrosteosis; Madelung's deformity (distal ulna)
4. Marfan S.

## UNCOMMON

1. Arthrogryposis (hip)
2. Bird-headed dwarfism (Seckel S.) (hip)
3. Campomelic dysplasia (hips, radial heads)
4. Cornelia de Lange S. (elbow)
5. Diastrophic dysplasia
6. Ehlers-Danlos S.
7. Fanconi S. (pancytopenia-dysmelia S.) (hip)
8. Farber's disease (lipogranulomatosis) (hip)
9. Fetal aminopterin S. (hip)
10. Frontometaphyseal dysplasia
11. Genu recurvatum (knee)
12. Geroderma osteodysplastica (hip)
13. Hereditary arthro-ophthalmopathy (Stickler S.)
14. Humero-spinal dysostosis (knee)
15. Keratoderma palmaris et plantaris familiaris (tylosis)
16. Kniest dysplasia (hip)
17. Larsen S. (elbow, knee, hip)
18. Mesomelic dysplasia (Werner)
19. Mietens-Weber S. (hip)
20. Mucopolysaccharidoses (eg, Morquio S.) (hip, elbow, fingers)
21. Noonan S. (elbow)
22. Oculo-dento-osseous dysplasia (hip)
23. Osteogenesis imperfecta
24. Otopalatodigital S. (elbow)
25. Pseudoachondroplasia (hip)
26. Riley-Day S. (hip)
27. Silver-Russell S. (hip, elbow)
28. Spondylo-epi-metaphyseal dysplasia with joint laxity
29. Whistling face S. (Freeman-Sheldon S.) (hip)
30. Winchester S.
31. XXXXX S.

*References:*
1. Jones KL: Smith's Recognizable Patterns of Human Malformation. Philadelphia:W.B. Saunders, 1988
2. Swischuk LE: Differential Diagnosis in Pediatric Radiology. Baltimore: Williams & Wilkins, 1984, pp 288-289
3. Taybi H, Lachman RS: Radiology of Syndromes, Metabolic Disorders, and Skeletal Dysplasias (ed 3) Chicago:Year Book Medical Publ, 1990, pp 872-873

## Gamut J-4

## MONOARTICULAR JOINT DISEASE

**COMMON**
1. Avascular necrosis (See B-51)
2. Gout
*3. Infectious arthritis (eg, pyogenic, tuberculous, fungal)
4. Osteoarthritis, secondary (eg, trauma, excess wear or mechanical stress, deformity or malignment)

**UNCOMMON**
1. Amyloidosis
2. Neuropathic (Charcot) joint (See J-8)
3. Pigmented villonodular synovitis
4. Pseudogout, other causes of chondrocalcinosis (occasionally)
*5. Reiter S.
*6. Rheumatoid monoarthritis (esp. juvenile); juvenile chronic arthritis
*7. Sympathetic joint effusion (eg, secondary to neoplasm in adjacent bone)
8. Synovial neoplasm (esp. synovioma), cyst, or other lesion (See J-20B)
9. Synovial osteochondromatosis

* Associated with marked periarticular demineralization.

# POLYARTICULAR JOINT DISEASE

## COMMON
1. Ankylosing spondylitis
2. Chondrocalcinosis (eg, pseudogout) (See J-24)
3. Gout
*4. Juvenile chronic arthritis
5. Osteoarthritis, primary or secondary (incl. erosive osteoarthritis)
6. Psoriatic arthritis
*7. Rheumatoid arthritis

## UNCOMMON
1. Acromegaly
2. AIDS (HIV) - associated arthritis
*3. Amyloidosis; familial Mediterranean fever
*4. Collagen disease$_g$ (eg, lupus erythematosus, scleroderma, CREST S., dermatomyositis, polyarteritis nodosa)
5. Enteropathic arthritis (eg, ulcerative colitis, Crohn's disease, Whipple's disease) (esp. sacroiliitis)
6. Hemochromatosis
*7. Hemophilia
8. Jaccoud's arthritis
9. Kashin-Beck disease
*10. Lyme disease
*11. Mixed connective tissue disease (MCTD)
12. Multicentric reticulohistiocytosis (lipoid dermatoarthritis)
13. Neuropathic arthropathy (Charcot joints)
14. Ochronosis
*15. [Regional migratory osteoporosis]
*16. Reiter S.
17. Relapsing polychondritis S.
18. Sarcoidosis
*19. Sjögren S.
*20. Smallpox

21. Viral synovitis, transient (eg, rubella, variola, mumps, serum hepatitis)
22. Wilson's disease

* Associated with periarticular demineralization.

## ARTHRITIS OCCURRING PREDOMINANTLY IN MEN

1. AIDS (HIV) - associated arthritis
2. Ankylosing spondylitis
3. Diffuse idiopathic skeletal hyperostosis (DISH)
4. Gout
5. Hemophilia
6. Ochronosis
7. Psoriatic arthritis
8. Reiter S.

## TRANSIENT ARTHRITIS[*]

1. Behcet S.
2. Dermatomyositis
3. Jaccoud's arthritis
4. Polyarteritis nodosa
5. Relapsing polychondritis
6. Sjögren S.
7. Viral (eg. rubella, mumps, serum hepatitis, AIDS)

* Transient episodes of arthritic symptoms and/or joint effusions that usually subside without residual joint damage.

### Reference:
1. Eisenberg RL: Clinical Imaging: An Atlas of Differential Diagnosis. Rockville, MD: Aspen Publishers, 1988, p 630

# RHEUMATOID-LIKE ARTHRITIS

**COMMON**
1. Ankylosing spondylitis
2. Erosive osteoarthritis, acute
3. Gout
4. Juvenile chronic arthritis (See J-6A)
5. Lupus erythematosus
6. Psoriatic arthritis
7. Reiter S.
8. Scleroderma; CREST S.

**UNCOMMON**
1. Dermatomyositis
2. Enteropathic arthritis
3. Hemochromatosis
4. Jaccoud's arthritis
5. Lipoid dermatoarthritis (reticulohistiocytoma)
6. Mixed connective tissue disease (MCTD)
7. Sjögren S.
8. [Sudeck's atrophy]

## Subgamut J-6A

# CLASSIFICATION OF JUVENILE CHRONIC ARTHRITIS

1. Juvenile-onset adult type (seropositive) rheumatoid arthritis
2. Seronegative chronic arthritis (Still's disease)
   a. Classic systemic disease
   b. Polyarticular disease
   c. Pauciarticular or monoarticular disease
3. Juvenile-onset ankylosing spondylitis

4. Psoriatic arthritis
5. Enteropathic arthritis
6. Miscellaneous arthritis

*Reference:*
1. Resnick D, Niwayama G: Diagnosis of Bone and Joint Disorders. Philadelphia: W.B. Saunders, 1981, p 1009

## Gamut J-7

# DEGENERATIVE ARTHRITIS IN A YOUNG ADULT (PREMATURE OSTEOARTHRITIS)

## COMMON
1. Acromegaly
2. Avascular necrosis (See B-51)
3. Chondromalacia of patella
4. Congenital dislocation of hip
5. Diffuse idiopathic skeletal hyperostosis (DISH, Forestier's disease)
6. [Erosive osteoarthritis]
7. Gout
8. Hemophilia
9. Infectious arthritis (pyogenic, tuberculous, smallpox)
10. Juvenile chronic arthritis
11. Neuropathic (Charcot) joint
12. Obesity; mechanical stress; malalignment
13. Pseudogout (calcium pyrophosphate dihydrate crystal deposition disease)
14. Rheumatoid arthritis (esp. juvenile)
15. Scoliosis
16. Spondylosis deformans
17. Thermal injury (burn, frostbite, electrical)
18. Trauma; postoperative

**UNCOMMON**

1. Amyloidosis, familial Mediterranean fever
2. Congenital bone dysplasias
3. Diabetes, juvenile
4. Ehlers-Danlos S.
5. Exostosis, intra-articular chondroma, dysplasia epiphysealis hemimelica (Trevor's disease)
6. Hemochromatosis
7. Hydroxyapatite deposition disease (HADD)
8. Idiopathic
9. Jackhammer operator's (driller's) disease of wrists
10. Kashin-Beck disease
11. Macrodystrophia lipomatosa
12. Multiple epiphyseal dysplasia (Fairbank)
13. Ochronosis (alkaptonuria)
14. Osteochondritis dissecans
15. Scheuermann's disease
16. Slipped capital femoral epiphysis
17. Spondyloepiphyseal dysplasia
18. Wilson's disease

*Reference:*

1. Greenfield GB: Radiology of Bone Diseases. (ed 5) Philadelphia: Lippincott, 1990

## Subgamut J-7A

# SECONDARY OSTEOARTHRITIS OF THE HIP

**COMMON**

1. Aseptic necrosis of femoral head
2. Athletic activity in adolescence; abnormal stress forces
3. Congenital dislocation of hip
4. Fracture
5. Legg-Perthes disease

6. Previous arthritis (eg, rheumatoid, pyogenic)
7. Slipped capital femoral epiphysis

## UNCOMMON

1. Acetabular dysplasia
2. Acromegaly
3. Endocrine disorders
4. Idiopathic coxa vara
5. Multiple epiphyseal dysplasia (Fairbank)
6. Obesity
7. Ochronosis (alkaptonuria)

*Reference:*
1. Greenfield GB: Radiology of Bone Diseases. (ed 5) Philadelphia: Lippincott, 1990

## Gamut J-8

# NEUROTROPHIC ARTHROPATHY (CHARCOT JOINT)

## COMMON

1. Diabetic myelopathy or neuropathy
2. Syphilis (tabes dorsalis)
3. Syringomyelia
4. Trauma to spinal cord or brain (eg, hemiplegia, paraplegia)

## UNCOMMON

1. Acrodystrophic neuropathy
2. Alcoholism
3. Amyloid neuropathy
4. Charcot-Marie-Tooth S.
5. Congenital disease involving spinal cord (eg, meningomyelocele, diastematomyelia, spina bifida vera)

6. Congenital indifference to pain
7. Cushing S.; systemic or local steroid therapy
8. Gangrene
9. Inflammatory disease of spinal cord (eg, arachnoiditis, acute myelitis, poliomyelitis)
10. Leprosy
11. Multiple sclerosis, other neurological diseases
12. Myelopathy of pernicious anemia
13. Neoplasm of spinal cord
14. Peripheral nerve injury
15. Postrenal transplant
16. Riley-Day S. (familial dysautonomia)

*References:*

1. Greenfield GB: Radiology of Bone Diseases. (ed 5) Philadelphia: Lippincott, 1990
2. Peitzman SJ, Miller JL, Ortega L, et al: Charcot arthropathy secondary to amyloid neuropathy. JAMA 1976;235:1345-1347
3. Resnick D, Niwayama G: Diagnosis of Bone and Joint Disorders. Philadelphia: W.B. Saunders, 1981, pp 2422-2447

## Gamut J-9

## NARROWED JOINT SPACE

**COMMON**

1. Ankylosing spondylitis
2. Avascular necrosis (See B-51)
3. Degenerative arthritis, primary or secondary (eg, post-traumatic)
4. Other chronic arthritides in their more advanced stages (eg, gout, juvenile chronic, enteropathic, neuropathic, lupus, scleroderma, tuberculous, fungal)
5. Psoriatic arthritis
6. Rheumatoid arthritis
7. Septic arthritis

**UNCOMMON**
1. Farber's lipogranulomatosis
2. Hemophilic arthropathy
3. Pigmented villonodular synovitis
4. Postoperative (eg, repair of slipped capital femoral epiphysis)
5. Pseudogout (calcium pyrophosphate dihydrate crystal deposition disease)
6. Reiter S.
7. Smallpox
8. Stickler S. (arthro-ophthalmopathy)
9. Winchester S.

*References:*
1. Resnick D, Niwyama G: Diagnosis of Bone and Joint Disorders. Philadelphia: W.B. Saunders, 1981
2. Swischuk LE: Differential Diagnosis in Pediatric Radiology. Baltimore: Williams & Wilkins. 1984, pp 285-287

## Gamut J-10

## WIDENED JOINT SPACE

**COMMON**
1. Congenital dislocation of hip or other joints
2. Hemarthrosis (eg, trauma, hemophilia or other bleeding disorder)
3. Joint laxity (eg, neuromuscular disorder)
4. Legg-Perthes disease, early
5. Pyogenic arthritis, early
6. Serous effusion (eg, rheumatoid arthritis, collagen disease$_g$, tuberculous arthritis)
7. Toxic (transient) synovitis, severe
8. Traumatic dislocation

## UNCOMMON

1. Acromegaly (cartilage hypertrophy)
2. Inflammatory synovial thickening
   a. Rheumatoid arthritis
   b. Gout
   c. Tuberculous or fungal arthritis
   d. Hemophiliac arthropathy
   e. Winchester S.
   f. Farber's lipogranulomatosis
   g. Pigmented villonodular synovitis
3. Ligamentum teres rupture; retained cartilage fragment (hip)
4. Neurotrophic arthropathy (atrophic type with bone resorption)
5. Synovial neoplasm

*Reference:*

1. Swischuk LE: Differential Diagnosis in Pediatric Radiology. Baltimore: Williams & Wilkins, 1984, pp 284-286

## Gamut J-11

## JOINT EFFUSION

## COMMON

1. Gout
2. Infectious arthritis (pyogenic, tuberculous, fungal, smallpox, Reiter S., Lyme disease)
3. Rheumatoid arthritis (incl. juvenile)
4. Synovitis (acute or chronic)
5. Trauma with hemorrhage

## UNCOMMON

1. Allergic reaction (eg, drugs, insect bite)
2. Bone neoplasm, primary or metastatic
3. Hemophilia

4. Juvenile chronic arthritis
5. Leukemia, lymphoma$_g$
6. Neuropathic (Charcot) joint
7. Pseudogout (calcium pyrophosphate dihydrate crystal deposition disease)
8. Rheumatic fever (acute)

*References:*
1. Greenfield GB: Radiology of Bone Diseases. (ed 5) Philadelphia: Lippincott, 1990
2. Oh KS, Ledesma-Medina J, Bender TM: Practical Gamuts and Differential Diagnosis in Pediatric Radiology. Chicago: Year Book Medical Publ., 1982, p 136
3. Resnick D, Niwayama G: Diagnosis of Bone and Joint Disorders. Philadelphia: W.B. Saunders, 1981

## Gamut J-12

## ARTHRITIS WITH OSTEOPOROSIS

### COMMON
1. Pyogenic arthritis
2. Rheumatoid arthritis

### UNCOMMON
1. AIDS (HIV)-associated arthritis
2. Amyloidosis; familial Mediterranean fever
3. Dermatomyositis, polymyositis
4. Enteropathic arthropathies
5. Fungal arthritis, mycetoma
6. Hemophilia
7. Juvenile chronic arthritis
8. Lupus erythematosus (late)
9. Lyme disease
10. Mixed connective tissue disease (MCTD)
11. [Regional migratory osteoporosis]
12. Reiter S. (acute)

13. Scleroderma
14. Sjögren S.
15. [Sudeck's atrophy]
16. Tuberculous arthritis

## Gamut J-13

# ARTHRITIS WITH LITTLE OR NO OSTEOPOROSIS

## COMMON
1. Ankylosing spondylitis
2. Diffuse idiopathic skeletal hyperostosis (DISH)
3. Gout
4. Neuropathic (Charcot) joint (See J-8)
5. Osteoarthritis (degenerative, traumatic, erosive)
6. Pseudogout (calcium pyrophosphate dihydrate crystal deposition disease)
7. Psoriatic arthritis

## UNCOMMON
1. Amyloidosis
2. Jaccoud's arthritis (post-rheumatic fever)
3. Lupus erythematosus (early)
4. Multicentric reticulohistiocytosis (lipoid dermatoarthritis)
5. Pigmented villonodular synovitis
6. Reiter S. (chronic or recurrent)
7. Sarcoidosis

## ARTHRITIS WITH MULTIPLE SUBLUXATIONS (USUALLY ULNAR DEVIATION IN THE HANDS)

**UNCOMMON**
1. Rheumatoid arthritis

**UNCOMMON**
*1. Ehlers-Danlos S.
*2. Jaccoud's arthritis (post-rheumatic fever)
*3. Juvenile chronic arthritis
*4. Lupus erythematosus
*5. Mixed connective tissue disease (MCTD)
*6. Neuropathic arthropathy with or without destruction
 7. Other advanced arthritis (eg, gouty, tuberculous, fungal$_g$, pyogenic)
 8. Psoriatic arthritis

\* Often without associated bone destruction.

## ARTHRITIS WITH "SWAN-NECK" DEFORMITY*

1. Jaccoud's arthritis
2. Lupus erythematosus
3. Psoriatic arthritis
4. Rheumatoid arthritis
5. Scleroderma

\* Extension at the PIP joint and flexion at the DIP joint of a finger.

*Reference:*
1. Burgener FA, Kormano M: Differential Diagnosis in Conventional Radiology. New York: Thieme Medical Publ, 1991, p 88

**Gamut J-16**

# ARTHRITIS ASSOCIATED WITH PERIOSTITIS

## COMMON
1. Juvenile chronic arthritis
2. Psoriatic arthritis
3. Pyogenic arthritis
4. Reiter S.

## UNCOMMON
1. AIDS (HIV)-associated arthritis
2. Enteropathic arthropathies (rarely)
3. Fungus disease$_g$, mycetoma
4. Hemophilia
5. Hypertrophic osteoarthropathy
6. Rheumatoid (esp. juvenile)
7. Smallpox
8. Tuberculosis

**Gamut J-17**

# CALCANEAL SPUR (PLANTAR SURFACE)

*1. Ankylosing spondylitis
 2. DISH
 3. Hypertrophic osteoarthritis (esp. from running or other chronic trauma)
 4. Idiopathic
*5. Psoriatic arthritis
*6. Reiter S.
*7. Rheumatoid arthritis

* Usually a fluffy rather than sharp spur.

*Reference:*
1. Sholkoff SD, Glickman MD, Steinbach HL: Roentgenology of Reiter's syndrome. Radiology 1970;97:497-503

## Gamut J-18

## CALCANEAL BONE RESORPTION (PLANTAR OR POSTERIOR SURFACE)

**COMMON**
1. Psoriatic arthritis
2. Reiter S.
3. Rheumatoid arthritis

**UNCOMMON**
1. Ankylosing spondylitis
2. Gout
3. Hyperparathyroidism
4. Multicentric reticulohistiocytosis (lipoid dermato-arthritis)
5. Osteomyelitis, decubitus ulcer

*Reference:*
1. Greenfield GB: Radiology of Bone Diseases. (ed 5) Philadelphia: Lippincott, 1990

## Gamut J-19

## ARTHRITIS WITH SOFT TISSUE NODULES

**COMMON**
1. Gout
2. Rheumatoid arthritis

**UNCOMMON**
1. Amyloidosis
2. Multicentric reticulohistiocytosis (lipoid dermatoarthritis)
3. Pigmented villonodular synovitis
4. Sarcoidosis

*Reference:*
1. Kinard RE, Vogler JB III, Helms CA: The nodular arthritides: The importance of soft tissue nodules in the evaluation of arthritic conditions. American Roentgen Ray Society Scientific Exhibit, Boston, 1985

## Gamut J-20

# SOFT TISSUE MASS ABOUT A JOINT

**COMMON**
1. Aneurysm, arteriovenous fistula
2. Bunion (esp. great toe)
3. [Fluid or blood in joint]
4. Ganglion
5. Gouty tophus
6. Infection (esp. abscess)
7. Myositis ossificans
8. Neurotrophic arthropathy (Charcot joint) (See J-8)
9. Synovial cyst (eg, Baker's cyst) (See J-20A)
10. Synovial hypertrophy secondary to arthritis
11. Synovial osteochondromatosis or chondromatosis

**UNCOMMON**
1. Amyloidosis
2. Chondroma, articular or para-articular
3. Hemangioma of synovium
4. Hydatid disease
5. Multiple reticulohistiocytosis (lipoid dermatoarthritis)

6. Neuroma
7. Parosteal sarcoma (esp. osteosarcoma or chondro-sarcoma); other parosteal neoplasm (See B-83)
8. Pigmented villonodular synovitis, giant cell tumor of tendon sheath, xanthoma
9. Synovioma
10. Synovitis, localized nodular

## Subgamut J-20A

## POPLITEAL (BAKER'S) CYST

**COMMON**
1. Internal derangement of knee (meniscal tear, cruciate tear, intra-articular loose body)
2. Osteoarthritis
3. Rheumatoid arthritis (incl. juvenile)

**UNCOMMON**
1. Arthritis, other (eg, septic, gout, pseudogout, lupus erythematosus, Reiter S.)
2. Chondromalacia of patella
3. Granulomatous synovitis (eg, tuberculosis, brucellosis)
4. Idiopathic (esp. in adolescent)
5. Osteochondritis dissecans
6. Pigmented villonodular synovitis
7. Sjögren S.

*References:*
1. Burleson RJ, Bicket WH, Dahlin DC: Popliteal cyst: A clinico-pathologic survey. J Bone Joint Surg 1956; 38:1265-1274
2. Gristina AG, Wilson PD: Popliteal cysts in adults and children: A review of 90 cases. Arch Surg 1964;88:357-363
3. Moore PT: Popliteal cysts. Semin Roentgenol 1982;17:3
4. Resnick D, Niwayama O: Diagnosis of Bone and Joint Diseases. Philadelphia: W.B. Saunders, 1981, pp 1156-1157
5. Weissman BN: Arthrography in arthritis. Radiol Clin North Am 1981;19:379-392

## BENIGN SYNOVIAL LESION INVOLVING A MAJOR JOINT

**COMMON**
1. Localized nodular synovitis
2. Pigmented villonodular synovitis (villonodular teno-synovitis, giant cell tumor of tendon sheath, xanthoma)
3. Synovial cyst (eg, Baker's cyst) (See J-20A)
4. Synovial hypertrophy secondary to arthritis or infection
5. Synovial osteochondromatosis or chondromatosis

**UNCOMMON**
1. Amyloidosis
2. Hemangioma
3. [Intracapsular chondroma]
4. Lipoma

## Gamut J-21

## BONE LESIONS INVOLVING BOTH SIDES OF A JOINT

**COMMON**
*1. Arthritic cysts or erosions (eg, degenerative arthritic cysts or geodes; gouty, rheumatoid, neuropathic or psoriatic erosions)
*2. Infection (esp. granulomatous—tuberculosis, fungus disease, sarcoidosis)
 3. Metastases
 4. Multiple myeloma

**UNCOMMON**

*1. Amyloidosis
 2. Angiomas
 3. Enchondromas; Ollier's disease; Maffucci S.
*4. Hemophilia
*5. Hydatid disease
*6. Jackhammer operator's disease (driller's disease, vibration S.)
 7. Multiple cartilaginous exostoses
 8. Osteopoikilosis; osteopathia striata
*9. Pigmented villonodular synovitis
*10. [Synovioma]

* With joint involvement.

# MULTIPLE FILLING DEFECTS IN THE KNEE OR OTHER JOINTS ON ARTHROGRAPHY

**COMMON**

1. Cartilage or bone fragments from trauma or degenerative joint disease
2. Rheumatoid arthritis
3. Synovial osteochondromatosis or chondromatosis

**UNCOMMON**

1. Blood clots; hemophilic arthritis
2. Gouty tophi
3. Lipoma arborescens
4. Neoplasm (eg, synovial hemangioma)
5. Pigmented villonodular synovitis
6. Tuberculosis

*Reference:*

1. Burgan DW: Lipoma arborescens of the knee: another cause of filling defects on a knee arthrogram. Radiology 1971;101: 583-584

---

Gamut J-23

# CALCIFIED LOOSE BODY IN A JOINT

## COMMON

1. [Chondrocalcinosis (eg, pseudogout) (See J-24)]
2. Degenerative arthritis with detached osteophyte or spur
3. Meniscus fragmentation with calcification
4. Neuropathic (Charcot) joint with debris (See J-8)
5. Osteochondrosis dissecans
6. Synovial osteochondromatosis
7. Trauma (eg, acute fracture with avulsed fragment in joint; loose bodies from old avulsed bone or cartilage fragments)

## UNCOMMON

1. [Dysplasia epiphysealis hemimelica (Trevor's disease) (unilateral intracapsular chondroma involving knee or ankle)]
2. Rheumatoid arthritis, chronic
3. Sequestrum from osteomyelitis, tuberculosis, or pyogenic arthritis
4. [Synovioma]

*Reference:*
1. Moldofsky PJ, Dalinka MK: Multiple loose bodies in rheumatoid arthritis. Skeletal Radiol 1979;4:219-222

## Gamut J-24

# CHONDROCALCINOSIS (CALCIFICATION IN ARTICULAR CARTILAGE)*

## COMMON

1. Calcium pyrophosphate dihydrate (CPPD) crystal deposition disease (pseudogout)

---

2. Degenerative or posttraumatic osteoarthritis
3. Hyperparathyroidism, primary or secondary (renal osteodystrophy)
4. Idiopathic (2% of normals, 3% of elderly)

**UNCOMMON**
1. Acromegaly
2. Chronic pyarthrosis, osteomyelitis
3. Diabetes
4. Gout
5. Hemochromatosis
6. Hydroxyapatite deposition disease (HADD)
7. Hypophosphatasia
8. Ochronosis (alkaptonuria)
9. Oxalosis
10. Wilson's disease

* Calcium may be calcium pyrophosphate, calcium hydroxyapatite, or calcium orthophosphate.

*References:*
1. Greenfield GB: Radiology of Bone Diseases. (ed 5) Philadelphia: Lippincott, 1990
2. Helms CA, et al: CPPD crystal deposition disease or pseudogout. Radiographics 1982;2:40
3. Jensen P: Chondrocalcinosis and other calcifications. Radiol Clin North Am 1988;26:1315-1325
4. Jensen PS, Putman CE: Current concepts with respect to chondrocalcinosis and the pseudogout syndrome. AJR 1975;123:531-539
5. Moskowitz RW, Garcia F: Chondrocalcinosis articularis (pseudogout syndrome). Arch Intern Med 1973;132:87-91
6. Murray RO, Jacobson HG, Stoker DJ: The Radiology of Skeletal Disorders. (ed 3) London: Churchill Livingstone, 1990

# PERIARTICULAR OR INTRA-ARTICULAR CALCIFICATION
## (See Gamuts J-23, J-24)

**COMMON**

1. Degenerative arthritis, loose body, "joint mouse"
2. Gout
*3. Hyperparathyroidism, primary or secondary (renal osteodystrophy)
4. Myositis ossificans
5. Neuropathic (Charcot) joint; paraplegia
6. Osteochondrosis dissecans ("joint mouse")
7. Peritendinitis calcarea (calcific synovitis, bursitis, tendinitis)
8. Posttraumatic (eg, Pellegrini-Stieda disease; avulsed fracture fragment; meniscus fragmentation with calcification)
9. Pseudogout (calcium pyrophosphate dihydrate crystal deposition disease); other causes of chondrocalcinosis (See J-24)
10. Scleroderma; CREST S.
11. Synovial osteochondromatosis
12. Vascular (eg, arteriosclerosis, aneurysm, varix)

**UNCOMMON**

1. Acromegaly
2. Burn
3. Calcinosis circumscripta (usually with collagen disease$_g$)
4. Calcinosis interstitialis universalis
5. Cerebrohepatorenal S. (Zellweger S.) (hip)
6. Chondrodysplasia punctata (Conradi's disease)
7. Dermatomyositis
8. Diabetes
9. Dysplasia epiphysealis hemimelica (Trevor's disease); intracapsular chondroma
10. Fluorosis

11. GM₁ gangliosidosis
12. Hematoma, traumatic or spontaneous; hemophilia
13. Hemochromatosis
14. Hemodialysis, chronic (therapy for renal failure with $1\text{-}\alpha\text{-}OHD_3$)
15. Hydroxyapatite crystal deposition disease (HADD)
16. Hypervitaminosis D
17. Hypoparathyroidism
18. Hypothyroidism (stippling before ossification)
19. Lupus erythematosus
20. Metastatic calcification
21. Milk-alkali S.
22. Mixed connective tissue disease (MCTD)
23. Multiple endocrine neoplasia, type 2
24. Ochronosis (alkaptonuria)
25. Osteochondroma; spur
26. Parosteal sarcoma (eg, osteosarcoma, chondrosarcoma)
27. Pyogenic arthritis
28. Rheumatoid arthritis
29. Sarcoidosis
30. Synovioma
31. Tuberculous arthritis (healed)
*32. Tumoral calcinosis (bursa)
33. Warfarin embryopathy
34. Werner S.
35. Widespread bone destruction (eg, metastatic disease)
36. Wilson's disease

* May show calcium-fluid levels.

*References:*

1. Greenfield GB: Radiology of Bone Diseases. (ed 5) Philadelphia: Lippincott, 1990
2. Resnick D, Niwayama G: Diagnosis of Bone and Joint Disorders. Philadelphia: W.B. Saunders, 1981, pp 1588-1591
3. Taybi H, Lachman RS: Radiology of Syndromes, Metabolic Disorders, and Skeletal Dysplasias. (ed 3) Chicago: Year Book Medical Publ, 1990, p 885

Gamut J-26

## LINEAR SIGNAL IN KNEE MENISCUS ON MRI

1. Degeneration
2. Frank tear
3. Intrasubstance tear
4. [Popliteus tendon sheath (pitfall)]
5. [Posterior ligaments of Humphry and Wrisberg (pitfall)]
6. Postoperative repair (scar)
7. [Transverse ligaments (pitfall)]
8. [Truncation artifact]

*Reference:*
1. Crues JV, et al: Chapter 63, In: Stark DD, Bradley WG (eds): Magnetic Resonance Imaging. (ed 2) St. Louis: CV Mosby, 1992

Gamut J-27

## INCREASED SIGNAL ON T2-WEIGHTED IMAGE AT MENISCO-CARTILAGE JUNCTION OF KNEE

1. Medial collateral ligament tear
2. Menisco-cartilage separation
3. [Normal fat]
4. Synovitis

## INCREASED SIGNAL IN SUPRASPINATUS TENDON ON PROTON DENSITY WEIGHTED IMAGE

1. Contusion
2. [Magic angle effect (nonthickened tendon)]
3. [Normal (fat between tendinous insertions)]
4. Tear
5. Tendinitis (thickened tendon)
6. Tendinosis (degeneration)

*Reference:*
1. Crues JV, et al: Chapter 64, In: Stark DD, Bradley WG (eds): Magnetic Resonance Imaging. (ed 2) St. Louis: CV Mosby, 1992

## INCREASED SIGNAL IN SUPRASPINATUS TENDON ON T2-WEIGHTED IMAGE

1. Partial tear or tendinitis (nondisplaced musculotendinous junction)
2. Post-traumatic contusion
3. Tear (displaced musculotendinous junction)

*Reference:*
1. Crues JV, et al: Chapter 64, In: Stark DD, Bradley WG (eds): Magnetic Resonance Imaging. (ed 2) St. Louis: CV Mosby, 1992

# S

# Soft Tissues

S

S

## SOFT TISSUE OSSIFICATION

**COMMON**
1. Myositis ossificans
2. Paraplegia; other neuropathic states; prolonged immobilization
3. Posttraumatic degenerative arthritis with ossified debris and loose bodies in and around a joint (esp. hip, knee, ankle)
4. Surgical scar; post–major joint replacement
5. Synovial osteochondromatosis (joint)

**UNCOMMON**
1. Burn, severe
2. Myositis (fibrodysplasia) ossificans progressiva
3. Osteosarcoma (soft tissue or parosteal)

## Gamut S-2

## CALCIFICATION IN THE MUSCLES AND SUBCUTANEOUS TISSUES
### (See Gamuts S-3 to S-8)

### Systemic

**COMMON**
1. Dermatomyositis
2. Gout; hyperuricemia
3. Hyperparathyroidism, primary or secondary (renal osteodystrophy)
4. Hypervitaminosis D
5. Paraplegia; poliomyelitis; immobilization osteoporosis
6. Scleroderma; CREST S.; acrosclerosis
7. Vascular, arterial or venous (See S-4)

## UNCOMMON

1. Basal cell nevus S. (Gorlin S.)
2. Calcinosis universalis
3. Calcium pyrophosphate dihydrate crystal deposition disease (pseudogout)
4. Carbon monoxide poisoning
5. Congenital fibromatosis
6. Copper deficiency, nutritional
7. Cystic fibrosis (eg, metastatic calcification)
8. Ehlers-Danlos S.
9. Epidermolysis bullosa
10. Fat necrosis (pancreatitis; Weber-Christian disease; neonatal subcutaneous fat necrosis-pseudosclerema)
11. Fibrogenesis imperfecta ossium
12. Fluorosis
13. Homocystinuria
14. Hypervitaminosis A (ligaments)
15. Hypoparathyroidism, pseudohypoparathyroidism, pseudopseudohypoparathyroidism
16. Idiopathic hypercalcemia (eg, Williams S.)
17. Leprosy (nerves)
18. Lipomatosis
19. Lupus erythematosus
20. Maffucci S.
21. Milk-alkali S.
22. Mixed connective tissue disease (MCTD)
23. Myositis (fibrodysplasia) ossificans progressiva
24. Oxalosis
25. Pachydermoperiostosis
26. Parasites (eg, cysticerci, guinea worms, *Loa loa,* hydatid cysts)
27. Progeria; Werner S.
28. Pseudoxanthoma elasticum
29. Rheumatoid arthritis, ankylosing spondylitis (ligaments)
30. Rothmund-Thomson S.
31. Widespread bone destruction with hypercalcemia (eg, metastases, myeloma, leukemia)

# Nonsystemic, Localized

## COMMON

1. Calcinosis circumscripta (esp. with scleroderma or other collagen disease)
2. Fracture with avulsed fragment
3. Idiopathic, physiologic
4. Injection or inoculation (eg, calcified sterile abscess or fat necrosis; antibiotic, bismuth, calcium gluconate, insulin, camphorated oil, or quinine injection; BCG vaccination)
5. Myositis ossificans (posttraumatic, postoperative - esp. after total hip or knee replacement, or in paraplegia - esp. hip); calcified hematoma
6. Peritendinitis calcarea (calcific bursitis or tendinitis)
7. Vascular, arterial or venous (See S-4)

## UNCOMMON

1. Epithelioma
2. Foreign body granuloma
3. Healing infection or abscess (eg, tuberculosis, pyogenic myositis or fibrositis)
4. Leprosy (nerves)
5. Melorheostosis
6. Neoplasm, benign (eg, hemangioma, lipoma, chondroma, fibromyxoma, leiomyoma, xanthoma)
7. Neoplasm, malignant (eg, soft tissue or parosteal osteosarcoma, chondrosarcoma, fibrosarcoma, liposarcoma; synovioma)
8. Parasite (eg, guinea worm, *Loa loa,* hydatid cyst)
9. Radiation therapy
10. Scar
11. Singleton-Merten S. (subungual, forearm)
12. Thermal injury (eg, burn, frostbite, electrical)
13. Tumoral calcinosis
14. Volkman's contracture

*References:*
1. Edeiken J, Dalinka M, Karasick D: Edeiken's Roentgen Diagnosis of Diseases of Bone. (ed 4) Baltimore: Williams & Wilkins, 1989

2. Gayler BW, Brogdon BG: Soft tissue calcifications in the extremities in systemic disease. Am J Med Sci 1965;590-605

3. Greenfield GB: Radiology of Bone Diseases. (ed 5) Philadelphia: Lippincott, 1990

4. Kuhn JP, Rosenstein BJ, Oppenheimer EH: Metastatic calcification in cystic fibrosis. Radiology 1970;97:59-64

5. Poznanski AK: The Hand in Radiologic Diagnosis. (ed 2) Philadelphia: W.B. Saunders, 1984, p 866

6. Stewart YL, Herling P, Dalinka MK: Calcification in soft tissues. JAMA 1983;250:78-81

7. Taybi H, Lachman RS: Radiology of Syndromes, Metabolic Disorders, and Skeletal Dysplasias. (ed 3) Chicago: Year Book Medical Publ, 1990, pp 893-894

8. Teplick JG, Haskin ME: Roentgenologic Diagnosis. (ed 3) Philadelphia: W.B. Saunders, 1976

## Gamut S-3

# CALCIFICATION IN A BURSA, TENDON, LIGAMENT, OR NERVE

### BURSA

1. Bursal osteochondromatosis
2. Calcific bursitis
3. Gout
4. Hyperparathyroidism
5. Hypervitaminosis D
6. Pseudogout
7. Tumoral calcinosis

### TENDON

1. Calcinosis universalis
2. De Quervain's disease (rare)
3. Diabetes
4. Ganglion (rare)
5. Gout
6. Ochronosis
7. Peritendinitis calcarea (esp. supraspinatus)
8. Pseudogout

## LIGAMENT

1. Ankylosing spondylitis
2. Calcifying aponeurotic fibroma
3. Degenerative change, physiologic (eg, Cooper's ligament, ligamentum nuchae)
4. Fluorosis
5. Hypervitaminosis A
6. Idiopathic
7. Myositis (fibrodysplasia) ossificans progressiva
8. Pellegrini-Stieda disease (medial collateral ligament of knee)
9. Renal osteodystrophy
10. Rheumatoid arthritis

## NERVE

1. Leprosy
2. Neurofibromatosis

*Reference:*
1. Greenfield GB: Radiology of Bone Diseases. (ed 5) Philadelphia: Lippincott, 1990

# VASCULAR CALCIFICATION

## COMMON

1. Aneurysm
2. Arteriosclerosis
3. Hemangioma; arteriovenous malformation
*4. Hyperparathyroidism, primary or secondary (renal osteodystrophy)
5. Mönckeberg's sclerosis (medial sclerosis)
6. Phleboliths (eg, normal, varicose veins, hemangioma, Maffucci S.)
7. Premature atherosclerosis
   a. Familial hyperlipemia

  b. Generalized (idiopathic) arterial calcification of infancy

  c. Osteogenesis imperfecta tarda

  d. Progeria

  e. Secondary hyperlipemia

   i. Cushing S.

   ii. Diabetes

   iii. Glycogen storage disease

   iv. Hypothyroidism

   v. Lipodystrophy

   vi. Nephrotic S.

   vii. Renal homotransplantation

  f. Werner S.

## UNCOMMON

 1. Buerger's disease

 2. Calcified thrombus (eg, vena cava, portal vein, left atrium, pulmonary artery, peripheral artery, Leriche S.)

 3. Cystic fibrosis

 4. Gout, hyperuricemia

 5. Homocystinuria

 *6. Hypervitaminosis D

 7. Hypoparathyroidism

 *8. Idiopathic hypercalcemia (Williams S.)

 *9. Immobilization

*10. Milk-alkali S.

 11. Ochronosis (alkaptonuria)

 12. Oxalosis

 13. Pseudoxanthoma elasticum

 14. Radiation therapy

 15. Raynaud's disease

*16. Sarcoidosis

 17. Takayasu's arteritis

 18. Thermal injury (eg, burn, frostbite)

*19. Widespread bone destruction (eg, metastatic disease)

\* Hypercalcemia.

*References:*

 1. Taybi H, Lachman RS: Radiology of Syndromes, Metabolic Disorders, and Skeletal Dysplasias. (ed 3) Chicago: Year Book Medical Publ, 1990, p 829

2. Teplick JG, Haskin ME: Roentgenologic Diagnosis. (ed 3) Philadelphia: W.B. Saunders, 1976

## Gamut S-5

# CALCIFICATION ABOUT THE FINGERTIPS

**COMMON**
1. Scleroderma (incl. CREST S., acrosclerosis)

**UNCOMMON**
1. Calcinosis circumscripta or universalis
2. Dermatomyositis
3. Epidermolysis bullosa
4. Lupus erythematosus
5. Mixed connective tissue disease (MCTD)
6. Raynaud's disease
7. Rothmund-Thomson S.

*References:*
1. Greenfield GB: Radiology of Bone Diseases. (ed 5) Philadelphia: Lippincott, 1990
2. Taybi H, Lachman RS: Radiology of Syndromes, Metabolic Disorders, and Skeletal Dysplasias. (ed 3) Chicago: Year Book Medical Publ, 1990, p 893

## Gamut S-6

# CALCIFICATION IN LYMPH NODES

**COMMON**
1. Histoplasmosis
2. Idiopathic
3. Tuberculosis

## UNCOMMON

1. BCG vaccination
2. Coccidioidomycosis
3. Filariasis
4. Granulomatous disease of childhood
5. Lymphoma (postradiation therapy)
6. Metastasis from osteosarcoma or other calcifying neoplasm (eg, ovarian, thyroid, colon)

*Reference:*

1. Greenfield GB: Radiology of Bone Diseases. (ed 5) Philadelphia: Lippincott, 1990

---

## Gamut S-7

# SOLITARY LARGE CALCIFIED SOFT TISSUE MASS ADJACENT TO BONE (See Gamuts S-1 to S-3, S-8)

## COMMON

1. Gouty tophus
2. Myositis ossificans
3. Osteochondroma

## UNCOMMON

1. Aneurysm
2. Calcifying aponeurotic fibroma
3. Ganglion (rarely)
4. Hemangioma
5. Hyperparathyroidism, primary or secondary
6. Hypervitaminosis D
7. Lipoma
8. Paraplegia
9. Parosteal osteoma or chondroma
10. Parosteal sarcoma
11. Soft tissue osteosarcoma or chondrosarcoma
12. Synovioma
13. Tumoral calcinosis

---

# SOFT TISSUE TUMOR WITH ASSOCIATED CALCIFICATION OR OSSIFICATION (See Gamut S-7)

## BENIGN

1. Benign mesenchymoma
2. Calcifying aponeurotic fibroma
3. Chondroma
4. Desmoid tumor
*5. Hemangioma (phleboliths)
6. Leiomyoma
*7. Lipoma
*8. [Myositis ossificans; calcified or ossified hematoma]
*9. [Synovial osteochondromatosis]
10. [Tumoral calcinosis]

## MALIGNANT

*1. Chondrosarcoma (conventional, mesenchymal)
2. Leiomyosarcoma
3. Liposarcoma
4. Malignant fibrous histiocytoma
5. Malignant schwannoma, neurofibrosarcoma
6. Osteosarcoma
*7. Synovioma (synovial sarcoma)

* Common.

### References:

1. Dorfman HD, Bhagavan BS: Malignant fibrous histiocytoma of soft tissue with metaplastic bone and cartilage formation: A new radiologic sign. Skeletal Radiol 1982; 8:145-150
2. Pringle J, Stoker DJ: Case report 110: Juvenile aponeurotic fibroma. Skeletal Radiol 1980;5:53-55

## Gamut S-9

# SOFT TISSUE MASS WITH UNDERLYING BONE EROSION OR DESTRUCTION

## COMMON
1. Abscess, cellulitis
2. Aneurysm (esp. aorta)
3. Carcinoma of skin or mouth
4. Decubitus ulcer
5. Gouty tophus
6. Rheumatoid arthritis

## UNCOMMON
1. Amyloidosis
2. Angioma; arteriovenous fistula
3. Carcinoma developing in sinus tract of osteomyelitis or tropical ulcer
4. Congenital fibromatosis
5. Fungus disease$_g$ (eg, actinomycosis, blastomycosis)
6. Ganglion
7. Glomus tumor
8. Hemophilia
9. Hyperkeratosis plantaris et palmaris
10. Kaposi sarcoma
11. Meningioma
12. Multicentric reticulohistiocytosis (lipoid dermatoarthritis)
13. Neurofibroma; neurofibromatosis
14. Neuroma (eg, Morton's neuroma of toe)
15. Parachordoma
16. [Parosteal sarcoma or other neoplasm (See B-83)]
17. Pigmented villonodular synovitis; giant cell tumor of tendon sheath
18. Sarcoma of soft tissues
19. Sebaceous or other cyst
20. Surfer's knot
21. Synovioma

# CLASSIFICATION OF SOFT TISSUE TUMORS

| BENIGN | MALIGNANT |
|---|---|

## Muscle

| | |
|---|---|
| Leiomyoma | Leiomyosarcoma |
| Leiomyoblastoma | Rhabdomyosarcoma |
| Rhabdomyoma | |

## Fat

| | |
|---|---|
| Lipoma | Liposarcoma |
| Lipomatosis | |
| Lipoblastoma | |
| Hibernoma | |

## Connective Tissue

| | |
|---|---|
| Fibroma | Fibrosarcoma |
| Benign fibrous histiocytoma | Malignant fibrous histiocytoma |

Fibromatoses
  Juvenile variants
    Angiofibroma
    Congenital generalized
      fibromatosis
    Fibromatous coli
    Juvenile aponeurotic
      fibroma
    Progressive myositis

  Adult variants
    Aggressive fibromatoses
    Idiopathic retroperitoneal fibrosis
    Keloid
    Myositis (fibrodysplasia)
      ossificans progressiva
    Palmar and plantar
      fibromatoses
    Pseudosarcomatous
      fasciitis

| BENIGN | MALIGNANT |
|---|---|

### Peripheral Nerve

| Schwannoma (neurilemoma), neurofibroma, neurofibromatosis | Malignant schwannoma (neurofibrosarcoma) |
|---|---|

### Sympathochromaffin Tissue

| Ganglioneuroma (differentiated) | Ganglioneuroblastoma |
|---|---|
| Pheochromocytoma | Neuroblastoma |
| | Malignant pheochromocytoma |
| | Neuroepithelioma |

### Carotid Body and Allied Structures

| Carotid body tumor | Malignant carotid body tumor |
|---|---|
| Paraganglioma | Malignant paraganglioma |

### Synovia

| Giant cell tumor of tendon sheath | Synovioma (synovial sarcoma) |
|---|---|
| | Clear-cell sarcoma of tendon sheath |
| Xanthoma | Fibrous xanthosarcoma |
| Ganglion | |
| Pigmented villonodular synovitis | |

### Angiomatous Tissue (Vascular or Lymphatic)

| Hemangioma | Angiosarcoma; hemangioendothelioma |
|---|---|
| Angiomatoses | |
| Glomus tumor | |
| Benign hemangiopericytoma | Malignant hemangiopericytoma |
| | Kaposi's sarcoma |
| Lymphangioma, cavernous; cystic hygroma | Lymphangiosarcoma |
| | Extranodal lymphoma |
| | Extramedullary plasmacytoma |

### Heterotopic Bone and Cartilage

| Myositis ossificans | Soft tissue osteosarcoma |
|---|---|
| Benign chondroma | Soft tissue chondrosarcoma |

**BENIGN**       **MALIGNANT**

## Uncertain or Mixed Tissue Origin

Granular cell myoblastoma    Malignant granular cell
Benign mesenchymoma             myoblastoma
Intramuscular myxoma         Alveolar soft-part sarcoma
                             Malignant mesenchymoma
                             Parachordoma
                             Malignant fibrous mesothelioma
                             Extraskeletal Ewing's sarcoma

## Others (Including Processes that May Mimic Neoplasm)

Inflammatory mass (eg,       Metastasis
   pyomyositis)              Malignant teratoma
Hematoma
Synovial cyst; popliteal
   cyst
Primary bone neoplasm
   invading soft tissue
Bursal swelling (incl.
   iliopsoas bursa)
Aneurysm
Arteriovenous malformation
   or fistula
Gardner S.
Accessory muscle mass
Wart, hyperkeratosis,
   other dermatological
   conditions
Traumatic neuroma

*Reference:*

1. Greenfield GB: Radiology of Bone Diseases. (ed 4) Philadelphia: Lippincott, 1986, pp 713-714

## Gamut S-11

# DISEASES AFFECTING MUSCLE TO FAT RATIO

## Diminution of Muscle: Cylinder Ratio (Below 0.64) (Decreased Muscle Mass, Often Increased Fat)

**COMMON**
1. Muscular dystrophy (dystrophia myotonica)
2. Paralysis (eg, poliomyelitis, meningomyelocele, brain damage)
3. [Steroid therapy, Cushing S. (increased subcutaneous fat)]

**UNCOMMON**
1. Amyotonia congenita (Oppenheim's disease)
2. Arthrogryposis multiplex congenita
3. Benign congenital hypotonia (Walton)
4. Disseminated lipogranulomatosis
5. Prader-Willi S.
6. Spinal atrophy, progressive (Werdnig-Hoffmann disease)
7. Spondyloepiphyseal dysplasia congenita

## Increase of Muscle: Cylinder Ratio (Over 0.72) Diminution in Subcutaneous Fat

**COMMON**
1. Malnutrition, cachexia, debilitating disease (eg, anorexia nervosa)

**UNCOMMON**
1. Diencephalic S.
2. Hyperthyroidism
3. Lipoatrophic diabetes (total lipodystrophy)

---

4. Mucopolysaccharidoses (eg, Hurler, Morquio)
5. Progeria; Werner S.
6. Renal tubular acidosis
7. Scleroderma, dermatomyositis

## Increase in Muscle Mass

**COMMON**
1. Exercise hypertrophy

**UNCOMMON**
1. Congenital muscular hypertrophy (de Lange)
2. Kocher-Debré-Sémélaigne S.
3. Muscle tumor or infection (pyomyositis)
4. Pseudohypertrophic muscular dystrophy

## Increase in Fat: Normal Muscle

**COMMON**
1. Exogenous obesity
2. Steroid therapy

**UNCOMMON**
1. Cushing S.
2. Laurence-Moon-Biedl S.
3. Prader-Willi S.

*References:*
1. Greenfield GB: Radiology of Bone Diseases. (ed 5) Philadelphia: Lippincott, 1990
2. Litt RE, Altman DH: Significance of the muscle cylinder ratio in infancy. AJR 1967;100:80-87
3. Swischuk LE: Differential Diagnosis in Pediatric Radiology. Baltimore: Williams & Wilkins, 1984, p 293-295

# THICKENING OF HEEL PAD (GREATER THAN 23 MM)

## COMMON
1. Acromegaly
2. Generalized edema (eg, congestive heart failure, deep vein thrombosis, lymphedema)
3. Infection of soft tissues (eg, mycetoma)
4. Normal variant; genetic (esp. black and Polynesian males)
5. Obesity; high body weight (over 200 pounds)
6. Trauma

## UNCOMMON
1. Dilantin therapy
2. Myxedema; thyroid acropachy
3. Occupational
4. Pachydermoperiostosis

*References:*
1. Greenfield GB: Radiology of Bone Diseases. (ed 5) Philadelphia: Lippincott, 1990
2. Kattan KR: Thickening of the heel pad associated with long-term Dilantin therapy. AJR 1975;124:52-56
3. Kho KM, Wright AD, Doyle FH: Heel pad thickness in acromegaly. Br J Radiol 1970;43:119-122

## Gamut S-13

# SOFT TISSUE EMPHYSEMA OR GAS

1. Gas abscess (pyomyositis from *Staph. aureus*)
2. Gas phlegmon, gas gangrene (clostridial infection)
3. Infiltration of air (eg, after fractured ribs with lung injury, fractured trachea or bronchi, tracheostomy, thoracotomy, open wound, hypodermoclysis)

*Reference:*
1. Greenfield GB: Radiology of Bone Diseases. (ed 5) Philadelphia: Lippincott, 1990

## Gamut S-14

# SWELLING OF THE INTERSTITIAL MARKINGS OF THE SOFT TISSUES ("RETICULATION" OF SOFT TISSUES)

## COMMON
1. Congestive heart failure
2. Edema, other causes
3. Infection of soft tissues (eg, cellulitis, tuberculosis, fungus disease$_g$, mycetoma)
4. Lymphatic obstruction; Milroy's disease
5. Neoplasm primary in soft tissues (eg, vascular or lymphatic tumor) or secondary to bone neoplasm
6. Osteomyelitis
7. Thermal injury (eg, burn, frostbite, electrical)
8. Trauma; spontaneous hemorrhage

## UNCOMMON
1. [Acromegaly]
2. Erythroblastosis fetalis
3. Infantile cortical hyperostosis (Caffey's disease)
4. Melorheostosis
5. Myositis (fibrodysplasia) ossificans progressiva (early)
6. Myxedema; thyroid acropachy
7. Nephrosis, nephritis
8. Neurofibromatosis
9. Sudeck's atrophy

*Reference:*
1. Greenfield GB: Radiology of Bone Diseases. (ed 5) Philadelphia: Lippincott, 1990

## Gamut S-15

# LYMPHANGIECTASIA
# (LYMPHATIC VESSEL DYSPLASIA)

1. Cirrhosis of liver
2. Filariasis
3. Infection (eg, tuberculosis, histoplasmosis, other fungi$_g$)
4. Neoplasm (lymphoma$_g$, lymphangioma, metastases to nodes)
5. Noonan S.
6. Primary congenital lymphatic dysplasia (isolated)
7. Traumatic, postoperative
8. Turner S.

*References:*
1. Brown LR, Reiman HM, Rosenow EC III, et al: Intrathoracic lymphangioma. Mayo Clin Proc 1986;61:882-892
2. Hoeffel JC, Juncker P, Remy J: Lymphatic vessels dysplasia in Noonan's syndrome. AJR 1980;134:399-401

## Gamut S-16

# LYMPHATIC OBSTRUCTION ON
# LYMPHANGIOGRAM (LYMPHEDEMA)

**COMMON**
1. Filariasis
2. [High pressure injection of contrast media]
3. Lymphoma$_g$ (esp. Hodgkin's)
4. Metastases to lymph nodes
5. Postoperative (eg, following excision of lymph nodes and damage to lymphatics, esp. radical mastectomy); lymphocyst, lymphocele
6. Trauma (peripheral lymphedema from extensive skin loss or burn; injury to cisterna chyli causing chylothorax)

**UNCOMMON**
1. Inflammation, lymphadenitis, phlebitis
2. Lymphangioma (esp. of thoracic duct)
3. [Primary lymphedema]
   a. Lymphedema congenita (eg, Milroy's disease; also seen with Turner S.)
   b. Lymphedema praecox (females, ages 9 to 25)
   c. Lymphedema tarda (after age 35)
4. Radiation therapy

*References:*

1. Escobar-Prieto A, Gonzalez G, Templeton AW, et al: Lymphatic channel obstruction: Patterns of altered flow dynamics. AJR 1971;113:366-375
2. Sutton D, Young JWR: A Short Textbook of Clinical Imaging. London: Springer-Verlag, 1990, pp 253-254

## Subgamut S-16A

# ROENTGEN SIGNS OF LYMPHATIC CHANNEL OBSTRUCTION

1. Backflow
2. Collateral circulation
3. Dilatation of lymph vessels
4. Extravasation
5. Stasis of lymph flow

## Gamut S-17

# FILLING DEFECT IN LYMPH NODE ON LYMPHANGIOGRAM

**COMMON**
1. Granulomatous disease (eg, sarcoidosis, tuberculosis, fungus disease$_g$)
2. Idiopathic

3. Lymphoma$_g$
4. Metastatic neoplasm (eg, carcinoma, melanoma, sarcoma)

**UNCOMMON**
1. Acute lymphadenitis (abscess)
2. Amyloidosis
3. Fatty replacement
4. Multiple myeloma
5. Normal anatomic hilum
6. Reactive hyperplasia of collagen disease$_g$ (eg, rheumatoid arthritis)
7. Sjögren S.

*References:*
1. Kuisk H: Technique of Lymphography and Principles of Interpretation. St Louis: Warren H Green, 1971
2. Wallace S, Jackson L, Dodd GD, Greening RR: Lymphangiographic interpretation. Radiol Clin North Am 1965;3: 467-485

# V

# Vertebral Column (Spine) and Its Contents

## ABNORMAL SIZE, SHAPE, OR HEIGHT OF VERTEBRAE

## ABNORMAL DENSITY OR DESTRUCTION OF VERTEBRAE

V

**V**

# CONGENITAL SYNDROMES WITH VERTEBRAL ABNORMALITY
## (See Gamuts V-12 to 16 and V-21 to 24)

## COMMON

1. Achondroplasia (narrow lumbar spinal canal, lower thoracic kyphosis, lumbar lordosis)
2. Cleidocranial dysplasia (spina bifida, kyphoscoliosis)
3. Cretinism, hypothyroidism (kyphosis, beaked, flat vertebrae)
4. Diastrophic dysplasia (kyphoscoliosis, platyspondyly, narrow lumbar spinal canal)
5. Klippel-Feil S. (cervical block vertebrae)
6. Mucopolysaccharidoses, esp. Morquio S. (atlanto-axial subluxation, narrow canal, kyphoscoliosis)
7. Multiple epiphyseal dysplasia (Fairbank) (hemivertebrae, platyspondyly)
8. Neurofibromatosis (kyphoscoliosis)
9. Osteogenesis imperfecta (scoliosis, fractured vertebrae)
10. Osteopetrosis (dense vertebrae, fractures)
11. Pseudoachondroplasia (kyphoscoliosis)
12. Spondyloepiphyseal dysplasia, all forms (kypho-scoliosis, platyspondyly)
13. Spondylometaphyseal dysplasia (kyphosis)
14. Thanatophoric dysplasia (platyspondyly, narrow spinal canal)
15. Trisomy 21 S. (Down S.) (atlanto-axial subluxation)

## UNCOMMON

1. Achondrogenesis (lumbar vertebrae appear absent)
2. Acrodysostosis (narrow spinal canal)
3. Arteriohepatic dysplasia (butterfly vertebrae, narrow spinal canal)
4. Asphyxiating thoracic dysplasia
5. Basal cell nevus S. (Gorlin S.)
6. Bird-headed dwarfism (Seckel S.) (kyphoscoliosis)

7. Campomelic dysplasia (hypoplastic cervical spine, kyphosis)
8. Cervico-oculo-acoustic S. (cervical segmentation malformation)
9. Chondrodysplasia punctata (Conradi's disease) (kyphoscoliosis, atlanto-axial subluxation)
10. Cockayne S.
11. Dysosteosclerosis (platyspondyly)
12. Dyssegmental dysplasia (short spine, ovoid or mis-shapen vertebrae)
13. Ehlers-Danlos S. (scoliosis, spondylolisthesis)
14. Enchondromatosis (Ollier's disease) (kyphoscoliosis)
15. Fetal alcohol S.
16. Focal dermal hypoplasia (Goltz S.)
17. Freeman-Sheldon S. (whistling face S.)
18. Geroderma osteodysplastica (platyspondyly)
19. GM$_1$ gangliosidosis; fucosidosis (platyspondyly)
20. Goldenhar S.
21. Hajdu-Cheney S. (kyphoscoliosis, osteoporosis)
22. Holt-Oram S.
23. Homocystinuria (kyphoscoliosis, osteoporosis, "cod-fish vertebrae")
24. Hyperphosphatasia (scoliosis, biconcave vertebrae)
25. Hypochondroplasia (narrow spinal canal, lordosis, platyspondyly)
26. Idiopathic hypercalcemia (Williams S.) (dense vertebrae, kyphoscoliosis)
27. Incontinentia pigmenti S.
28. Kniest dysplasia (platyspondyly, lordosis, kypho-scoliosis, narrow spinal canal)
29. Larsen S. (cervical kyphosis)
30. Marfan S. (scoliosis, spondylolisthesis)
31. Marshall S. (platyspondyly)
32. Metaphyseal chondrodysplasias (Jansen, McKusick) (atlanto-axial instability)
33. Metaphyseal dysplasia (Pyle's disease) (platyspondyly)
34. Metatropic dysplasia (kyphoscoliosis, platyspondyly, atlanto-axial subluxation)
35. Nail-patella S. (osteo-onychodysplasia) (spina bifida)

36. Narrow lumbar spinal canal S.
37. Oculo-mandibulo-facial S. (Hallermann-Streiff S.) (spina bifida)
38. Oculovertebral S. (hemivertebrae, block vertebrae)
39. Osteochondromuscular dystrophy (Schwartz-Jampel S.) (kyphoscoliosis, platyspondyly)
40. Osteodysplasty (Melnick-Needles S.) (increased vertebral height, anterior concavity)
41. Osteoglophonic dwarfism (platyspondyly, narrow spinal canal)
42. Otopalatodigital S. (posterior spinal defects)
43. Parastremmatic dwarfism (kyphoscoliosis, platyspondyly)
44. Patterson S. (pseudoleprechaunism)
45. Popliteal web S. (spina bifida)
46. Prader-Willi S. (kyphosis)
47. Progeria
48. Radial aplasia-thrombocytopenia S.
49. Rothmund-Thomson S. (flat, elongated vertebrae)
50. Rubinstein-Taybi S.
51. Shawl scrotum S. (hypoplastic C1, subluxation C1-C2)
52. Short rib-polydactyly S. (misshapen, poorly ossified vertebrae, coronal clefts)
53. Smith-McCort S. (platyspondyly)
54. Spondylocostal dysostosis (fused, absent, butterfly, or hemivertebrae; kyphoscoliosis)
55. Spondylo-epi-metaphyseal dysplasia (kyphoscoliosis)
56. Spondyloperipheral dysplasia (platyspondyly)
57. Stickler S. (arthro-ophthalmopathy)
58. Trisomy 13 S.
59. Trisomy 18 S.

*References:*

1. Felson B, (ed): Dwarfs and other little people. Semin Roentgenol 1973;8:258-259
2. Jones KL: Smith's Recognizable Patterns of Human Malformation. Philadelphia: W.B. Saunders, 1988
3. Kozlowski K, Beighton P: Gamut Index of Skeletal Dysplasias. Berlin: Springer-Verlag, 1984, p 41

4. Taybi H, Lachman RS: Radiology of Syndromes, Metabolic Disorders, and Skeletal Dysplasias. (ed 3) Chicago: Year Book Medical Publ, 1990

## Gamut V-2

# NONSPINAL CONDITIONS ASSOCIATED WITH VERTEBRAL ANOMALIES

## COMMON

1. Cloacal abnormality
2. Congenital heart disease
3. Genitourinary abnormality
4. Neurofibromatosis
5. Sprengel's deformity

## UNCOMMON

1. Neurenteric cyst; duplication cyst
2. Venolobar S. (eg, scimitar S., lobar agenesis)

## Gamut V-3

# KYPHOSIS

## COMMON

1. Congenital spinal anomaly (eg, fused vertebrae, hemivertebra, spina bifida with meningocele, bony bar)
2. Congenital syndromes (esp. achondroplasia, chondro-dystrophies, storage diseases, neurofibromatosis) (See V-1)
3. Fracture, traumatic or pathologic; dislocation

4. Idiopathic
5. Infection (eg, spinal osteomyelitis or tuberculosis—Pott's disease)
6. Neoplasm of spine, primary or metastatic; multiple myeloma
7. Neuromuscular disorder with hypotonia (eg, cerebral palsy, muscular dystrophy, myasthenia gravis)
8. [Normal in infants (thoracolumbar; C2-3 angulation)]
9. Osteoporosis (esp. senile or postmenopausal) (See B-44)
10. Paget's disease
11. Paralysis (eg, poliomyelitis, paraplegia)
12. Posture, faulty or occupational (upper thoracic, changes with position)
13. Rheumatoid or ankylosing spondylitis
14. Scheuermann's disease (juvenile kyphosis)

## UNCOMMON
1. Acromegaly; excessive endocrine growth
2. Charcot spine
3. Cretinism, hypothyroidism
4. Generalized weakness
5. Osteomalacia, rickets
6. Radiation therapy atrophy
7. Syringomyelia

*Reference:*
1. Schmorl G, Junghanns H: The Human Spine in Health and Disease. (ed 2) New York: Grune and Stratton, 1971, pp 344-362

## Gamut V-4

## SCOLIOSIS

### COMMON
1. Chest wall abnormality (eg, asymmetric chest, congenital rib anomalies, Sprengel's deformity)

  2. Congenital spinal anomaly (eg, fusion of posterior elements, unilateral bar, meningomyelocele, segmentation anomaly, wedge vertebra, hemivertebra, Klippel-Feil S.)

  3. Congenital syndromes (esp. Marfan S., homocystinuria, osteogenesis imperfecta, storage diseases, neurofibromatosis) (See V-1)

  4. Idiopathic

  5. Infection (eg, spinal tuberculosis, osteomyelitis)

  6. Leg shortening or amputation; pelvic tilt; foot deformity

  7. Neoplasm, intraspinal or extraspinal, primary or metastatic; multiple myeloma

  8. Neuromuscular disorder with hypotonia (eg, cerebral palsy, muscular dystrophy, Friedreich's ataxia)

  9. Osteoporosis (See B-44)

10. Paralysis (eg, poliomyelitis, paraplegia, hemiparesis, hemiplegia)

11. Postoperative (eg, thoracoplasty, pneumonectomy)

12. [Postural-changes with position]

13. Pulmonary or pleural disease, unilateral (eg, fibrosis, fibrothorax, empyema, hypoplastic lung)

14. Spasm (eg, retroperitoneal, psoas, or abdominal abscess, inflammation, or hemorrhage; ureteral or renal calculus)

15. Trauma (fracture, subluxation)

**UNCOMMON**

  1. Congenital heart disease (eg, ASD, tetralogy)

  2. Neurenteric cyst, duplication cyst

  3. Osteoid osteoma

  4. Radiation therapy atrophy

  5. Rickets

  6. Syringomyelia

*Reference:*

  1. Schmorl G, Junghanns H: The Human Spine in Health and Disease. (ed 2) New York: Grune and Stratton, 1971, pp 364-374

## Gamut V-5

# PARASPINAL SOFT TISSUE MASS

**COMMON**
1. Abscess
2. Aortic aneurysm; tortuous aorta
3. [Esophageal dilatation; achalasia]
4. Hematoma, traumatic or spontaneous
5. [Hiatal hernia]
6. Idiopathic; anatomic variant
7. Lymphadenopathy, any cause
8. Lymphoma$_g$, leukemia
9. Metastatic neoplasm
10. Myeloma
11. Neurogenic tumor (neurofibroma, neurilemoma, ganglioneuroma, neuroblastoma); intraspinal tumor of hourglass type
12. [Osteoarthritis (spondylosis deformans); other arthritis with spur formation; DISH; extruded disk]
13. Osteomyelitis of spine with abscess (eg, tuberculous, sarcoid, fungal$_g$, brucella, salmonella, other bacterial); nonspecific spondylitis
14. [Pleural effusion, empyema]
15. [Pneumonia, atelectasis]

**UNCOMMON**
1. Amyloidosis
2. Bochdalek hernia
3. Bronchogenic cyst
4. Chemodectoma
5. Dilated azygos system (eg, superior or inferior vena cava obstruction); mediastinal varices
6. Eosinophilic granuloma of vertebra
7. Extramedullary hematopoiesis (esp. in thalassemia)
8. Hydatid disease
9. Hydroureter; retrocaval ureter
10. Meningocele, all types
11. [Mesothelioma]

---

12. Mustard operation for transposition of great vessels
13. Neoplasm of spine, primary (eg, giant cell tumor, chordoma, sarcoma)
14. Neurenteric cyst, duplication cyst
15. Other posterior mediastinal or retroperitoneal neoplasm
16. Paget's disease (uncalcified osteoid)
17. Pancreatic pseudocyst or neoplasm
18. Pheochromocytoma; other adrenal neoplasm
19. Retroperitoneal fibrosis
20. Rhabdomyosarcoma, other soft tissue sarcoma
21. Sequestration, extrapulmonary
22. Splenosis
23. Thoracic kidney

*References:*

1. Gupta SK, Mohan V: The thoracic paraspinal line: Further significance. Clin Radiol 1979;30:329-335
2. Greenfield GB: Radiology of Bone Diseases. (ed 5) Philadelphia: Lippincott, 1990
3. Polansky SM, Culham JAG: Paraspinal densities developing after repair of transposition of the great arteries. AJR 1980; 134:394-396

## Gamut V-6

# CERVICAL SPINE INJURIES: MECHANISM OF INJURY

**FLEXION**

1. Anterior subluxation
2. Bilateral interfacetal dislocation
3. Clay-shoveler's fracture
4. Flexion teardrop fracture
5. Simple wedge fracture

**FLEXION-ROTATION**

1. Rotatory dislocation with interlocking
2. Unilateral interfacetal dislocation

## EXTENSION-ROTATION
1. Pillar fracture

## VERTICAL COMPRESSION
1. Bursting fracture
    a. Burst fracture, lower cervical vertebrae
    b. Fracture of occipital condyle
    c. Jefferson fracture of atlas

## EXTENSION
1. Extension teardrop fracture
2. Hangman's fracture (deceleration, hyperextension)
3. Hyperextension fracture-dislocation
4. Posterior dislocation of atlas with fractured odontoid
5. Posterior neural arch fracture of atlas

## SHEARING
1. Fracture of odontoid process

## LATERAL FLEXION

*References:*
1. Bonakdarpour A: Cervical Spine Trauma. American Roentgen Ray Society Refresher Course, Washington, 1986
2. Harris JH Jr: The Radiology of Acute Cervical Spine Trauma. Baltimore: Williams & Wilkins, 1978
3. Kattan KR: Trauma and No-trauma of the Cervical Spine. Springfield, IL: CC Thomas, 1975

**Gamut V-7**

# CERVICAL SPINE INJURIES: STABILITY

## Stable

1. Anterior subluxation
2. Burst fracture (lower cervical vertebrae)

3. Clay-shoveler's fracture
4. Dens fractures, types I and III
5. Pillar fracture
6. Posterior neural arch fracture of atlas
7. Simple wedge fracture
8. Unilateral interfacetal dislocation

## Unstable

1. Bilateral interfacetal dislocation
2. Dens fracture, type II
3. Extension teardrop fracture (stable in flexion, unstable in extension)
4. Flexion teardrop fracture
5. Hangman's fracture
6. Hyperextension fracture-dislocation
7. Jefferson fracture of atlas

*References:*
1. Bonakdarpour A: Cervical Spine Trauma. American Roentgen Ray Society Refresher Course, Washington, 1986
2. Harris JH Jr: The Radiology of Acute Cervical Spine Trauma. Baltimore: Williams & Wilkins, 1978
3. Kattan KR: Trauma and No-trauma of the Cervical Spine. Springfield, IL: CC Thomas, 1975

## Gamut V-8

# ATLANTO-AXIAL SUBLUXATION OR INSTABILITY

## COMMON
1. Incompetence of transverse atlanto-axial ligament (congenital, traumatic, or hyperemic condition)
2. [Normal widening of C1-dens distance in children (up to 4-5 mm)]
3. Rheumatoid arthritis; juvenile chronic arthritis

4. Trauma (with fracture of odontoid or torn transverse ligaments)

## UNCOMMON

1. Absent anterior arch of atlas
2. Absent, hypoplastic, or separate odontoid process (os odontoideum)
3. Ankylosing spondylitis
4. Atlanto-occipital fusion
5. Behcet S.
6. Block vertebra C2-C3
7. Congenital syndromes (esp. Down S., Morquio S.) (See V-8A)
8. Gout
9. Lupus erythematosus; CREST S.
10. Pseudogout
11. Psoriatic arthritis
12. Reiter S.
13. Retropharyngeal or nasopharyngeal infection or abscess (child)
14. Tuberculosis

*References:*

1. Elliott S: The odontoid process in children—is it hypoplastic? Clin Radiol 1988;39:391-393
2. Kattan KR: Trauma and No-trauma of the Cervical Spine. Springfield, IL: CC Thomas, 1975
3. Koss JC, Dalinka MK: Atlantoaxial subluxation in Behcet's syndrome. AJR 1980;134:392-393
4. Martel W: The occipito-atlanto-axial joints in rheumatoid arthritis and ankylosing spondylitis. Am J Roentgenol, 1961; 86:223-240
5. Swischuk LE: Differential Diagnosis in Pediatric Radiology. Baltimore: Williams & Wilkins, 1984, p 433-434
6. Wortzman G, Dewar FP: Rotary fixation of the atlantoaxial joint: rotational atlantoaxial subluxation. Radiology 1968; 90:479-487

## Subgamut V-8A

# CONGENITAL SYNDROMES WITH ATLANTO-AXIAL SUBLUXATION OR INSTABILITY*

**COMMON**
1. Chondrodysplasia punctata (Conradi's disease)
2. Marfan S.
3. Mucopolysaccharidoses (eg, Morquio S.)
4. Trisomy 21 S. (Down S.)

**UNCOMMON**
1. Aarskog S.
2. Diastrophic dysplasia
3. Dyggve-Melchior-Clausen S.
4. Klippel-Feil S.
5. Metaphyseal chondrodysplasia (McKusick)
6. Metatropic dysplasia
7. Mucolipidosis III
8. Patterson S. (pseudoleprechaunism)
9. Pseudoachondroplasia
10. Spondyloepiphyseal dysplasia
11. Winchester S.

*Congenital laxity of ligaments and associated hypoplasia of dens and C1.

*References:*
1. Rosenbaum DM, Blumhagen JD, King HA: Atlanto-occipital instability in Down syndrome. AJR 1986; 146:1269-1272
2. Taybi H, Lachman RS: Radiology of Syndromes, Metabolic Disorders, and Skeletal Dysplasias. (ed 3) Chicago: Year Book Medical Publ, 1990, p 879

## Gamut V-9

# ODONTOID (DENS) ABSENCE, HYPOPLASIA, OR FRAGMENTATION

## COMMON

1. Craniovertebral anomaly (eg, occipitalization of atlas, atlanto-axial fusion, os odontoideum)
2. Klippel-Feil S.
3. Morquio S.
4. Rheumatoid arthritis; ankylosing spondylitis
5. Trauma
6. Trisomy 21 S. (Down S.)

## UNCOMMON

1. Achondroplasia
2. Chondrodysplasia punctata (Conradi's disease)
3. Diastrophic dysplasia
4. Dyggve-Melchior-Clausen S.
5. Kniest dysplasia
6. Metaphyseal chondrodysplasia (McKusick)
7. Metastasis
8. Metatropic dysplasia
9. Mucopolysaccharidoses, other (esp. Hurler S.); mucolipidosis III; fucosidosis
10. Multiple epiphyseal dysplasia (Fairbank)
11. Resorption after cervical spine trauma in infancy
12. Smith-McCort S.
13. Spondylo-epi-metaphyseal dysplasia
14. Spondyloepiphyseal dysplasia congenita
15. Tuberculous spondylitis

*References:*
1. Elliott S: The odontoid process in children—is it hypoplastic? Clin Radiol 1988; 39:391-393
2. Epstein BS: The Spine. Philadelphia: Lea & Febiger, 1976
3. Garber JN: Abnormalities of the atlas and axis vertebrae—congenital and traumatic. J Bone Joint Surg 1964;46A: 1782-1791
4. Gwinn JL, Smith JL: Acquired and congenital absence of the odontoid process. AJR 1962;88:424-431

5. Kozlowski K, Beighton P: Gamut Index of Skeletal Dysplasias. Berlin: Springer-Verlag, 1984, p 47
6. Schlesinger S: Small or hypoplastic dens. Semin Roentgenol 1986;21:241-242
7. Swischuk LE: Differential Diagnosis in Pediatric Radiology. Baltimore: Williams & Wilkins, 1984, p 433
8. Taybi H, Lachman RS: Radiology of Syndromes, Metabolic Disorders, and Skeletal Dysplasias. (ed 3) Chicago: Year Book Medical Publ, 1990, p 880
9. Wackenheim A: Roentgen Diagnosis of the Craniovertebral Region. Berlin: Springer-Verlag, 1974, pp 363-366

## Gamut V-10

# CRANIOVERTEBRAL JUNCTION ABNORMALITY

## Congenital

### BONE ABNORMALITY, ASYMPTOMATIC

1. Asymmetric atlanto-axial joint
2. Asymmetric atlanto-occipital joint
3. Posterior atlas arch defect
4. Rachischisis of C 1
5. Third occipital (tertiary) condyle

### BONE ABNORMALITY, SYMPTOM-PRODUCING

1. Atlanto-axial fusion or malsegmentation
2. Atlanto-occipital fusion (occipitalization of atlas); hypoplasia of occipital condyle
3. Basilar invagination
4. Odontoid dysplasia with atlanto-axial dislocation; os odontoideum (separate odontoid); hypoplasia or aplasia of dens
5. Stenosis of foramen magnum

### CERVICOMEDULLARY ANOMALY

1. AV malformation
2. Chiari malformations
3. Hydromyelia

# Acquired

## BONE LESION
1. Fibrous dysplasia
2. Inflammatory disease
3. Neoplasm of skull base (primary or metastatic)
4. Paget's disease
5. Posttraumatic or degenerative lesion

## EXTRAMEDULLARY LESION
1. Aneurysm
2. Cyst (eg, arachnoid cyst, epidermoid cyst)
3. Neoplasm (eg, meningioma, neurofibroma, lipoma)

## INTRAMEDULLARY LESION
1. Glioma
2. Hemangioblastoma
3. Syringomyelia

*Reference:*
1. Guinto FC Jr, Kumar R, Mirfakhree M: Radiological Society of North America Scientific Exhibit, Washington, 1984

## Gamut V-11

# FUSION OF THE CERVICAL SPINE

## COMMON
1. Ankylosing spondylitis
2. Block vertebrae, congenital or acquired (eg, trauma, surgery, tuberculosis or other infection)
3. Juvenile chronic arthritis (Still's disease)
4. Rheumatoid arthritis
5. Synostosing intervertebral osteochondrosis; DISH

## UNCOMMON
1. Klippel-Feil S.
2. Myositis (fibrodysplasia) ossificans progressiva
3. Psoriatic arthritis

*References:*
1. Connor JM, Smith R: The cervical spine in fibrodysplasia ossificans progressiva. Br J Radiol 1982;55:492-496
2. Dihlmann VW, Friedmann G: Die röntgenkriterien der juvenilrheumatischen zervikalsynostose im erwachsenen-alter. Fortschr Röntgenstr 1977;126:536-541

## Gamut V-12

# VERTEBRAL MALSEGMENTATION (SUPERNUMERARY, ABSENT, PARTIALLY FORMED, OR BLOCK VERTEBRAE)

## COMMON

1. Chondrodysplasia punctata (Conradi's disease)
2. Diastematomyelia
3. Isolated anomaly
4. Klippel-Feil S.
5. Meningomyelocele

## UNCOMMON

1. Aicardi S.
2. Arteriohepatic S. (Alagille S.)
3. Basal cell nevus S. (Gorlin S.)
4. Cat's cry S. (cri du chat S.)
5. Caudal dysplasia S.
6. Cervico-oculo-acoustic S. (Wildervanck S.)
7. Dyssegmental dysplasia
8. Femoral hypoplasia-unusual facies S.
9. Fetal alcohol S.
10. Focal dermal hypoplasia (Goltz S.)
11. Goldenhar S.
12. Holt-Oram S.
13. Incontinentia pigmenti
14. Larsen S.

15. LEOPARD S.
16. Multiple pterygium S.
17. MURCS association
18. Noonan S.
19. Poland S.
20. Robinow S.
21. Split notochord S.
22. Spondylocostal dysostosis
23. Tethered cord S.
24. Trisomy 8 S.
25. Trisomy 18 S.
26. VATER association

*References:*
1. Kozlowski K, Beighton P: Gamut Index of Skeletal Dysplasias. Berlin: Springer-Verlag, 1984, p 45
2. Taybi H, Lachman RS: Radiology of Syndromes, Metabolic Disorders, and Skeletal Dysplasias. (ed 3) Chicago: Year Book Medical Publ, 1990, p 881

## Gamut V-13

## CORONAL CLEFT VERTEBRAE

**COMMON**
1. Chondrodysplasia punctata (Conradi's disease)
2. Kniest dysplasia
3. Metatropic dysplasia
4. Normal variant (esp. in lower thoracic–upper lumbar spine of premature male infant)

**UNCOMMON**
1. Atelosteogenesis
2. Dyssegmental dysplasia
3. Fibrochondrogenesis
4. Humerospinal dysostosis
5. Malsegmentation of spine

6. Micrognathic dwarfism (Weissenbacher-Zweymuller S.)
7. Trisomy 13 S.

*References:*
1. Fielden P, Russell JGB: Coronally cleft vertebra. Clin Radiol 1970;21:327-328
2. Kozlowski K, Beighton P: Gamut Index of Skeletal Dysplasias. Berlin: Springer-Verlag, 1984, p 46
3. Rowley KA: Coronal cleft vertebra. J Fac Radiol 1955; 6:267-274
4. Swischuk LE: Differential Diagnosis in Pediatric Radiology. Baltimore: Williams & Wilkins, 1984, pp 398-399
5. Taybi H, Lachman RS: Radiology of Syndromes, Metabolic Disorders, and Skeletal Dysplasias. (ed 3) Chicago: Year Book Medical Publ, 1990, p 880
6. Wollin DG, Elliott GB: Coronal cleft vertebrae and persistent notochordal derivatives of infancy. J Can Assoc Radiol 1961;12:78-81

## Gamut V-14

# PROMINENT ANTERIOR CANAL (CENTRAL VEIN GROOVE) OF A VERTEBRAL BODY

**COMMON**
1. Hypothyroidism
2. Normal (up to age 7)
3. Sickle cell anemia$_g$

**UNCOMMON**
1. Gaucher's disease
2. Leukemia, lymphoma$_g$
3. Metastatic neuroblastoma
4. Osteopetrosis
5. Progeria
6. Thalassemia major

*References:*
1. Greenfield GB: Radiology of Bone Diseases. (ed 5) Philadelphia: Lippincott, 1990
2. Mandell GA, Kricum ME: Exaggerated anterior vertebral notching. Radiology 1979;131:367-369
3. Swischuk LE: Differential Diagnosis in Pediatric Radiology. Baltimore: Williams & Wilkins, 1984, pp 399-400

## Gamut V-15

# CONGENITAL PLATYSPONDYLY

**COMMON**
1. Hypothyroidism, juvenile; cretinism
2. Morquio S.
3. Osteogenesis imperfecta congenita
4. Spondyloepiphyseal dysplasia, all forms
5. Thanatophoric dysplasia

**UNCOMMON**
1. Achondrogenesis
2. Achondroplasia (homozygous)
3. Cephaloskeletal dysplasia (Taybi-Linder S.)
4. Diastrophic dysplasia
5. Dyggve-Melchior-Clausen S.
6. Dysosteosclerosis
7. Ehlers-Danlos S.
8. Geroderma osteodysplastica
9. $GM_1$ gangliosidosis; fucosidosis
10. Homocystinuria
11. Hyperphosphatasia
12. Hypochondroplasia
13. Hypophosphatasia, severe
14. [Idiopathic juvenile osteoporosis]
15. Kniest dysplasia
16. Larsen S.
17. Marshall S.
18. Metatropic dysplasia

19. Oculo-mandibulo-facial S. (Hallermann-Streiff S.)
20. Osteochondromuscular dystrophy (Schwartz-Jampel S.)
21. Osteoglophonic dwarfism
22. Parastremmatic dwarfism
23. Pseudoachondroplasia
24. Rothmund-Thomson S.
25. Short rib–polydactyly S., type 1 (Saldino-Noonan)
26. Smith-McCort S.
27. Spondylo-epi-metaphyseal dysplasia
28. Spondylometaphyseal dysplasia (Kozlowski)
29. Spondyloperipheral dysplasia

*References:*
1. Kozlowski K; Platyspondyly in childhood. Pediatr Radiol 1974;2:81-88
2. Kozlowski K, Beighton P: Gamut Index of Skeletal Dysplasias. Berlin: Springer-Verlag, 1984, p 43
3. Swischuk LE: Differential Diagnosis in Pediatric Radiology. Baltimore: Williams & Wilkins, 1984, pp 403-404
4. Taybi H, Lachman RS: Radiology of Syndromes, Metabolic Disorders, and Skeletal Dysplasias. (ed 3) Chicago: Year Book Medical Publ, 1990, p 880

## Gamut V-16

## ANISOSPONDYLY[*]

1. Campomelic dysplasia
2. Homocystinuria
3. Kniest dysplasia
4. Osteogenesis imperfecta
5. Spondylo-epi-metaphyseal dysplasia
6. Spondyloepiphyseal dysplasia
7. Spondylometaphyseal dysplasia
8. Stickler S. (arthro-ophthalmopathy)

[*] Irregular flattening of two or more vertebral bodies in the presence of other normal vertebrae.

*Reference:*
1. Kozlowski K, Beighton P: Gamut Index of Skeletal Dysplasias. Berlin: Springer-Verlag, 1984, p 44

## Gamut V-17

## SOLITARY COLLAPSED VERTEBRA (INCLUDING VERTEBRA PLANA) (See Gamut V-18)

**COMMON**

*1. Eosinophilic granuloma (histiocytosis $X_g$)
*2. Fracture, traumatic or pathologic
*3. Hemangioma
 4. Hyperparathyroidism, brown tumor
*5. Lymphoma$_g$, leukemia,
*6. Metastasis (incl. neuroblastoma)
 7. Myeloma, plasmacytoma
 8. [Normal developmental variant (eg, C5 or C6 or a thoracic vertebra reduced in height)]
 9. Osteomyelitis (eg, tuberculous, fungal$_g$, pyogenic, brucellar, typhoid, syphilitic)
10. Osteoporosis (eg, senile, postmenopausal) (See B-44)
*11. Paget's disease
12. Steroid therapy; Cushing S.


**UNCOMMMON**

1. Amyloidosis
2. Benign bone tumor, other (eg, giant cell tumor, aneurysmal bone cyst)
3. Chordoma
4. Hydatid disease
5. Neuropathy (eg, diabetes, syphilis, congenital indifference to pain)
6. Osteomalacia
7. Sarcoidosis

8. Sarcoma (eg, Ewing's, osteosarcoma, chondrosarcoma)
9. Scheuermann's disease
*10. Traumatic ischemic necrosis (eg, Kümmell's disease)

*May produce vertebra plana.


## Gamut V-18

# MULTIPLE COLLAPSED VERTEBRAE
## (See Gamut V-15)

### COMMON

1. Fractures, traumatic or pathologic
2. Hyperparathyroidism, primary or secondary
3. Metastases
4. Multiple myeloma
5. Neuropathy (eg, diabetes, syphilis, congenital indifference to pain)
6. Osteomalacia (See B-46)
7. Osteomyelitis (eg, tuberculous, fungal$_g$, pyogenic, brucellar, syphilitic)
8. Osteoporosis (eg, senile, postmenopausal, idiopathic juvenile; hypogonadism; prolonged immobilization) (See B-44)
9. Scheuermann's disease
10. Sickle cell anemia, other anemias$_g$
11. Steroid therapy; Cushing S.


### UNCOMMON

1. Amyloidosis
2. Congenital fibromatosis
3. Convulsions (eg, tetanus, tetany, hypoglycemia, shock therapy)
4. Gaucher's disease
5. Hemangiomatosis (vanishing bone disease)
6. Histiocytosis X$_g$
7. Hydatid disease

8. Hyperphosphatasia
9. Hypophosphatasia
10. Lymphoma_g, leukemia
11. Osteogenesis imperfecta
12. Osteolysis (Hajdu-Cheney S.)
13. Paget's disease
14. [Platyspondyly, esp. dwarf syndromes (eg, Morquio S., spondyloepiphyseal dysplasia, pseudoachondroplasia, thanatophoric dysplasia) (See V-15)]
15. Radiation therapy
16. Rheumatoid arthritis

## Gamut V-19

# BICONCAVE ("FISH") VERTEBRAE (INCLUDING STEP-LIKE VERTEBRAE)

**COMMON**
1. Metastatic disease
2. Osteomalacia, rickets (See B-46)
3. Osteoporosis (eg, senile, postmenopausal, malnutrition, steroid therapy, hyperparathyroidism) (See B-44)
*4. Renal osteodystrophy
*5. Schmorl's nodes
*6. Sickle cell anemia

**UNCOMMON**
*1. Gaucher's disease
*2. Homocystinuria
3. Lymphoma_g
4. Osteogenesis imperfecta
*5. Other anemias_g (eg, thalassemia major, hereditary spherocytosis, iron deficiency)

*"Step-like" vertebra with H-shaped or Lincoln log configuration may occur.

*References:*

1. Greenfield GB: Radiology of Bone Diseases. (ed 5) Philadelphia: Lippincott, 1990
2. Rohlfing BM: Vertebral end-plate depression: Report of two patients without hemoglobinopathy. AJR 1977;128:599-600
3. Schwartz AM, Homer MJ, McCauley RGK: Step-off vertebral body: Gaucher's disease versus sickle cell hemoglobinopathy. AJR 1979;132:81-85
4. Swischuk LE: Differential Diagnosis in Pediatric Radiology. Baltimore: Williams & Wilkins, 1984, pp 407-408
5. Westerman MP, Greenfield GB, Wong PWK: "Fish vertebrae," homocystinuria, and sickle cell anemia. JAMA 1974; 230:261-262
6. Ziter FMH Jr: Central vertebral end-plate depression in chronic renal disease: Report of two cases. AJR 1979; 132:809-811

## Gamut V-20

## WEDGED VERTEBRAE*

1. Chronic hyperflexion of spine; muscular hypotonia
2. Congenital syndromes with thoracolumbar wedging (eg, achondroplasia, hypothyroidism, mucopolysaccharidoses)
3. Hemivertebra
4. Kyphosis (See V-3)
5. Normal variant (minimal wedging in thoracic spine)
6. Pathological fracture in weakened vertebra (eg, metastasis, myeloma, primary neoplasm)
7. Rotoscoliosis (lateral wedging)
8. Scheuermann's disease
9. Trauma (compression fracture)
10. Tuberculosis (gibbus); other chronic infection of spine

*Primarily anterior wedging unless otherwise indicated.

*Reference:*

1. Swischuk LE: Differential Diagnosis in Pediatric Radiology. Baltimore: Williams & Wilkins, 1984, p 411

## Gamut V-21

# BEAKED OR HOOK-SHAPED VERTEBRAE IN A CHILD

## COMMON

1. Achondroplasia (central anterior wedging)
2. Cretinism, hypothyroidism (inferior beak)
3. Mucopolysaccharidoses (esp. Morquio S.–central beak, Hunter S.–inferior beak, Hurler S.)
4. Neuromuscular disease with generalized hypotonia (eg, Werdnig-Hoffmann disease, Niemann-Pick disease, phenylketonuria, mental retardation)
5. Normal variant in infants (thoracolumbar junction, C2-3 angulation)
6. Scheuermann's disease
7. Trauma, acute or chronic; battered child S. (hyperflexion-compression spinal injury)

## UNCOMMON

1. Diastrophic dysplasia
2. Dyggve-Melchior-Clausen S.
3. Immunodeficiency (severe combined) and adenosine deaminase deficiency
4. Marshall S.
5. Mucolipidoses; fucosidosis; mannosidosis
6. Neurofibromatosis (dysplastic vertebrae)
7. Pseudoachondroplasia
8. Spondyloepiphyseal dysplasia
9. Trisomy 21 S. (Down S.)

*References:*
1. Swischuk LE: The beaked, notched, or hooked vertebra; its significance in infants and young children. Radiology 1970; 95:661-664
2. Swischuk LE: Differential Diagnosis in Pediatric Radiology. Baltimore: Williams & Wilkins, 1984, pp 412-413
3. Taybi H, Lachman RS: Radiology of Syndromes, Metabolic Disorders, and Skeletal Dysplasias. (ed 3) Chicago: Year Book Medical Publ, 1990, pp 879-880

## Gamut V-22

## CUBOID VERTEBRAE

**COMMON**
1. Achondroplasia
2. Normal variant (cervical spine and thoracolumbar junction)

**UNCOMMON**
1. Diastrophic dysplasia
2. Hypochondroplasia
3. Mucopolysaccharidoses
4. Short-rib polydactyly syndromes (eg, Saldino-Noonan S., Majewski S.)
5. Thanatophoric dysplasia

*Reference:*
1. Swischuk LE: Differential Diagnosis in Pediatric Radiology. Baltimore: Williams & Wilkins, 1984, p 406

## Gamut V-23

## ROUND VERTEBRAE

**COMMON**
1. Hypothyroidism, untreated
2. Normal in neonate (esp. thoracolumbar junction) or child with delayed appearance of ring epiphyses
3. Vertebral body underdevelopment (eg, meningomyelocele)

**UNCOMMON**
1. Bone dysplasias with "pear shaped" vertebrae (eg, Morquio S.; spondyloepiphyseal dysplasia; Dyggve-Melchior-Clausen S.)

2. Short rib-polydactyly syndromes (eg, Saldino-Noonan S.; Majewski S.)

*Reference:*

1. Swischuk LE: Differential Diagnosis in Pediatric Radiology. Baltimore: Williams & Wilkins, 1984, pp 409-410

## Gamut V-24

## TALL VERTEBRAE

### COMMON

1. [Block vertebra]
2. Hypotonia (eg, neuromuscular disorders, mental retardation); non–weight bearing
3. Rubella S.
4. Trisomy 21 S. (Down S.)

### UNCOMMON

1. Freeman-Sheldon S. (whistling face S.)
2. Marfan S., arachnodactyly
3. Osteodysplasty (Melnick-Needles S.)
4. Proteus S.
5. Spondylocostal dysplasia

*References:*

1. Gooding CA, Neuhauser EBD: Growth and development of the vertebral bodies in the presence and absence of normal stress. AJR 1965;93:388-393
2. Kozlowski K, Beighton P: Gamut Index of Skeletal Dysplasias. Berlin: Springer-Verlag, 1984, p 44
3. Swischuk LE: Differential Diagnosis in Pediatric Radiology. Baltimore: Williams & Wilkins, 1984, p 408
4. Taybi H, Lachman RS: Radiology of Syndromes, Metabolic Disorders, and Skeletal Dysplasias. (ed 3) Chicago: Year Book Medical Publ, 1990, p 881

Gamut V-25

## FUSED OR BLOCK VERTEBRAE

### Congenital

1. Focal dermal hypoplasia (Goltz S.) (anterior fusion)
2. Isolated anomaly (esp. C2-3)
3. Klippel-Feil S.
4. With spinal dysraphism

### Acquired

1. Ankylosing spondylitis
2. Infection (esp. tuberculosis)
3. Rheumatoid arthritis (esp. juvenile)
4. Scheuermann's disease
5. Surgical fusion
6. Trauma, severe

*Reference:*
1. Swischuk LE: Differential Diagnosis in Pediatric Radiology. Baltimore: Williams & Wilkins, 1984, pp 415-416

## Gamut V-26

## ENLARGEMENT OF ONE OR MORE VERTEBRAE

### COMMON
1. Acromegaly; gigantism
2. Paget's disease

### UNCOMMON
1. Benign bone tumor (eg, giant cell tumor, hemangioma, aneurysmal bone cyst, osteoblastoma)

2. Compensatory enlargement from non–weight bearing (eg, paralysis)
3. Congenital (eg, block vertebra)
4. Fibrous dysplasia
5. Hydatid disease
6. Hyperphosphatasia

*References:*
1. Epstein BS: The Spine. (ed 4) Philadelphia: Lea & Febiger, 1976
2. Greenfield GB: Radiology of Bone Diseases. (ed 5) Philadelphia: Lippincott, 1990

## Gamut V-27

## "SQUARING" OF ONE OR MORE VERTEBRAL BODIES

**COMMON**
1. Ankylosing spondylitis
2. Paget's disease

**UNCOMMON**
1. Normal variant
2. Psoriatic arthritis
3. Reiter S.
4. Rheumatoid arthritis

*Reference:*
1. Jacobson HG: Personal communication

## Gamut V-28

# SPOOL-SHAPED VERTEBRAE (ANTERIOR AND POSTERIOR SCALLOPING)

## COMMON

1. Hypotonia
2. Neurofibromatosis
3. Normal (occasionally mild in lumbar spine)

## UNCOMMON

1. Mucopolysaccharidoses
2. Osteodysplasty (Melnick-Needles S.)
3. Trisomy 21 S. (Down S.); other trisomies

*Reference:*

1. Swischuk LE: Differential Diagnosis in Pediatric Radiology. Baltimore: Williams & Wilkins, 1984, p 414

## Gamut V-29

# ANTERIOR GOUGE DEFECT (SCALLOPING) OF ONE OR MORE VERTEBRAL BODIES

## COMMON

1. Aneurysm of aorta
2. Lymphoma$_g$, chronic leukemia
3. Lymphadenopathy from metastases or inflammation
4. Normal variant (lower thoracic, upper lumbar)
5. Tuberculosis

## UNCOMMON

1. Adjacent intra-abdominal neoplasm or cyst
2. Cockayne S.

3. Glycogen storage disease
4. Neurofibromatosis (dysplastic vertebra)
5. Osteodysplasty (Melnick-Needles S.)
6. Trisomy 21 S. (Down S.)

*Reference:*
1. Swischuk LE: Differential Diagnosis in Pediatric Radiology. Baltimore: Williams & Wilkins, 1984, pp 401-402

## Gamut V-30

# EXAGGERATED CONCAVITY (SCALLOPING) OF THE POSTERIOR SURFACE OF ONE OR MORE VERTEBRAL BODIES

**COMMON**
1. Achondroplasia
2. Increased intraspinal pressure
3. Neoplasm of spinal canal (eg, ependymoma, dermoid, lipoma, neurofibroma, meningioma)
4. Neurofibromatosis with or without neurofibroma ("dural ectasia"); congenital expansion of the subarachnoid space ("intraspinal meningocele")
5. Normal variant (physiologic scalloping—esp. L4, L5)

**UNCOMMON**
1. Acromegaly
2. Communicating hydrocephalus, severe
3. Cyst of spinal canal
4. Hydatid disease
5. Other congenital syndromes
   a. Cockayne S.
   b. Diastrophic dysplasia
   c. Dyggve-Melchior-Clausen S.
   d. Ehlers-Danlos S. (dural ectasia)
   e. Marfan S. (dural ectasia)

    f.  Metatropic dysplasia

    g.  Mucopolysaccharidoses
       (eg, Hurler, Hunter, Morquio)

    h.  Osteogenesis imperfecta tarda

    i.  Smith-McCort S.

    j.  Thanatophoric dysplasia

6.  Spinal dysraphism, meningomyelocele

7.  Syringomyelia, hydromyelia

*References:*

1. Greenfield GB: Radiology of Bone Diseases. (ed 5) Philadelphia: Lippincott, 1990

2. Heard G, Payne EE: Scalloping of the vertebral bodies in von Recklinghausen's disease of the nervous system (neurofibromatosis). J Neurol Neurosurg Psychiatry 1962;25: 345-351

3. Howieson J, Norrell HA, Wilson CB: Expansion of the subarachnoid space in the lumbosacral region. Radiology 1968;90:488-492

4. Kozlowski K, Beighton P: Gamut Index of Skeletal Dysplasias. Berlin: Springer-Verlag, 1984, p 46

5. Leeds NE, Jacobson HG: Plain film examination of the spinal canal. Semin Roentgenol 1972;7:179-196

6. Mitchell GE, Lourie H, Berne AS: The various causes of scalloped vertebrae with notes on their pathogenesis. Radiology 1967;89:67-74

7. Salerno NR, Edeiken J: Vertebral scalloping in neurofibromatosis. Radiology 1970;97:509-510

8. Swischuk LE: Differential Diagnosis in Pediatric Radiology. Baltimore: Williams & Wilkins, 1984, pp 401-402

## Gamut V-31

# INCREASED BAND(S) OF DENSITY IN THE SUBCHONDRAL ZONES OF VERTEBRAE (INCLUDING RUGGER JERSEY SPINE)

## COMMON

1. Compression fracture

2. Hypercorticism, Cushing S., steroid therapy

*3. Hyperparathyroidism, primary or esp. secondary
   (renal osteodystrophy)
*4. Osteopetrosis
 5. Paget's disease
 6. Sclerosing spondylosis in the elderly

**UNCOMMON**

 1. Growth arrest lines
 2. Heavy metals (eg, thorotrast, lead)
 3. Hypoparathyroidism, pseudohypoparathyroidism
*4. Idiopathic hypercalcemia (Williams S.)
 5. Leukemia, treated
*6. Myeloid metaplasia (myelosclerosis)
 7. Radiation therapy

*May have the appearance of a "rugger jersey."

---

**Gamut V-32**

## BONE-IN-BONE OR SANDWICH VERTEBRA

**COMMON**

 1. Osteopetrosis
 2. Paget's disease
 3. Physiologic in newborn
 4. Renal osteodystrophy, healing

**UNCOMMON**

 1. Chronic illness (growth arrest lines)
 2. Hypercalcemia; hypervitaminosis D
 3. Lead poisoning, chronic
 4. Radiation therapy
 5. Thorotrast

*Reference:*

1. Swischuk LE: Differential Diagnosis in Pediatric Radiology.
   Baltimore: Williams & Wilkins, 1984, p 391

---

# INCREASED VERTICAL (PIN-STRIPE) TRABECULATION OF ONE OR MORE VERTEBRAL BODIES*

## COMMON

1. Anemia, primary$_g$
2. Hemangioma
3. Osteoporosis
4. Paget's disease

## UNCOMMON

1. Lymphoma$_g$, leukemia
2. Metastatic disease (esp. carcinomatosis)
3. Multiple myeloma (esp. myelomatosis)

*Due to loss of the minor bony trabeculae, with the remaining major trabeculae aligned vertically for support.

## Gamut V-34

# FOCAL AREA OF SCLEROSIS IN A VERTEBRA

## COMMON

1. Bone island
2. Fracture (compression or healing)
3. Idiopathic
4. Osteoblastic metastasis
5. Sclerosis of apophyseal joints due to arthritis or malalignment
6. Spondylosis, chronic sclerosing (sclerosing osteitis)

## UNCOMMON

1. Enostoma, osteoma
2. Histiocytosis X$_g$, healed

3. Lymphoma$_g$
4. Osteoblastoma
5. Osteoid osteoma
6. Osteomyelitis, chronic (eg, tuberculosis, brucellosis, typhoid)
7. Sarcoidosis
8. Sarcoma (esp. osteosarcoma)
9. Sclerotic pedicle (See V-41)
10. Tuberous sclerosis

*Reference:*
1. Swischuk LE: Differential Diagnosis in Pediatric Radiology. Baltimore: Williams & Wilkins, 1984, p 392

## Gamut V-35

# DENSE SCLEROTIC VERTEBRA, SOLITARY OR MULTIPLE (INCLUDING IVORY VERTEBRA)

## COMMON
*1. Fluorosis
2. Fracture (compression or healing)
*3. Lymphoma$_g$
*4. Myelosclerosis (myeloid metaplasia)
*5. Osteoblastic metastasis
6. Osteomyelitis, chronic sclerosing (eg, tuberculosis, syphilis, brucellosis, typhoid)
*7. Paget's disease
8. Renal osteodystrophy

## UNCOMMON
1. Hemangioma
2. Hypervitaminosis D
3. Idiopathic (eg, nondiscogenic sclerosis)
4. Idiopathic hypercalcemia (Williams S.)

---

5. Mastocytosis
6. Multiple myeloma (rare)
7. Osteoblastoma
8. Osteoma, enostoma, bone island
*9. Osteopetrosis
10. Radiation therapy; radium poisoning
11. Rickets, healing
12. Sarcoidosis
13. Sarcoma (eg, osteosarcoma; chondrosarcoma; Ewing's sarcoma)
14. Sickle cell anemia$_g$
15. Spondylosis, chronic sclerosing; intervertebral disc disease
16. Tuberous sclerosis

*Can cause "ivory" vertebra(e).

*Reference:*
1. Jacobson HG, Siegelman SS: Some miscellaneous solitary bone lesions. Semin Roentgenol 1966;1:314-335

## Gamut V-36

## SPINAL OSTEOPENIA (LOSS OF DENSITY)

**COMMON**
1. Anemia$_g$ (esp. sickle cell anemia, thalassemia)
2. Carcinomatosis
3. Hyperparathyroidism, primary or secondary (renal osteodystrophy)
4. Multiple myeloma
5. Osteomalacia (See B-46)
6. Osteoporosis (esp. senile or postmenopausal; prolonged immobilization)(See B-44)
7. Steroid therapy; Cushing S.

**UNCOMMON**
1. Acromegaly
2. Amyloidosis

3. Fibrogenesis imperfecta ossium
4. Gaucher's disease; Niemann-Pick disease
5. Homocystinuria
6. Hyperthyroidism
7. Hypogonadism (eg, Fröhlich's S.; Turner S.)
8. Leukemia, lymphoma$_g$
9. Osteogenesis imperfecta

*Reference:*
1. Greenfield GB: Radiology of Bone Diseases. (ed 5) Philadelphia: Lippincott, 1990

## Gamut V-37

## LYTIC LESION OF THE SPINE

**COMMON**
1. Hemangioma
2. Histiocytosis X$_g$ (esp. eosinophilic granuloma)
3. Metastasis (incl. neuroblastoma)
4. Myeloma, plasmacytoma
5. Osteomyelitis, spondylitis (eg, tuberculous, sarcoid, fungal, brucellar, other bacterial)
6. Paget's disease
7. Rheumatoid arthritis
8. [Schmorl's nodes]

**UNCOMMON**
1. Aneurysmal bone cyst
2. Brown tumor of hyperparathyroidism
3. Chondroid lesion
4. Chordoma, notochordal remnant
5. Fibrous dysplasia
6. Giant cell tumor
7. Gout
8. Hemangiopericytoma

9. Hydatid disease
10. Intraspinal neoplasm with erosion of vertebra (eg, neurofibroma, meningioma)
11. Lymphoma_g
12. [Meningocele, diastematomyelia]
13. Nonossifying fibroma
14. Osteoblastoma
15. Sarcoma (eg, Ewing's, osteolytic osteosarcoma, chondrosarcoma, fibrosarcoma, malignant fibrous histiocytoma, rhabdomyosarcoma)
16. Traumatic ischemic necrosis (Kümmell's disease)

## Gamut V-38

# CYST-LIKE EXPANSILE LESION OF THE BODY AND/OR APPENDAGES OF A VERTEBRA

**COMMON**
1. Aneurysmal bone cyst
2. Hemangioma
3. Osteoblastoma

**UNCOMMON**
1. Chondroid lesion
2. Fibrous dysplasia
3. Giant cell tumor
4. Gout
5. Hemangiopericytoma
6. Hydatid cyst
7. Metastasis
8. Myeloma, plasmacytoma

# ABNORMAL SIZE OR SHAPE OF A VERTEBRAL PEDICLE

## ABSENT OR HYPOPLASTIC PEDICLE
1. Congenital absence or hypoplasia
2. Destroyed pedicle (See V-40)
3. Mucopolysaccharidoses (esp. Hunter S.)
4. Neurofibromatosis
5. [Poorly visualized pedicles C2-C5]
6. Radiation therapy

## ENLARGED PEDICLE
1. Compensatory hypertrophy with contralateral deficiency of neural arch
2. Neoplasm (eg, osteoblastoma, hemangioma)

## DYSPLASTIC PEDICLE
1. Diastematomyelia
2. Klippel-Feil S.
3. Meningomyelocele
4. Neurofibromatosis
5. Other congenital anomaly

## FLATTENED PEDICLE
1. Intraspinal expanding neoplasm or cyst; AV malformation
2. Normal (eg, upper lumbar spine)
3. Syringomyelia, hydromyelia

## Gamut V-40

# VERTEBRAL PEDICLE EROSION OR DESTRUCTION

## COMMON

1. Intraspinal neoplasm or cyst (esp. neurofibroma, meningioma)
2. Metastasis
3. Tuberculosis, fungus$_g$, or other infectious disease

## UNCOMMON

1. Benign bone tumor (eg, aneurysmal bone cyst, giant cell tumor, hemangiopericytoma)
2. [Congenital absence]
3. Eosinophilic granuloma (histiocytosis $X_g$)
4. Hydatid disease
5. Lymphoma$_g$
6. Multiple myeloma
7. Syringomyelia
8. Vertebral artery aneurysm or tortuosity (cervical spine); AV malformation

## Gamut V-41

# VERTEBRAL PEDICLE SCLEROSIS

## COMMON

1. Metastasis (osteoblastic)
2. Osteoblastoma
3. Osteoid osteoma
4. Stress-induced
    a. Congenital absence or hypoplasia of contralateral posterior elements
    b. Malalignment of apophyseal joints
    c. Spondylolisthesis

**UNCOMMON**
1. Idiopathic
2. Lymphoma$_g$
3. Osteosarcoma; Ewing's sarcoma
4. Paget's disease
5. Posttraumatic (healed fracture)

*References:*
1. Pettine K, Klassen R: Osteoid osteoma and osteoblastoma of the spine. J Bone Joint Surg 1986;68A:354-361
2. Swischuk LE: Differential Diagnosis in Pediatric Radiology. Baltimore: Williams & Wilkins, 1984, p 396
3. Wilkinson RH, Hall JE: The sclerotic pedicle: Tumor or pseudotumor? Radiology 1974;111:683-688

## Gamut V-42

# SMALL OR NARROW INTERVERTEBRAL FORAMEN

**COMMON**
1. Degenerative or posttraumatic arthritis with hypertrophic bony ridging and spurring

**UNCOMMON**
1. Diastematomyelia
2. Fused vertebra
3. Klippel-Feil S.
4. Meningomyelocele
5. Posterior subluxation of cervical spine
6. Unilateral bar with scoliosis

*Reference:*
1. Swischuk LE: Differential Diagnosis in Pediatric Radiology. Baltimore: Williams & Wilkins, 1984, pp 418-419

## Gamut V-43

# ENLARGED INTERVERTEBRAL FORAMEN

**COMMON**
1. Neurofibroma

**UNCOMMON**
1. Congenital absence or hypoplasia of pedicle or neural arch
2. Dermoid, teratoma
3. Dejerine-Sottas S. (hypertrophic interstitial neuropathy)
4. Dural ectasia (eg, idiopathic, Marfan S., Ehlers-Danlos S.)
5. Fibroma of spinal ligaments
6. Hydatid disease
7. Lipoma
8. Lymphoma$_g$
9. Meningioma
10. Metastasis to spine or nerve
11. Neuroblastoma, ganglioneuroma
12. Neurofibromatosis (bony dysplasia, dural ectasia, lateral thoracic meningocele)
13. Posttraumatic (eg, fracture; traumatic avulsion of nerve root with "diverticulum"); postsurgical
14. Primary neoplasm of spine or spinal cord (eg, chordoma)
15. Spondylolysis
16. Vertebral artery aneurysm or tortuosity (eg, coarctation of aorta)

*References:*
1. Anderson RE, Shealy CN: Cervical pedicle erosion and rootlet compression caused by a tortuous vertebral artery. Radiology 1970;96:537-538
2. Danziger J, Bloch S: The widened cervical intervertebral foramen. Radiology 1975;116:671-674
3. Patel DV, Ferguson RJL, Schey WL: Enlargement of the intervertebral foramen, an unusual cause. AJR 1978;131: 911-913
4. Swischuk LE: Differential Diagnosis in Pediatric Radiology. Baltimore: Williams & Wilkins, 1984, pp 418-419

# DEFECTIVE OR DESTROYED POSTERIOR NEURAL ARCHES

## Congenital Defects

1. Defect in posterior arch of C1 (rarely C2 or other vertebrae)
2. Diastematomyelia
3. Meningocele, meningomyelocele, sacral dimple
4. [Normal synchondroses between body and arches]
5. Spina bifida occulta (usually L5 or S1)

## Acquired Defects or Destruction

1. Fracture with hyperextension injury (eg, hangman's fracture of C2)
2. Histiocytosis $X_g$
3. Hydatid disease
4. Metastasis
5. Multiple myeloma
6. Osteomyelitis
7. Primary neoplasm of spine (eg, hemangioma, aneurysmal bone cyst, osteoblastoma, sarcoma)
8. Spondylolysis, spondylolisthesis (pars interarticularis defects or fatigue fractures)

*Reference:*
1. Swischuk LE: Differential Diagnosis in Pediatric Radiology. Baltimore: Williams & Wilkins, 1984, pp 396-398

# SPINA BIFIDA OCCULTA OR APERTA

## Spina Bifida Occulta*

**COMMON**
1. Isolated anomaly

**UNCOMMON**
1. Dermoid; epidermoid cyst
2. Diastematomyelia
3. Filum terminale lipoma
4. Lipomeningocele
5. Tethered cord S.

* Skin-covered defect in posterior neural arch, commonly seen in the lower lumbar spine or upper sacrum and rarely associated with neurologic defect by itself.

## Spina Bifida Aperta*

1. Meningocele
2. Meningomyelocele
3. Myeloschisis
4. Myelocystocele

* Incomplete fusion of posterior elements of vertebrae and overlying soft tissues, almost always associated with neurologic defect.

*Reference:*
1. Dahner W: Radiology Review Manual. Baltimore: Williams & Wilkins, 1991, p 95

# SACRAL AGENESIS OR DEFORMITY

## Agenesis or Hypoplasia

1. Caudal regression S. or mermaid S. (usually in infants of diabetic mothers)
2. Teratoma, presacral

## Deformity (Curved or Sickle-Shaped Sacrum)

1. Imperforate anus
2. Meningocele (anterior, lateral, or intrasacral)
3. Teratoma, presacral
4. Tethered cord (often with spinal lipoma)

*Reference:*
1. Swischuk LE: Differential Diagnosis in Pediatric Radiology. Baltimore: Williams & Wilkins, 1984, pp 435-436

## Gamut V-46

## SACROILIAC JOINT DISEASE (EROSION, WIDENING, SCLEROSIS AND/OR FUSION)

**COMMON**
+*1. Ankylosing spondylitis
 *2. Infectious arthritis or osteomyelitis (eg, pyogenic, tuberculous)
+3. [Osteitis condensans ilii]
  4. Osteoarthritis, degenerative or posttraumatic
  5. Rheumatoid arthritis (incl. juvenile)

**UNCOMMON**
+1. Agenesis (caudal dysplasia)
 2. Bone neoplasm, primary (eg, chordoma, sarcoma) or metastatic
 3. Enteropathic arthritis due to inflammatory bowel disease (eg, ulcerative colitis, Crohn's disease, Whipple's disease)
 4. Familial Mediterranean fever
*5. Gaucher's disease
 6. Gout

+7. Hyperparathyroidism, primary or secondary (renal osteodystrophy)
+8. Leukemia
+9. Multicentric reticulohistiocytosis (lipoid dermatoarthritis)
*10. Occupational acro-osteolysis (eg, polyvinylchloride osteolysis)
*11. Paraplegia, paralysis
 12. Pseudogout (CPPD crystal deposition disease)
 13. Pseudohypoparathyroidism
*14. Psoriatic arthritis
*15. Reiter S.
*16. Relapsing polychondritis
 17. Sacroiliitis circumscripta

+Bilateral symmetrical.
*Fusion of sacroiliac joint(s) may occur.

### References:

1. Burgener FA, Kormano M: Differential Diagnosis in Conventional Radiology. (ed 2) New York: Thieme Medical Publ, 1991, p183
2. Resnik CS, Resnick D: Radiology of disorders of the sacroiliac joints. JAMA 1985;253:2863-2866

## Gamut V-47

# SACROCOCCYGEAL OR PRESACRAL MASS
## (See Gamut V-48)

### COMMON

1. Abscess (eg, rectal perforation from trauma or surgery; sinus tract from Crohn's disease, ulcerative colitis, amebiasis, schistosomiasis, tuberculosis, or lymphogranuloma venereum)
2. Bone cyst or neoplasm, benign (eg, aneurysmal bone cyst, giant cell tumor)

3. Carcinoma of prostate
4. Hematoma; fracture
5. Malignant neoplasm of sacrum (eg, chordoma, sarcoma, metastasis, myeloma)
6. [Normal variant; pelvic surgery]
7. Teratoma; dermoid cyst

## UNCOMMON

1. Arachnoid, extradural, or perineural cyst
2. [Ectopic kidney]
3. Hamartoma
4. Hydatid cyst
5. Hydroureter; urinoma
6. Intraspinal neoplasm, other (eg, ependymoma, lipoma)
7. Lymphocele
8. Lymphoma$_g$
9. Meningocele, anterior sacral
10. Neurenteric cyst
11. Neurogenic tumor
12. Osteomyelitis of sacrum
13. Ovarian cyst or neoplasm; tubovarian abscess
14. Rectal duplication
15. Spindle cell tumor$_g$

*References:*
1. Epstein BS: The Spine. (ed 4) Philadelphia: Lea & Febiger, 1976
2. Lombardi G, Passerini A: Spinal Cord Diseases: A Radiologic and Myelographic Analysis. Baltimore: Williams & Wilkins, 1964
3. Silverman FN (ed): Caffey's Pediatric X-ray Diagnosis. (ed 8) Chicago: Year Book Medical Publ, 1985
4. Werner JL, Taybi H: Presacral masses in childhood. AJR 1970;109:403-410

## Gamut V-48

# PRIMARY NEOPLASM OF THE SACRUM
## (See Gamut V-47)

## Benign

**COMMON**
1. Giant cell tumor

**UNCOMMON**
1. Aneurysmal bone cyst
2. Osteoblastoma
3. Osteochondroma
4. Osteoma

## Malignant

**COMMON**
1. Chordoma

**UNCOMMON**
1. Chondrosarcoma
2. Ewing's sarcoma
3. Fibrosarcoma; malignant fibrous histiocytoma
4. Lymphoma$_g$
5. Malignant giant cell tumor
6. Neurogenic sarcoma
7. Osteosarcoma
8. Paget's sarcoma
9. Plasmacytoma
10. Radiation-induced sarcoma
11. Spindle cell neoplasm$_g$

*Reference:*
1. Smith J: International Skeletal Society Lecture. Philadelphia, 1984

## Gamut V-49

# NARROW DISK SPACES

**COMMON**
1. Ankylosing spondylitis
2. Block vertebra, congenital or acquired (See V-25)
*3. Degenerative disk disease (usually associated with osteoarthritis)
*4. Herniated disk
5. Kyphosis, scoliosis (severe)
*6. Neuropathic arthropathy (eg, diabetes, syringomyelia, tabes dorsalis)
*7. Osteomyelitis (eg, pyogenic, tuberculous, sarcoid, brucellar, typhoid)
*8. Rheumatoid arthritis; other inflammatory arthritis
9. Scheuermann's disease

**UNCOMMON**
1. Cockayne S.
2. Discitis, spondyloarthritis (childhood)
3. Kniest dysplasia
4. Morquio S.
5. Neoplasm (rarely)
*6. Ochronosis (alkaptonuria)
*7. Pseudogout (CPPD crystal deposition disease)
8. Spondyloepiphyseal dysplasia
*9. Trauma (flexion-rotation injury)

*Often with adjacent sclerosis of the vertebral margins.

*Reference:*
1. Swischuk LE: Differential Diagnosis in Pediatric Radiology. Baltimore: Williams & Wilkins, 1984, pp 424-426

## Gamut V-50

# WIDE DISK SPACES

1. Acromegaly
2. Biconcave vertebrae, other causes (See V-19)
3. Gaucher's disease
4. Osteomalacia (See B-46)
5. Osteoporosis (See B-44)
6. Platyspondyly (esp. Morquio S., osteogenesis imperfecta, cretinism) (See V-15)
7. Sickle cell anemia
8. Trauma (hyperextension injury to spine)

## Gamut V-51

# CALCIFICATION OF ONE OR MORE INTERVERTEBRAL DISKS

**COMMON**

1. Degenerative spondylosis
2. Idiopathic (eg, transient calcification in children; persistent type in adults)
3. Ochronosis (alkaptonuria)
4. Posttraumatic
5. Spinal fusion (eg, congenital block vertebra, Klippel-Feil S., myositis ossificans progressiva, surgical fusion)

**UNCOMMON**

1. Aarskog S.
2. Ankylosing spondylitis
3. Cockayne S.
4. Diffuse idiopathic skeletal hyperostosis (DISH)
5. Gout
6. Hemochromatosis

7. Homocystinuria
8. Hypercalcemia
9. Hyperparathyroidism
10. Hypervitaminosis D
11. Hypophosphatasia
12. Infection (eg, brucellosis)
13. Paraplegia; poliomyelitis
14. Pseudogout (CPPD crystal deposition disease)
15. Rheumatoid spondylitis (incl. juvenile chronic arthritis)
16. Spondyloepiphyseal dysplasia tarda

*References:*
1. Dussault RG, Kaye JJ: Intervertebral disk calcification associated with spine fusion. Radiology 1977;125:57-61
2. Edeiken J, Dalinka M, Karasick D: Edeiken's Roentgen Diagnosis of Diseases of Bone. (ed 4) Baltimore: Williams & Wilkins, 1989
3. Greenfield GB: Radiology of Bone Diseases. (ed 5) Philadelphia: Lippincott, 1990
4. Kozlowski K, Beighton P: Gamut Index of Skeletal Dysplasias. Berlin: Springer-Verlag, 1984, pp 48-49
5. Mainzer F: Herniation of the nucleus pulposus. A rare complication of intervertebral-disk calcification in children. Radiology 1973;107:167-170
6. Murray RO, Jacobson HG, Stoker D: The Radiology of Skeletal Disorders. (ed 3) Edinburgh: Churchill Livingstone, 1990
7. Swischuk LE: Differential Diagnosis in Pediatric Radiology. Baltimore: Williams & Wilkins, 1984, p 427
8. Taybi H, Lachman RS: Radiology of Syndromes, Metabolic Disorders, and Skeletal Dysplasias. (ed 3) Chicago: Year Book Medical Publ, 1990, p 880
9. Weinberger A, Myers AR: Intervertebral disc calcification in adults: a review. Semin Arthritis Rheum 1978;18:69-75

## Gamut V-52

# GAS IN AN INTERVERTEBRAL DISK (VACUUM DISK)

**COMMON**
1. Degenerative disk disease; spondylosis deformans

**UNCOMMON**
1. Fractured vertebra
2. Osteomyelitis of vertebra (rare)
3. Osteonecrosis with vertebral collapse (Kümmell's disease)
4. Schmorl's nodes (on CT)

*Reference:*
1. Greenfield GB: Radiology of Bone Diseases. (ed 5) Philadelphia: Lippincott, 1990

## Gamut V-53

# SYNDROMES WITH A NARROW SPINAL CANAL (NARROW INTERPEDICULAR DISTANCE): SPINAL STENOSIS

**COMMON**
1. Achondroplasia, hypochondroplasia
2. Acromegaly
3. Diastrophic dysplasia
4. Klippel-Feil S.

**UNCOMMON**
1. Acrodysostosis
2. Acromesomelic dysplasia
3. Arteriohepatic S. (Alagille S.)

4. Cauda equina S. (narrow lumbar spinal canal S.)
5. Dyschondrosteosis
6. Gordon S.
7. Kniest dysplasia
8. Osteoglophonic dwarfism
9. Pseudogout
10. Pseudohypoparathyroidism, pseudopseudohypoparathyroidism
11. Smith-McCort S.
12. Thanatophoric dysplasia
13. Weill-Marchesani S.

*References:*

1. Kozlowski K, Beighton P: Gamut Index of Skeletal Dysplasias. Berlin: Springer-Verlag, 1984, pp 47-48
2. Taybi H, Lachman RS: Radiology of Syndromes, Metabolic Disorders, and Skeletal Dysplasias. (ed 3) Chicago: Year Book Medical Publ, 1990, p 880

## Gamut V-54

# WIDE SPINAL CANAL (INCREASED INTERPEDICULAR DISTANCE) (See Gamuts V-55 and V-58)

**COMMON**

1. Intraspinal neoplasm (eg, ependymoma, astrocytoma, neurofibroma, lipoma) or cyst
2. Meningocele, meningomyelocele
3. [Rotation of vertebra due to scoliosis or poor radiographic positioning]

**UNCOMMON**

1. AV malformation
2. Diastematomyelia
3. Idiopathic

4. Marfan S.
5. Mucopolysaccharidoses (esp. Hurler S., Hunter S., Morquio S.)
6. Neurofibromatosis, dural ectasia
7. Otopalatodigital S.
8. Syringomyelia, hydromyelia
9. Tethered cord S.

## Gamut V-55

# INTRAMEDULLARY LESION (WIDENING OF SPINAL CORD ON MYELOGRAPHY, CT, OR MRI)

## COMMON

1. [Extrinsic compression (eg, by cervical ridge, herniated disk, large extramedullary or extradural tumor)]
2. Inflammation (eg, abscess; myelitis—viral or bacterial; multiple sclerosis)
3. Intramedullary tumor (esp. ependymoma and astrocytoma; also ganglioglioma, hemangioblastoma, primary melanoma)
4. Syringomyelia, hydromyelia (see V-55A)

## UNCOMMON

1. AV malformation, angioma
2. Dermoid; teratoma; epidermoid
3. Diastematomyelia
4. Granuloma (eg, sarcoidosis, tuberculosis)
5. Hematoma, contusion, or edema of cord; anti-coagulant therapy
6. Lipoma
7. Lymphoma$_g$
8. Metastasis (eg, breast, lung, melanoma); drop metastasis through the central canal (eg, medulloblastoma)
9. Myelomeningocele

10. [Postradiation myelopathy]
11. [Spinal cord atrophy (See V-56)]

*References:*
1. Epstein BS: Spinal canal mass lesions. Radiol Clin North Am 1966;4:185-202
2. Epstein BS: The Spine: A Radiological Text and Atlas. (ed 4) Philadelphia: Lea & Febiger, 1976
3. Lewtas N: The Spine and Myelography. In: Sutton D (ed), Textbook of Radiology and Imaging. (ed 4) Edinburgh: Churchill Livingstone, 1987
4. Moseley IF: Myelography. In: du Boulay GH (ed), A Textbook of Radiological Diagnosis. (ed 5) London: HK Lewis, 1984
5. Stevens JM: The Spine and Spinal Cord. In: Sutton D, Young JWR (eds): A Short Textbook of Clinical Imaging. London: Springer-Verlag, 1990, pp 806-811

## Subgamut V-55A

# CAUSES OF SYRINGOMYELIA OR HYDROMYELIA

1. Arachnoiditis
2. Chiari I, Chiari II (Arnold Chiari) malformation
3. Herniation of cerebellar tonsils through foramen magnum due to posterior fossa mass
4. Posttraumatic
5. Spinal stenosis
6. Tumor (rostral or caudal to cyst; intra- or extramedullary)

*Reference:*
1. Houghton V, et al: Chapter 40, In: Stark DD, Bradley WG (eds): Magnetic Resonance Imaging. (ed 2) St. Louis: CV Mosby, 1992

Gamut V-56

# SPINAL CORD ATROPHY

## COMMON
1. Multiple sclerosis
2. Posttraumatic
3. Spondylosis; disk hernation (esp. cervical)
4. Syringomyelia, hydromyelia (after collapse)

## UNCOMMON
1. Amyotrophic lateral sclerosis
2. AV malformation of cord
3. Friedreich's ataxia
4. Ischemia with cord infarction
5. Other motor neuron disease or motor and sensory neuropathies
6. Postradiation therapy myelopathy
7. Subacute combined degeneration
8. Tabes dorsalis

*Reference:*
1. Stevens JM: The Spine and Spinal Cord. In: Sutton D, Young JWR (eds): A Short Textbook of Clinical Imaging. London: Springer-Verlag, 1990, p 811

## Gamut V-57

# SMALL SPINAL CORD

## FOCALLY SMALL CORD
1. Bony spinal stenosis
2. Collapsed syrinx
3. Compression due to herniated disk, epidural tumor, or extramedullary mass (eg, arachnoid cyst)
4. Multiple sclerosis

5. Myelomalacia
6. Postinfarction of cord
7. Postradiation therapy myelopathy
8. Postsurgical
9. Posttraumatic

## DIFFUSELY SMALL CORD

1. Atrophy
2. Collapsed syrinx
3. Cord tethering
4. Cord transection
5. Kyphoscoliosis
6. Multiple sclerosis (diffuse)
7. Postoperative (caudal to level of previous surgery)
8. Postradiation therapy myelopathy

*References:*

1. Houghton V, et al: Chapter 40, In: Stark DD, Bradley WG (eds): Magnetic Resonance Imaging. (ed 2) St. Louis: CV Mosby, 1992
2. Shoukimas GM: Chapter 41, In: Stark DD, Bradley WG (eds): Magnetic Resonance Imaging. (ed 2) St. Louis: CV Mosby, 1992

## Gamut V-58

# INTRADURAL, EXTRAMEDULLARY LESION (ON MYELOGRAPHY, CT, OR MRI)

## COMMON

1. Arachnoiditis (see V-58A)
2. Meningioma
3. Metastasis, esp. leptomeningeal seeding from CNS tumor (eg, medulloblastoma, glioblastoma, pinealoma, ependymoma) or hematogenous from lung, breast, melanoma, lymphoma$_g$
4. Neurofibroma

**UNCOMMON**

1. Arachnoid cyst
2. Cysticercosis (cysts)
3. Dermoid, teratoma; neuroectodermal cyst; epidermoid cyst
4. Ependymoma of conus medullaris
5. Granuloma (eg, tuberculoma; fungal—aspergilloma; sarcoid)
6. Hemangioblastoma; hemangiopericytoma
7. Lipoma (lipomyeloschisis)
8. Meningocele
9. [Tortuosity of nerve roots]
10. Vascular malformation; angioma; varices

*Reference:*

1. Stevens JM: The Spine and Spinal Cord. In: Sutton D, Young JWR (eds): A Short Textbook of Clinical Imaging. London: Springer-Verlag, 1990, pp 802-806

## Subgamut V-58A

### ARACHNOIDITIS

1. Cysticercosis
2. Pantopaque myelography
3. Postoperative
4. Posttraumatic
5. Spinal meningitis (eg, bacterial, tuberculous, fungal, sarcoid, HIV 1 infection)

# EXTRADURAL LESION (ON MYELOGRAPHY, CT, OR MRI)

## COMMON
1. Dermoid, teratoma, epidermoid
2. Epidural metastasis (eg, lymphoma$_g$)
3. Epidural scar (eg, after disk surgery)
4. Fracture fragment or dislocation from vertebral trauma
5. Hematoma, traumatic or spontaneous
6. Herniated disk
7. [Iatrogenic (needle point defect, extradural injection of Pantopaque)]
8. Ligamentum flavum thickening; intraspinal ligament - ossification (eg, DISH; primary—esp. in Japanese)
9. Lipomatosis (obesity, steroid therapy, Cushing S.)
10. Meningioma (with intradural component)
11. Metastasis (esp. carcinoma of lung, breast, prostate, colon)
12. Neurogenic tumor (eg, neurofibroma)
13. Osteomyelitis, epidural abscess (esp. tuberculous, pyogenic)
14. Spinal stenosis; spondylosis; osteophyte
15. Vertebral neoplasm with intraspinal extension (eg, sarcoma, myeloma, chordoma, hemangioma, giant cell tumor, aneurysmal bone cyst, osteoblastoma, osteochondroma)

## UNCOMMON
1. Amyloidosis
2. Arachnoid cyst
3. Arachnoiditis (See V-58A)
4. Epidural granuloma (eg, tuberculous, fungal$_g$, sarcoid)
5. Extramedullary hematopoiesis
6. Lipoma
7. Osteoporosis with fracture and granulation tissue

8. Paget's disease (uncalcified osteoid)
9. Parasitic infection (eg, cysticercosis, hydatid disease, schistosomiasis)
10. Retroperitoneal neoplasm extending through intervertebral foramen (eg, neuroblastoma, lymphoma$_g$)

*References:*

1. Du Boulay GH (ed): A Textbook of X-Ray Diagnosis by British Authors. Neuroradiology. London: AK Lewis, 1984
2. Epstein BS: Spinal canal mass lesions. Radiol Clin North Am 1966;4:185-202
3. Houghton V, et al: Chapter 40, In: Stark DD, Bradley WG (eds): Magnetic Resonance Imaging. (ed 2) St. Louis: CV Mosby, 1992
4. Shoukimas GM: Chapter 41, In: Stark DD, Bradley WG (eds): Magnetic Resonance Imaging. (ed 2) St. Louis: CV Mosby, 1992
5. Stevens JM: The Spine and Spinal Cord. In: Sutton D, Young JWR (eds): A Short Textbook of Clinical Imaging. London: Springer-Verlag, 1990, pp 791-802
6. Taveras JM, Wood EH: Diagnostic Neuroradiology. (ed 2) Baltimore: Williams & Wilkins, 1976

## Gamut V-60

# EXTRADURAL LESION WITH NORMAL ADJACENT BONE

## At Level of Disk Only

1. Disk bulge
2. Disk extrusion
3. Disk protrusion
4. Epidural scar (eg, after disk surgery)
5. Marginal osteophyte

## Not Necessarily at Level of Disk

1. Arachnoid cyst
2. Conjoined root sleeve

3. Epidural abscess
4. Epidural granuloma (eg, tuberculous, fungal, sarcoid, schistosomal)
5. Epidural hematoma
6. Epidural lipomatosis (obesity, steroid therapy, Cushing S.)
7. Epidural metastasis
8. Extruded or sequestered disk
9. Lipoma (spinal dysraphism)
10. Lymphoma
11. Neurogenic tumor (eg, neurofibroma) or meningioma with extradural component
12. "Pseudomass" at dens due to C1-2 subluxation in rheumatoid arthritis, etc.
13. Root sleeve diverticulum
14. Root sleeve ectasia
15. Synovial cyst from facet joint
16. Tarlov (perineural) cyst

*Reference:*

1. Shoukimas GM: Chapter 41, In: Stark DD, Bradley WG (eds): Magnetic Resonance Imaging. (ed 2) St. Louis: CV Mosby, 1992

## Gamut V-61

# SPINAL BLOCK (ON MYELOGRAPHY, CT, OR MRI)

**COMMON**

1. Fracture, traumatic or pathologic
2. Hemorrhage (traumatic, spontaneous, anticoagulant therapy)
3. Herniated disk
4. Metastasis or contiguous spread of malignancy
5. Neoplasm of spine, primary (eg, sarcoma, myeloma, chordoma, giant cell tumor)

6. Neurogenic tumor (esp. neurofibroma)
7. Spinal stenosis

## UNCOMMON

1. Abscess, epidural
2. Achondroplasia
3. Arachnoiditis (See V-58A)
4. Cyst of spinal canal (eg, congenital, arachnoid, dermoid, cysticercus, hydatid)
5. Fibrous dysplasia
6. Granuloma (eg, tuberculosis, schistosomiasis)
7. Hemangioma of vertebra
8. Intramedullary lesion, large (eg, syringomyelia, ependymoma, lipoma)
9. Klippel-Feil S.
10. Lipoma of canal
11. Lymphoma$_g$
12. Meningioma
13. Osteomyelitis of spine
14. Paget's disease

*References:*

1. Greenfield GB: Radiology of Bone Diseases. (ed 5) Philadelphia: Lippincott, 1990
2. O'Carroll MP, Witcombe JB: Primary disorders of bone with "spinal block." Clin Radiol 1979;30:299-306

## Gamut V-62

# TORTUOUS FILLING DEFECT ON LUMBAR MYELOGRAPHY

## COMMON

1. Nerve root elongation, redundancy, or displacement (eg, spinal stenosis or arthrosis, disk herniation, achondroplasia)

**UNCOMMON**

1. Arachnoiditis (See V-58A)
2. Extradural or intradural neoplasm
3. Multiple lesions at same or adjacent levels
4. Vascular abnormality (eg, AV malformation, venous angioma, varices)

*Reference:*

1. Cronquist S, Thulin C-A: Significance of tortuous filling defects at lumbar myelography. Acta Radiologica Diag 1979; 20:561-568

---

## Gamut V-63

# FOCAL VERTEBRAL BODY ABNORMALITY WITH DECREASED SIGNAL ON T1-WEIGHTED IMAGE AND INCREASED SIGNAL ON T2-WEIGHTED IMAGE

1. Acute fracture
2. [Flow artifact from aorta or iliac arteries]
3. GCSF (granulocyte colony stimulating factor) therapy
4. Infection (from osteomyelitis or diskitis)
5. Marrow replacement
6. Multiple myeloma
7. Osseous metastasis
8. Primary bone tumor (eg, Ewing's, lymphoma, osteosarcoma)
9. Type I degenerative endplate changes

*Reference:*

1. Shoukimas GM: Chapter 41, In: Stark DD, Bradley WG (eds): Magnetic Resonance Imaging. (ed 2) St. Louis: CV Mosby, 1992

## Gamut V-64

# FOCAL VERTEBRAL BODY ABNORMALITY WITH HIGH SIGNAL ON T1-WEIGHTED IMAGE

### LOW SIGNAL ON T2-WEIGHTED IMAGE
1. Fat island
2. Fatty replacement following radiation
3. Type II degenerative endplate changes

### HIGH SIGNAL ON T2-WEIGHTED IMAGE
1. Fat island on fast/turbo spin echo images
2. Hemangioma

*References:*
1. Ross JS, et al: Chapter 42, In: Stark DD, Bradley WG (eds): Magnetic Resonance Imaging. (ed 2) St. Louis: CV Mosby, 1992
2. Shoukimas GM: Chapter 41, In: Stark DD, Bradley WG (eds): Magnetic Resonance Imaging. (ed 2) St. Louis: CV Mosby, 1992

## Gamut V-65

# DIFFUSE VERTEBRAL BODY ABNORMALITIES ON MRI

### BRIGHT ON T1-WEIGHTED IMAGES
1. Aplastic anemia
2. Postradiation

### INTERMEDIATE ON T1-WEIGHTED IMAGES
1. Diffuse marrow replacement by tumor (multiple myeloma, diffuse metastatic disease)
2. [Menstruating woman]

3. Myelophthistic marrow replacement (Gaucher's disease)
4. [Normal elderly with osteoporosis]
5. Polycythemia vera

## DARK ON T1-WEIGHTED IMAGES
1. Myelofibrosis
2. Osteopetrosis
3. Renal osteodystrophy
4. Sclerotic metastases (eg, prostate)

*Reference:*
1. Pomeranz SJ: Gamuts and Pearls in MRI. Richmond: Wm Byrd Press, 1990

## Gamut V-66

## INTRAMEDULLARY LESION, CSF INTENSITY

1. Hydromyelia (See V-55A)
2. Post-traumatic cystic myelomalacia
3. Syringomyelia (See V-55A)
4. [Truncation artifact]
5. Tumor cyst (cystic neoplasm)

*Reference:*
1. Houghton V, et al: Chapter 40, In: Stark DD, Bradley WG (eds): Magnetic Resonance Imaging. (ed 2) St. Louis: CV Mosby, 1992

# INTRAMEDULLARY LESION, DARK ON T1-WEIGHTED IMAGE, BRIGHT ON T2-WEIGHTED IMAGE, WITHOUT MASS EFFECT

1. Acute disseminated encephalomyelitis (ADEM)
2. Arteriovenous malformation
3. Cord edema (eg, due to herniated disk)
4. [CSF motion artifact]
5. Devic's syndrome (demyelination of cord and optic neuritis)
6. Gliosis
7. Multiple sclerosis
8. Small glioma
9. Small nonhemorrhagic contusion
10. Subacute infarct
11. [Truncation artifact]

*Reference:*
1. Houghton V, et al: Chapter 40, In: Stark DD, Bradley WG (eds): Magnetic Resonance Imaging. (ed 2) St. Louis: CV Mosby, 1992

## Gamut V-68

# INTRAMEDULLARY LESION, DARK ON T1-WEIGHTED AND BRIGHT ON T2-WEIGHTED IMAGES, WITH MASS EFFECT

**COMMON**
1. Acute contusion
2. Acute disseminated encephalomyelitis (ADEM)
3. Astrocytoma

4. Ependymoma
5. Hemangioblastoma
6. Leptomeningeal carcinomatosis (eg, breast)
7. Myelitis

**UNCOMMON**
1. Acute infarct
2. Acute tumefactive multiple sclerosis
3. Drop metastasis down central canal (eg, medulloblastoma)
4. Lymphoma
5. Radiation necrosis
6. Spinal meningitis

*References:*
1. Houghton V, et al: Chapter 40, In: Stark DD, Bradley WG (eds): Magnetic Resonance Imaging. (ed 2) St. Louis: CV Mosby, 1992
2. Shoukimas GM: Chapter 41, In: Stark DD, Bradley WG (eds): Magnetic Resonance Imaging. (ed 2) St. Louis: CV Mosby, 1992

## Gamut V-69

# INTRAMEDULLARY LESION, DARK ON T1 AND T2-WEIGHTED IMAGES, WITH MASS EFFECT

1. Focal calcification
2. Hemosiderin from old bleed (eg, from cavernous angioma or AVM)
3. [Metallic artifact from previous surgery]
4. Osseous spur in diastematomyelia

### Gamut V-70

## INTRAMEDULLARY LESION, BRIGHT ON T1-WEIGHTED IMAGE

### BRIGHT ON T2-WEIGHTED IMAGE
1. Late subacute hematomyelia (extracellular met-hemoglobin from tumor, AVM, trauma)
2. Proteinaceous cyst (eg, from tumor)

### DARK ON T2-WEIGHTED IMAGE
1. Early subacute hematomyelia (intracellular met-hemoglobin from tumor, AVM, trauma)

### Gamut V-71

## EXTRAMEDULLARY, INTRADURAL LESION WITH CSF INTENSITY

1. Arachnoid cyst
2. Cysticercosis
3. Multicystic arachnoiditis

### Gamut V-72

## EXTRAMEDULLARY, INTRADURAL LESION , DARK ON T1-WEIGHTED IMAGE, BRIGHT ON T2-WEIGHTED IMAGE, WITHOUT MASS EFFECT

1. [Flow artifact]
2. Fungal meningitis
3. Small drop metastases

*References:*
1. Houghton V, et al: Chapter 40, In: Stark DD, Bradley WG (eds): Magnetic Resonance Imaging. (ed 2) St. Louis: CV Mosby, 1992
2. Shoukimas GM: Chapter 41, In: Stark DD, Bradley WG (eds): Magnetic Resonance Imaging. (ed 2) St. Louis: CV Mosby, 1992

## Gamut V-73

## EXTRAMEDULLARY, INTRADURAL LESION, DARK ON T1-WEIGHTED IMAGE, BRIGHT ON T2-WEIGHTED IMAGE, WITH MASS EFFECT

1. Arachnoiditis
2. Black epidermoid
3. Dermoid (cystic)
4. Exophytic glioma (apparent extramedullary)
5. Large drop metastases
6. Meningioma
7. Neurilemoma/schwannoma
8. Neurofibroma

*References:*
1. Houghton V, et al: Chapter 40, In: Stark DD, Bradley WG (eds): Magnetic Resonance Imaging. (ed 2) St. Louis: CV Mosby, 1992
2. Ross JS, et al: Chapter 42, In: Stark DD, Bradley WG (eds): Magnetic Resonance Imaging. (ed 2) St. Louis: CV Mosby, 1992
3. Shoukimas GM: Chapter 41, In: Stark DD, Bradley WG (eds): Magnetic Resonance Imaging. (ed 2) St. Louis: CV Mosby, 1992

# SOURCES OF DROP METASTASES TO SPINAL SUBARACHNOID SPACE

## CNS Sources

**COMMON**
1. Astrocytoma
2. Ependymoma
3. Glioblastoma multiforme
4. Medulloblastoma

**UNCOMMON**
1. Choroid plexus carcinoma
2. Pineoblastoma
3. Pineocytoma
4. Teratoma

## Non-CNS Sources

1. Metastatic carcinoma (esp. breast, lung)
2. Metastatic lymphoma
3. Metastatic melanoma

*Reference:*
1. Shoukimas GM: Chapter 41, In: Stark DD, Bradley WG (eds): Magnetic Resonance Imaging. (ed 2) St. Louis: CV Mosby, 1992

## Gamut V-74

# EXTRAMEDULLARY, INTRADURAL LESION, BRIGHT ON T1-WEIGHTED IMAGE, DARK ON T2-WEIGHTED IMAGE

1. Dermoid (fatty)
2. Fatty filum
3. Lipoma
4. Pantopaque
5. White epidermoid

*Reference:*
1. Shoukimas GM: Chapter 41, In: Stark DD, Bradley WG (eds): Magnetic Resonance Imaging. (ed 2) St. Louis: CV Mosby, 1992

## Gamut V-75

# EXTRAMEDULLARY, INTRADURAL SIGNAL VOID

1. Arteriovenous malformation
2. [CSF flow artifact]
3. [Metallic artifact]

# Abbreviations

| | |
|---|---|
| ADEM | acute disseminated encephalomyelitis |
| AIDS | acquired immune deficiency S. |
| AP | anteroposterior |
| AV(M) | arteriovenous (malformation) |
| CNS | central nervous system |
| CPPD | calcium pyrophosphate dihydrate crystal deposition disease |
| CREST S. | calcinosis-Raynaud's-sclerodactyly-telangiectasia |
| CSF | cerebrospinal fluid |
| DIP | distal interphalangeal (joint) |
| DISH | diffuse idiopathic skeletal hyperostosis |
| eg | for example |
| esp | especially |
| g | consult Glossary |
| HADD | hydroxyapatite deposition disease |
| HIV | human immunodeficiency virus |
| ie | that is |
| incl | including |
| L | left |
| MCTD | mixed connective tissue disease |
| occas | occasionally |
| PA | posteroanterior |
| PIP | proximal interphalangeal (joint) |
| R | right |
| S. | syndrome |
| TORCH | toxoplasmosis, rubella, cytomegalovirus, herpes simplex fetal infections |
| VATER S. | vertebral (or vascular) anomalies; anal anomalies (or auricular defects); tracheoesophageal fistula; esophageal atresia (or ring); renal anomalies (or radial defects, rib anomalies) |

# Glossary

ANEMIA, PRIMARY - erythroblastosis, hemolytic anemia, pyruvate kinase deficiency, sickle cell disease and variants,
spherocytosis, thalassemia and variants

ANEURYSM - arteriosclerotic, arteriovenous (incl. fistula, malformation), dissecting, false, mycotic, poststenotic, syphilitic
(See ANGIOMA)

ANGIOMA - arteriovenous malformation, cirsoid aneurysm,
hemangioma (incl. capillary, cavernous), varices

ARTERIOVENOUS MALFORMATION (AVM) - See
ANEURYSM

BLEEDING OR CLOTTING DISORDER - anticoagulant effect, coagulopathy (eg, disseminated intravascular type-
DIC), hemophilia, purpura (eg, Henoch-Schönlein),
thrombocytopenia

COLLAGEN DISEASE - dermatomyositis, lupus erythematosus, polyarteritis nodosa, scleroderma, mixed connective tissue disease (MCTD), CREST S.
(calcinosis-Raynaud's-sclerodactyly-telangiectasia)

FAT EMBOLISM - incl. diffuse embolization of fatty bone marrow (after fracture), amniotic fluid, or oily contrast medium

FUNGUS DISEASE - actinomycosis, blastomycosis, coccidioidomycosis, cryptococcosis (torulosis), histoplasmosis,
duboisii, nocardiosis, paracoccidiomycosis (South American
blastomycosis), sporotrichosis

GLYCOGEN STORAGE DISEASE - von Gierke (Type I),
Pompe (Type II), Cori (Type III), McArdle (Type V)

HISTIOCYTOSIS X - eosinophilic granuloma, Hand-Schüller-
Christian disease, Letterer-Siwe's disease (nonlipid histiocytosis)

IMMUNOLOGIC DISORDERS - agammaglobulinemia (Bru-
ton S.) or dysgammaglobulinemia, AIDS, ataxia-telangiecta-
sis S. Bloom S., Buckley S., combined deficiency S.,
DiGeorge S., chronic granulomatous disease of childhood,
Job S.

LYMPHOMA - includes Burkitt's lymphoma, Hodgkin's disease, non-Hodgkin's lymphoma, leukemia (all varieties, including chloroma)

MUCOPOLYSACCHARIDOSES - also mucolipidoses and other lysosomal storage diseases (See B-1)

MUSCULAR DISORDERS - See NEUROMUSCULAR DISORDERS

NEOPLASMS, BENIGN - chondroma, hamartoma, hemangioma, hemangiopericytoma, lipoma, pseudotumor, teratoma

NEUROGENIC NEOPLASM - ganglioneuroma and para-ganglioneuroma, ganglioneuroblastoma, neurilemoma, neuroblastoma, neurofibroma, neurosarcoma, schwannoma

NEUROMUSCULAR DISORDERS - amyotonia congenita, amyotrophic lateral sclerosis, cerebral palsy, Duchenne S., meningomyelocele, muscular dystrophy, myasthenia gravis, myotonic dystrophy, parkinsonism, poliomyelitis, visceral myopathy, Werdnig-Hoffmann disease

PARALYSIS - bulbar paralysis, paraplegia, peripheral paralysis, poliomyelitis, quadriplegia

# General References

The following books and articles provided invaluable source material in the preparation of this book. Their excellent tables and lists formed a nucleus for many of the gamuts.

Burgener FA, Kormano M: Differential Diagnosis in Conventional Radiology. (ed 2) New York: Thieme Medical Publ, 1991

DuBoulay GH: Principles of X-ray Diagnosis of the Skull. (ed 2) London: Butterworths, 1980

Edeiken J, Dalinka M, Karasick D: Edeiken's Roentgen Diagnosis of Diseases of Bone. (ed 4) Baltimore: Williams & Wilkins, 1989

Eisenberg RL: Clinical Imaging: An Atlas of Differential Diagnosis. (ed 2) Rockville, MD: Aspen Publ, 1992

Epstein BS: The Spine. (ed 4) Philadelphia: Lea & Febiger, 1976

Felson B (ed): Dwarfs and other little people. Semin Roentgenol, 1973

Grainger RG, Allison DJ: Diagnostic Radiology. (ed 2) Edinburgh: Churchill Livingstone, 1992

Greenfield GB: Radiology of Bone Diseases. (ed 5) Philadelphia: Lippincott, 1990

Jones KL: Smith's Recognizable Patterns of Human Malformation. (ed 3) Philadelphia: W.B. Saunders, 1988

Koslowski K, Beighton P: Gamut Index of Skeletal Dysplasias: An Aid to Radiodiagnosis. New York: Springer-Verlag, 1984

Kreel L: Outline of Radiology. New York: Appleton-Century-Crofts, 1971

Murray RO, Jacobson HG, Stoker D: The Radiology of Skeletal Disorders. (ed 3) London: Churchill Livingstone, 1989

Newton TH, Potts DG: Radiology of the Skull and Brain. St. Louis: C.V. Mosby, 1971

Poznanski AK: The Hand in Radiologic Diagnosis. (ed 2) Philadelphia: W.B. Saunders, 1984

Ravin CE, Cooper C (eds): Review of Radiology. Philadelphia: W.B. Saunders, 1990

Reeder MM, Palmer PES: The Radiology of Tropical Diseases. Baltimore: Williams & Wilkins, 1981

Resnick D, Niwayama G: Diagnosis of Bone and Joint Disorders. Philadelphia: W.B. Saunders, 1981

Silverman FN (ed): Caffey's Pediatric X-ray Diagnosis: An Integrated Imaging Approach. (ed 8) Chicago: Year Book Medical Publ, 1985

Stark DD, Bradley WG (eds): Magnetic Resonance Imaging. (ed 2) St. Louis: CV Mosby, 1992

Sutton D, Young JWR (eds): A Short Textbook of Clinical Imaging. London: Springer-Verlag, 1990

Swischuk LE: Differential Diagnosis in Pediatric Radiology. Baltimore: Williams & Wilkins, 1984

Swischuk LE: Imaging of the Newborn, Infant, and Young Child. (ed 3) Baltimore: Williams & Wilkins, 1989

Taveras JM, Wood EH: Diagnostic Neuroradiology. (ed 2) Baltimore: Williams & Wilkins, 1976, vol 1

Taybi H, Lachman RS: Radiology of Syndromes, Metabolic Disorders, and Skeletal Dysplasias. (ed 3) Chicago: Year Book Medical Publ, 1990

Teplick JG, Haskin ME: Roentgenologic Diagnosis. (ed 3) Philadelphia: W.B. Saunders, 1976

Wilson JD, et al: Harrison's Principles of Internal Medicine. (ed 12) New York: McGraw-Hill, 1991

# Index

---

**K**nee

bright intramedullary signal on T2-weighted image of, with
intact cortex, 250

high intramedullary signal on T2-weighted image of, with
disrupted cortex, 250

menisco-cartilage junction of, increased signal on T2-weighted
image at, 360

meniscus, linear signal in, on MRI, 360

multiple filling defects in, on arthrography, 355

Knock-knees, 252–253

Kyphosis, 394–395

**L**arge

bones of one hand, 211, 212

calcified soft tissue mass adjacent to bone, solitary, 372–373

destructive bone lesion, 116–117

epiphyses, 53–54

hands for age, 210–211

Late-onset dwarfism, 26–27

Laxity, joint, congenital syndromes with, 334–335

Legs, bow, 251–252

Lesions, bone (*see* Bone, lesions)

Lethal forms of dwarfism, 25–26

Ligament

calcification in, 368–369

insertions, proliferation of new bone at, 154–155

Limb

asymmetry in size of, 38–40

localized accelerated maturation, elongation, or overgrowth of,
40–41

Limbs, short, congenital syndromes with, 28–30

Long

bones

erosion of medial aspect of proximal metaphyses of, 70

short, with pronounced metaphyseal flaring, 66

fingers, 199–200

lesions of ribs, 281

thin bones, 34–35

Loose body, calcified, in joint, 356

Looser's zones, 162

Lower extremities, gamuts, 12–13

Lucent (*see also* Radiolucent)

center, dense cortex with, 55–56

defects in bones of hands, wrists, feet, or ankles, well- defined
solitary or multiple, 216–217

lesion, of bone surrounded by marked sclerotic reaction or rim,
109–110